Neuro-Ophthalmology

Desmond P. Kidd

Neuro-Ophthalmology

Illustrated Case Studies

Springer

Desmond P. Kidd
Department of Clinical Neurosciences
Royal Free Hospital
London
UK

ISBN 978-1-4471-2409-2 ISBN 978-1-4471-2410-8 (eBook)
DOI 10.1007/978-1-4471-2410-8

Library of Congress Control Number: 2017933279

Printed on acid-free paper

This Springer imprint is published by Springer Nature
The registered company is Springer-Verlag London Ltd.
The registered company address is: 236 Gray's Inn Road, London WC1X 8HB, United Kingdom

For Catherine and Iain

Foreword

This is an educational entertainment, not a textbook. Neurologists and ophthalmologists often approach neuro-ophthalmology with apprehension since it requires a little extra learning to understand the principles, yet having done so it proves to be not only reasonably straightforward but also remarkably fascinating and stimulating. The purpose here, therefore, is to allow the reader to acquire extra knowledge about the subject relatively easily and without the need to spend hours of study, simply by reading a number of clinical cases. Each case is set out in a realistic scenario, with the history and examination first, then a pause for consideration leading to investigations. The results of these are set out and where necessary a further pause follows to allow the reader to reflect on the information provided before the denouement arrives. A short summary of important points which allow an understanding of where our knowledge of the pathogenesis and treatment of the disease currently exists finishes each case.

There are 50 cases, each of which is real and none of which has been altered, which have been picked because they are interesting or provide good examples of the clinical or radiological or pathological aspects of the disease, and allow a reasonably comprehensive run through the major topics of neuro-ophthalmology. We start at the orbit and work backwards. There is also an appendix which gives background information if required, and tips on how best to perform the neuro-ophthalmic examination.

I wish to thank the production team at Springer Verlag, in particular Joanna Renwick, who was very patient as the project evolved haphazardly from a multi-author collaboration to the work of an overworked and rather harassed but nonetheless very keen neuro-ophthalmologist.

Contents

Part I
The Orbit and Muscles

Case 1

History

This 47 year old lady presented to the emergency department of her local hospital with a two week history of diminishing vision in the left eye. There was no pain and no other symptom. Owing to congenital toxoplasmosis the vision in her right eye had always been poor. There was no diplopia. An MRI scan of the brain had been adjudged to be normal and she was referred to the Neuro-ophthalmology service.

Her past medical history was remarkable only for a longstanding seizure disorder well controlled on Carbamazepine SR 1200 mg per day. There were no other symptoms, and no symptoms on systematic enquiry.

Examination

The central visual acuities were 6/36 on the right (unchanged from previously) and 6/36 on the left. Color vision was normal on the right and reduced 6/17 on the left. There was a 2 mm left sided axial proptosis. The eye movements were full but there was a small exophoria −12 L/R for distance and −18 L/R for near. The ocular media were clear and the discs were normal. There was a macular scar in keeping with previous toxoplasmosis on the right side. The left visual field was constricted (Fig. 1.1a).

D.P. Kidd, *Neuro-Ophthalmology*, DOI 10.1007/978-1-4471-2410-8_1

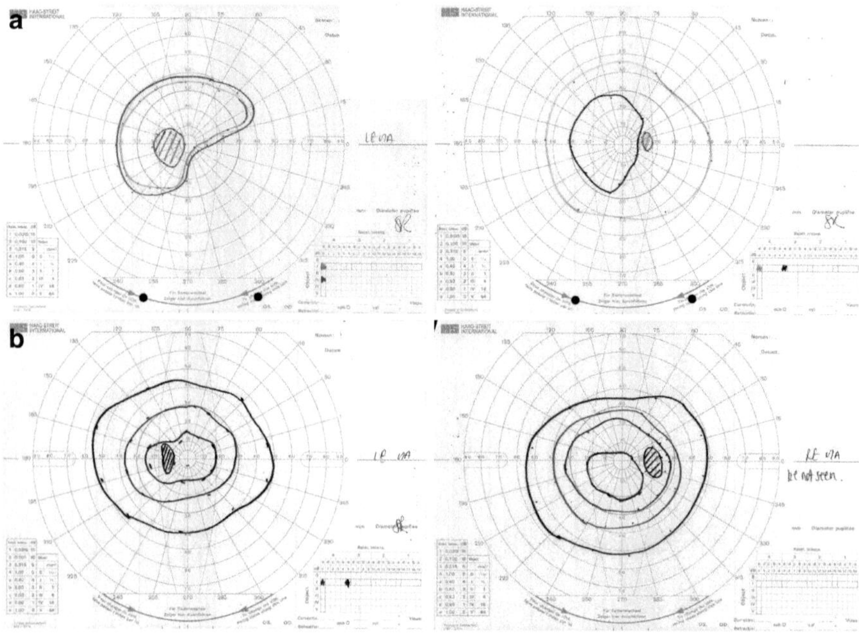

Fig. 1.1 Goldman visual fields (**a**) showing constriction on both sides at presentation and (**b**) with improvement following treatment

Evaluation

This is an emergency; the patient presents with an escalating problem with double vision and a reduction in the acuity of her good eye. The presence of proptosis makes an anteriorly placed lesion highly likely, and the development of an optic neuropathy implies that the orbit is under pressure. The most common causes of a subacute orbital lesion are shown in the table. In this case inflammatory, infective and neoplastic lesions would be the most likely with this subacute and escalating clinical syndrome. A regular MRI scan of the brain is not sufficient to evaluate orbital disease; only one or two axial sections are seen and coronal and sagittal orbital views are necessary (Fig. 1.2).

Blood and imaging investigations were carried out immediately, and following this she was admitted to hospital for the treatment noted below on the same day.

Investigations

FBC and biochemical screening were normal. The ESR was 9 and CRP 3. Thyroid function was normal.

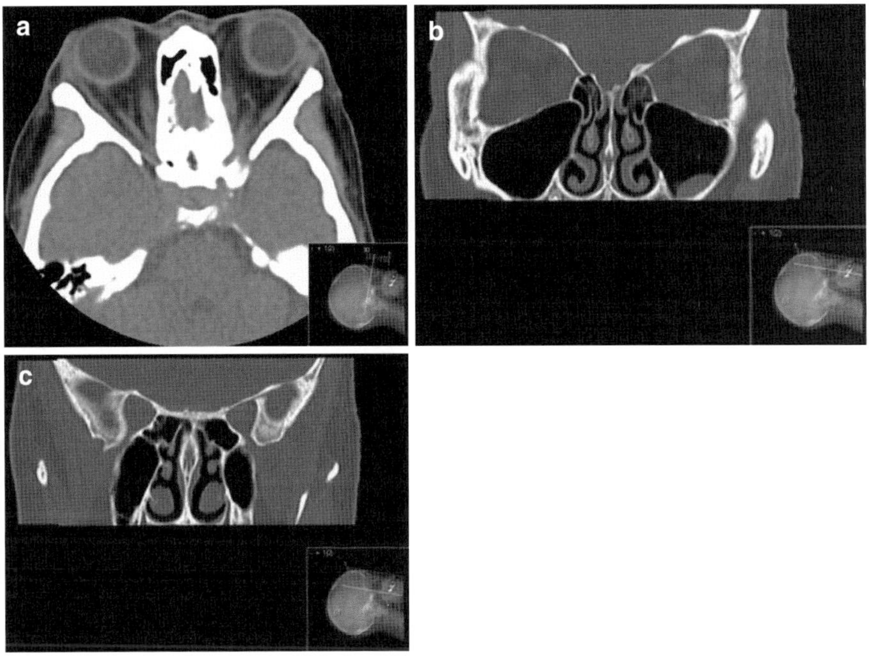

Fig. 1.2 CT scan of orbits: coronal and axial scans (**a**, **b**), showing a rather symmetrical bilateral proptosis caused by enlargement of the rectus muscles on both sides, which does not extend anteriorly to involve the tendons, but which does extend back to cause crowding on both sides (**c**), at the orbital apex on both sides, but worse on the left where compression of the optic nerve may be seen. Inflammatory change is seen within the orbital fat. The lacrimal glands are not enlarged and the superior ophthalmic veins not distended

The CT scan of orbits showed clear evidence for enlargement of the rectus muscles within the orbit, causing proptosis on the left and compression of the left optic nerve at the orbital apex. The oblique muscles were not affected and the tendons also spared (Table 1.1). The findings are in keeping with thyroid orbitopathy. The thyroid peroxisomal antibodies were subsequently found to be raised at 556 IUM/l (0–99).

She was treated with high dose intravenous steroids; 5 g of methylprednisolone. Her vision continued to deteriorate for 2 days then improved and stabilized at 6/24. She was referred for irradiation of the orbit and this took place a month later; she received 25 Gy in 15 fractions over 21 days.

Her vision improved to 6/9 with normal color vision; the field enlarged (Fig. 1.1b).

Discussion

Thyroid orbitopathy is an inflammatory condition in which a T cell mediated immune response develops leading to inflammation within the orbital structures, including the muscles and the orbital fat. A subacute proptosis develops associated with restriction of eye movements, lid retraction and eye dryness with irritation, tearing and redness

[1–3]. Untreated, the condition becomes chronic leading to the development of fibrosis within the muscles, which become permanently restricted and atrophic [3].

All patients possess anti-thyrotrophin receptor antibodies; their level correlates with the clinical features in Graves' disease and thyroid dermopathy, and are associated with a more poor prognosis [4]. 5 % of patients with thyroid orbitopathy are euthyroid, as in this case, and this is associated with a lower titer of anti-thyrotropin receptor antibody.

There is a clear relationship between the severity of the disease and a poor response to immunosuppression with cigarette smoking, and this too correlates with the severity of cigarette consumption.

How orbital inflammation develops in Graves' disease is as yet undefined, although there are experimental data showing that orbital fibroblasts express thyrotropin receptor antigen [4].

Treatment involves corticosteroids at high dose, either continuous oral or (as is my preference) brief high dose intravenous steroids, then orbital irradiation [5–7]. There is evidence to suggest that both together is more effective than either on its own [5]. New biological treatments blocking IL-1, IL-6 and TNFα, and B cell depletion with Rituximab [4] are undergoing treatment trials at present. Orbital decompressive surgery is required in only rare cases nowadays, when the above measures fail [5, 6].

Table 1.1 Common orbital lesions

Vascular:	Capillary hemangioma
	Cavernous hemangioma
	Lymphangioma
	Orbital varix
	Arteriovenous malformation
	Carotico-cavernous fistula
Choristomas and cysts:	Dermoid
	Epidermoid
	Meningocoele
	Encephalocoele
Inflammation:	Sinus mucocoele
	Dacroadenitis
	Orbital myositis
	Idiopathic orbital inflammatory disease
	Thyroid orbitopathy
Neoplasia:	Lacrimal adenoma
	Schwannoma of V
	Optic nerve sheath meningioma
	Optic nerve glioma
	Sphenoid wing meningioma
	Rhabdomyosarcoma
	Lymphoma
Metastatic carcinoma:	Hematogenous
	Direct invasion
	E.g. melanoma, squamous cell carcinoma
Infection:	Orbital cellulitis
	Abscess

Data from [1, 2]

References

1. Rose GE, Verity D. Orbital disease. In: Kidd DP, Biousse V, Newman NJ, editors. Neuro-ophthalmology. Philadelphia: Butterworth Heinemann Elsevier; 2008. p. 82–8.
2. Rose GE, Verity D. Neuro-ophthalmology of orbital disease. In: Kennard C, Leigh RJ, editors. Handbook of neurology; neuro-ophthalmology. 102nd ed. Amsterdam: Elsevier BV; 2011. p. 479–81.
3. Utiger RD. Pathogenesis of Graves' ophthalmopathy. N Engl J Med. 1992;326:1172–3.
4. Bahn RS. Graves' ophthalmopathy. N Engl J Med. 2010;362:726–38.
5. Prabhu RS, Liebman L, Wojno T, Hayek B, Hall WA, Crocker I. Clinical outcomes of radiotherapy as initial local therapy for Graves' ophthalmopathy and predictors of the need for post-radiotherapy decompressive surgery. Radiat Oncol. 2012;7:95.
6. Matthieson C, Thompson JS, Thompson D, Farris B, Wilkes B, Ahmad S, Herman T, Bogardus Jr C. The efficacy of radiation therapy in the treatment of Graves' orbitopathy. Int J Radiat Oncol Biol Phys. 2012;82:117–23.
7. Hahn E, Laperriere N, Millar AM, Oestreicher J, McGowan H, Krema H, Gill H, DeAngelis D, Hurwitz J, Tucker N, Simpson R, Chung C. Orbital radiation therapy for Graves' ophthalmopathy: measuring clinical efficacy and impact. Pract Radiat Oncol. 2014;4:233–9.

Case 2

History

This 37 year old man presented to the emergency department of the hospital with a 6 day history of double vision which was associated with a mild periorbital ache on the right. The double vision was horizontal, and worse when looking to the right. This did not worsen but on the day prior to admission he had noticed a reduction in vision on the right side. He felt his vision to be normal on the left, and described the problem on the right as being a general blurredness. There was no pain within the eye, nor any pain elicited by eye movement.

There were no constitutional symptoms nor a preceding viral illness, and no prior neurological symptoms. He took no regular treatment. He had an office based job and had not travelled over the previous year.

Examination

The higher cognitive functions were normal. His central visual acuity was 6/12 N8 3/17 on the right, and 6/5 N5 17 on the left. There was a mild right relative afferent pupillary defect. There was a small and mild central field loss on the right. The eye movements were limited on the right in horizontal gaze and there was a mild right lateral rectus weakness. There were no other abnormal neurological signs.

He was afebrile and the systemic examination was normal.

D.P. Kidd, *Neuro-Ophthalmology*, DOI 10.1007/978-1-4471-2410-8_2

Evaluation

This 37 year old man presents with a unilateral disorder with pain, double vision and reduced visual acuity. This would suggest an anteriorly placed single lesion within the orbit or just behind. The examination shows evidence for an optic neuropathy and a sixth neuropathy (or lateral rectus restriction). The signs of an orbital lesion involve diplopia and optic neuropathy but there is usually proptosis, although in this case the disorder had only just presented itself so conceivably the pathological process was not yet so advanced as to occupy much space. The physical signs of a lesion at the orbital apex include all of the above, and in addition there is an ophthalmic division trigeminal neuropathy (see Appendix 3).

The history is short and the clinical syndrome subacute, so the initial investigation should consider infective, inflammatory and neoplastic causes. In the first instance this should include investigations for orbital cellulitis, thyroid orbitopathy, orbital inflammatory disease, lymphoma and metastasis.

Investigations

Screening blood tests were normal; the ESR was 6, the white cell count not raised. CK, ACE and immunoglobulins were normal. Thyroid function tests were normal. Thyroid peroxidase and acetyl choline receptor antibodies were negative. ANCA negative.

An MRI scan showed engorgement of the orbit on the right due to enlargement of the muscles therein (Fig. 2.1). The tendon sheaths were also involved. The superior ophthalmic vein was engorged. There was a resultant proptosis.

A CSF examination was normal.

An ENT examination of the posterior nasal space showed no abnormality. Serological tests for mucormycosis, aspergillus and cysticercosis were negative.

Management

During investigation his visual acuity deteriorated to 6/24. A right lateral rectus biopsy was performed, which showed an infiltration of lymphocytes but no granulomas and no vasculitis. He received treatment with 3 g of intravenous methylprednisolone, followed by an oral steroid taper over 8 months. The clinical signs and MRI abnormalities returned to normal and he has remained well since.

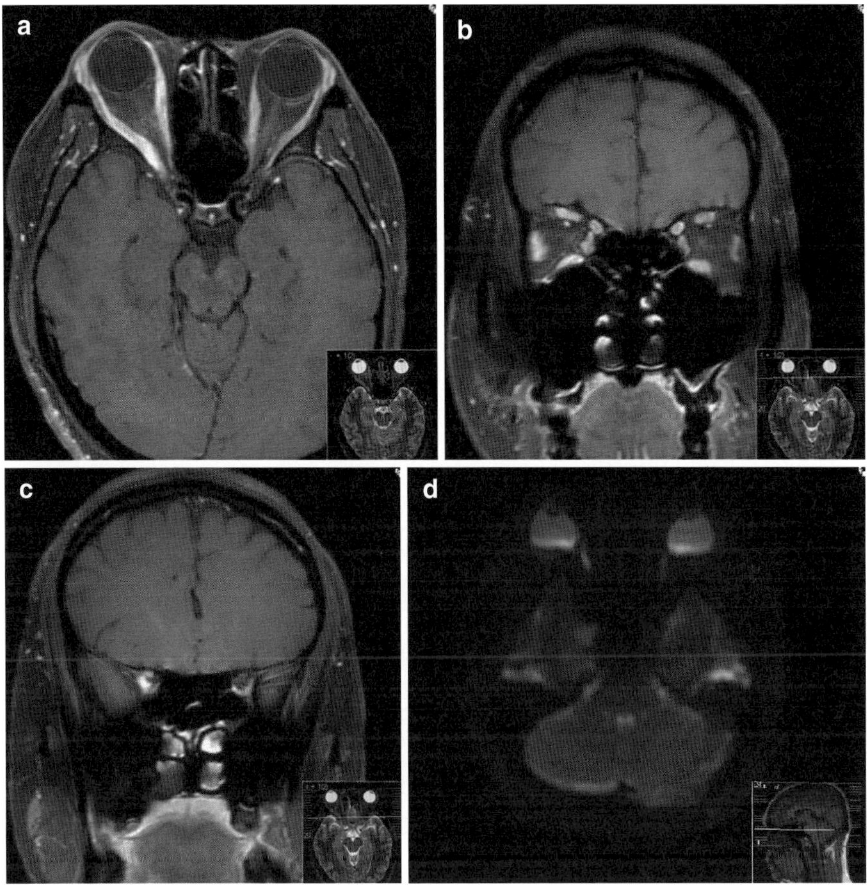

Fig. 2.1 T1 weighted axial and coronal MRI following contrast injection: (**a**, **b**, **c**): there is a mild proptosis on the right side. There is enlargement of the right lateral and medial rectus muscles which exhibit high signal intensity. Note that the tendon insertions are also involved. There are less marked changes in the other muscles on the right and also on the left. The superior ophthalmic vein is dilated. The optic nerve – sheath complex also exhibits high signal. ADC map (**d**), showing of the orbit showing restricted diffusion within the right lateral rectus muscle

Discussion

The clinical features pointed to a lesion within the orbit; pain, diplopia and reduced acuity are all important features. The clinical syndrome was similar to that of patient 1; she did not notice diplopia owing to her longstanding maculopathy, but the disorder presented in the same way.

Blood investigations and serological tests did not suggest a systemic disorder or infection, and thyroid and acetyl choline receptor antibodies were negative. CSF showed no evidence for meningitis (inflammatory or infective), and an ENT exam showed no evidence for nasopharyngeal carcinoma (which is more common in people of Chinese descent than Caucasians) and intercurrent infective sinus disease.

Imaging showed a unilateral disorder in which the orbit was under pressure due to enlargement of the muscles. This caused proptosis and engorgement of the superior ophthalmic vein, and the optic neuropathy due to compression of the nerve at the orbital apex. Importantly the tendons were involved, which is against dysthyroid eye disease (see Case 1).

Orbital cellulitis is uncommon, more prevalent in children complicating sinus infection, but can be difficult to identify before sight threatening complications arise [1]. Imaging cannot reliably distinguish between orbital infection, inflammation or malignancy, although one study found that using diffusion weighted imaging infection was more bright on DWI than inflammation, which in turn was more bright than lymphoma [2].

Orbital inflammatory disease may arise through a number of different pathological processes (Table 2.1) [3, 4]. Thyroid orbitopathy is by far and away the most common, in which an inflammatory infiltrate develops in the orbital muscles (characteristically the recti and not the obliques, and with sparing of the tendon insertions) and the orbital fat leading to proptosis, extraocular muscle weakness and restriction, and, if orbital pressure is high at the apex and the proptosis stretches the optic nerve, optic neuropathy.

Granulomatous inflammatory disease such as sarcoidosis, granulomatosis with polyangiitis (GPA) (formerly ANCA-positive vasculitis) and Churg-Strauss syndrome are also associated with orbital inflammation, and the more rare causes such as Erdheim-Chester disease, in which histiocytic inflammation develops, and fibrosclerotic orbital disease in which an inflammatory infiltration with marked fibrosis develops, may also cause the disorder.

The emerging and as yet incompletely understood entity of IgG4 related disease has recently been shown to be associated with orbital inflammation, particularly that

Table 2.1 Differential diagnosis of orbital inflammatory disease

Idiopathic orbital inflammatory disease
Sarcoidosis
Granulomatosis with polyangiitis (GPA)
Erdheim-Chester disease
Churg-Strauss syndrome
Systemic lupus erythematosus
Sjogren's syndrome
Polyarteritis nodosa
Associated with Crohn's disease, scleroderma
Giant cell arteritis
Neoplasia: lymphoma, metastatic leukemia and lymphoma. Metastatic epithelial disease and melanoma, rhabdomyosarcoma
Infection: paranasal sinus and dental infections, direct following trauma or surgery

associated with lacrimal gland involvement. This is a systemic disorder causing inflammation and fibrosis of many tissues including the liver and pancreas, the thyroid, kidneys and lungs [4, 5]. A recent review [4] has stated that 60 % have isolated lacrimal disease or associated lymphadenopathy and/or salivary gland involvement (Mickulicz's syndrome) whilst 25 % have extraocular muscle disease and the remainder orbital soft tissue involvement. Commonly seen on orbital MRI is enlargement of the infraorbital nerve.

Imaging including CT and MRI show the features, and FDG-PET show high uptake lesions. The pathology is of an intense inflammatory infiltration of lymphocytes, plasma cells and abundant eosinophils. Fibrosis is often seen. Immunostaining reveals CD20 positive T cells and staining of IgG4 plasma cells is abundant [6].

Treatment is with corticosteroids and, with relapsing or treatment resistant disease, immune suppressants. Rituximab is reported to work well in severe cases.

Orbital myositis is now accepted as an uncommon subtype of this group of disorders [7] accounting for 8 % of disease subtypes. Patients present with orbital pain and diplopia, then proptosis. The horizontal recti are said to be affected more often than the vertical or the obliques. Unilateral involvement occurs in 80 % of adults and bilateral disease is more common in children.

References

1. Murphy C, Livingstone I, Foot B, Murgatroyd H, MacEwen CJ. Orbital cellulitis in Scotland: current incidence, aetiology, management and outcomes. Br J Ophthalmol. 2014;98:1575–8.
2. Kapur R, Sepahdari AR, Mafee MF, Putterman AM, Aakalu V, Wendel LJ, Setabutr P. MR imaging of orbital inflammatory syndrome, orbital cellulitis, and orbital lymphoid lesions: the role of diffusion-weighted imaging. AJNR. 2009;30:64–70.
3. Gordon LK. Orbital inflammatory disease: a diagnostic and therapeutic challenge. Eye. 2006;20:1196–206.
4. Rosenbaum JT, Choi DS, Wilson DJ, Grossniklaus HE, Sibley CH, Harrington CA, Planck SR. Molecular diagnosis of orbital inflammatory disease. Exp Mol Pathol. 2015;98(2):225–9. epub Jan 14.
5. Lindfield D, Attfield F, McElvanney A. Systemic immunoglobulin G4 (IgG4) disease and idiopathic orbital inflammation; removing "idiopathic" from the nomenclature? Eye. 2012;26: 623–9.
6. McNabb AA, McKelvie P. IgG4-related ophthalmic disease part II: clinical aspects. Ophthal Plast Reconstruct Surg. 2015;31(3):167–78. epub Jan 5.
7. Fraser CL, Skalicky SE, Gurbaxani A, McCluskey P. Ocular myositis. Curr Allergy Asthma Rep. 2013;13:315–21.

Case 3

History

This 56 year old lady was referred by her local Neurologist with a 2 year history of a painful feeling of fullness around and behind the left eye. This progressively worsened; at times it would keep her awake at night. More recently she had noticed intermittent double vision.

At the local hospital the neurological and ophthalmic examinations had been considered to be normal. Blood tests had been normal, including acetylcholine receptor antibodies, the ESR was 17. An MRI scan of the brain was reported to be normal. A single fiber EMG showed no abnormalities within frontalis.

Her past medical history was remarkable only for diet controlled type 2 diabetes. There was no hypertension. There was no history of trauma.

Examination

She saw 6/6 in both eyes with normal color vision and symmetrical pupillary responses. The fields were full. An orthoptic assessment revealed a slight underaction (6 diopters) of inferior rectus on the left. There was a 3 mm proptosis and the eyelids were puffy. There was injection of the conjunctiva on the left. The ocular examination was otherwise normal save for a mild symmetrical blepharitis. The discs were normal and the retinal veins not engorged.

D.P. Kidd, *Neuro-Ophthalmology*, DOI 10.1007/978-1-4471-2410-8_3

Evaluation

It was considered inconceivable that the scan could be normal and arrangements were made for it to be reviewed. The history is typical for an orbital mass lesion; dysthyroid eye disease (see Case 1) would be a common cause and may be unilateral or markedly asymmetrical, orbital cavernomas are common in women and present precisely thus. Meningioma of the sphenoid region (see Case 24) is also common in this clinical context, and indeed more common in women of the middle years. Such a long history would make an inflammatory cause such as idiopathic orbital inflammatory disease, infection such as mucocoele or pyocoele, and metastatic disease, less likely. If the MRI did not show a mass lesion then uncommon vascular causes would be considered, for example orbital venous engorgement.

Investigations

A further MRI was undertaken which showed a left sided proptosis, with enlargement of the medial, lateral and superior rectus muscles on that side only. Dilated veins were seen within the left middle cranial fossa (Fig. 3.1).

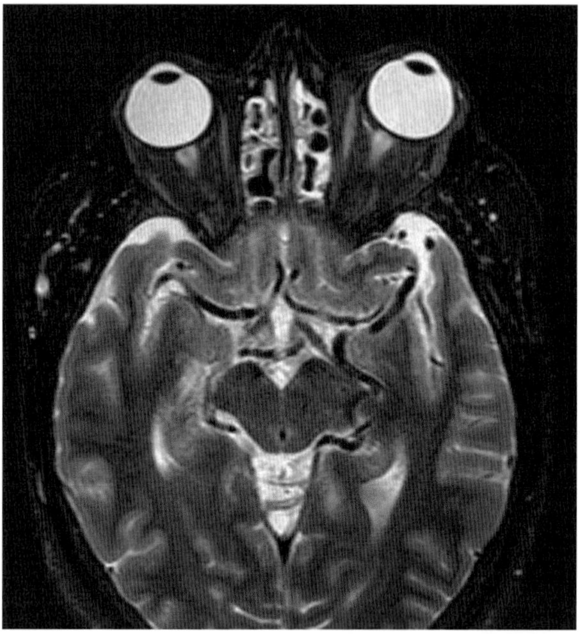

Fig. 3.1 Axial T2 weighted MRI of orbit showing enlargement of the rectus muscles on the left side, an axial proptosis and enlarged veins within the left temporal lobe, extending back to the brainstem

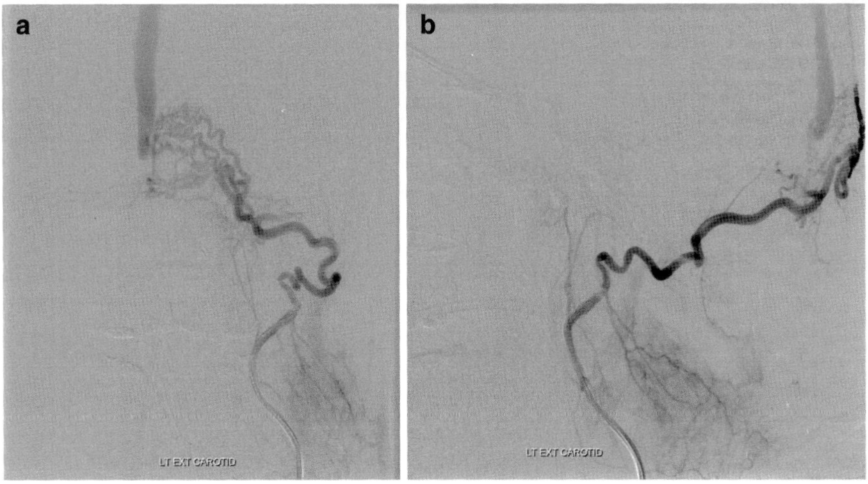

Fig. 3.2 Arteriogram showing numerous fistulae arising from the external carotid artery and enlarged veins (courtesy of Dr Peter Cowley, Consultant Neuroradiologist, Royal Free Hospital and National Hospital for Neurology and Neurosurgery)

A CT of the region showed no bony erosion and no calcification.

An intra-arterial angiogram showed a high flow dural arteriovenous shunt which arose through fistulae arising from several branches of the external carotid artery with venous drainage into the superior sagittal sinus and deep cerebral veins (Fig. 3.2).

Onyx embolization of the main occipital artery feeders was undertaken on both sides and she improved, with resolution of her symptoms. Since other fistulae remain she is being monitored in the neurovascular clinic.

Discussion

Dural carotid-cavernous fistulas are acquired arteriovenous malformations between the cavernous sinus and meningeal branches of the internal carotid artery, the external carotid artery and branches from both arteries. They can develop at any age, but are much more common in middle aged or elderly women. They are associated with pregnancy, atherosclerosis and hypertension, Ehlers-Danlos syndrome and trauma (including surgery). It is thought that they develop after thrombosis of the cavernous sinus leads to the development of collateral venous outflow. The clinical syndrome produced depends on the pressure within the shunt and whether the venous outflow is anterior, posterior or both [1].

Posteriorly draining fistulas: it stands to reason that venous pressure will not increase within the orbit under this circumstance, and such fistulas, which drain into the superior and inferior petrosal sinuses, are often asymptomatic. However there are reports of rare complications, due it seems to venous engorgement, of isolated trigeminal and facial neuropathies, and ocular motor nerve palsies (*i.e.* III, IV and/or VI), which may present acutely, with headache, and involve the pupil leading to the supposition that the cause is an aneurysm of the posterior communicating artery. Brain stem venous congestion and also intracerebral hemorrhage has also been reported (reviewed in [1]).

Sometimes there is a change in flow and drainage becomes predominately anterior, and the clinical features change.

Anteriorly draining fistulas: these drain into the superior and inferior ophthalmic veins, leading to venous congestion within the orbit. Pressure within them is not as high as in direct carotico-cavernous fistulas complicating intracavernous carotid artery aneurysms (see Case 23) and the clinical features therefore develop subacutely and often chronically. There is conjunctival injection, which, if corkscrew in appearance, is said to be pathognomonic for the condition [2], and there may be eyelid swelling and proptosis. Angle closure glaucoma may develop and signs of a venous stasis retinopathy with "dot and blot" retinal hemorrhage, choroidal effusion, folds and detachment, and optic disc swelling.

As this case proves, MR and CT angiographic imaging does not always allow the disorder to be ascertained with certainty; oftentimes it may only be revealed at catheter angiography of internal and external carotid arteries.

20–50 % resolve spontaneously, or after catheter angiography, or after pressure changes in air flight [3]. Otherwise endovascular treatment is indicated in those with sight threatening venous stasis retinopathy, central retinal vein occlusion and glaucoma.

References

1. Miller NR. Carotid-cavernous sinus fistulas. In: Miller NR, Newman NJ, editors. Walsh and Hoyt's clinical neuro-ophthalmology. 6th ed. Philadelphia: Lippincott Williams and Wilkins; 2005. p. 2283–93.
2. Miller NR. Dural carotid-cavernous fistulas: epidemiology, clinical presentation and management. Neurosurg Clin N Am. 2012;23:179–92.
3. Liu HM, Wang YH, Chen YF, Cheng JS, Yip PK, Tu YK. Long-term clinical outcome of spontaneous carotid cavernous sinus fistulae supplied by dural branches of the internal carotid artery. Neuroradiology. 2001;43:1007–14.

Case 4

History

An 89-year-old lady presented to her local ophthalmic department with diplopia. She was noted to have impaired abduction on the left; the remainder of the examination was unremarkable, and, in view of her hypertension and age, the diplopia was attributed to a microvascular cause. There were early signs of improvement, but this was short-lived and she developed periocular pain. Over the following 3 months this became severe, and she noted a progressive visual loss on the left side. She was referred to the Neuro-ophthalmology department of the Royal Free Hospital.

Examination

There was a left proptosis. Visual acuity was 6/12 on the right with normal color vision and on the left there was only perception of hand movements. The left disc was pale.

There was a complete left ptosis and the ipsilateral pupil was dilated with no response to light or accommodation. There was some downwards movement of the left eye, but no other movements.

She had impaired sensation over the left forehead with an absent corneal reflex.

D.P. Kidd, *Neuro-Ophthalmology*, DOI 10.1007/978-1-4471-2410-8_4

Evaluation

This elderly lady presents with a rapidly progressive painful ophthalmoparesis with proptosis and visual loss. The IIIrd and VIth nerves are also affected; the IVth seems to remain functional. The presence of proptosis implies an anteriorly placed disorder either within the orbit or at the orbital apex.

Neoplastic causes would include secondary tumor and lymphoma; a more slowly growing lesion such as sphenoid ridge meningioma would not appear so quickly and would not be associated with neuropathic pain of this severity. A vascular cause such as a high flow anterior carotico-cavernous fistula would be associated with conjunctival chemosis and retinal venous congestion. Inflammatory lesions such as idiopathic orbital inflammation, orbital myositis, thyroid orbitopathy and sarcoidosis would be unlikely at this age. Giant cell arteritis at this age can present with pain, visual loss and ophthalmoparesis, but would not be associated with proptosis. Infections in the sinuses leading to orbital cellulitis should certainly be considered, although would be more subacute than this history of 3 months.

A neoplastic cause would considered most likely, and imaging arranged after screening blood investigations (including ESR) were unremarkable.

Investigation

Magnetic resonance imaging showed an enhancing lesion in the orbital apex extending anteriorly along the superior aspect of the orbit and the track of the ophthalmic division of the trigeminal nerve, and posteriorly to involve the cavernous sinus and in to Meckel's cave (Fig. 4.1).

On closer inspection of the left brow area, there was a suspicious lesion of the skin, from which biopsies were obtained in the dermatology clinic.

The histological examination revealed a moderately differentiated squamous cell carcinoma (Fig. 4.2).

Palliative radiotherapy was offered in the Dermatology department.

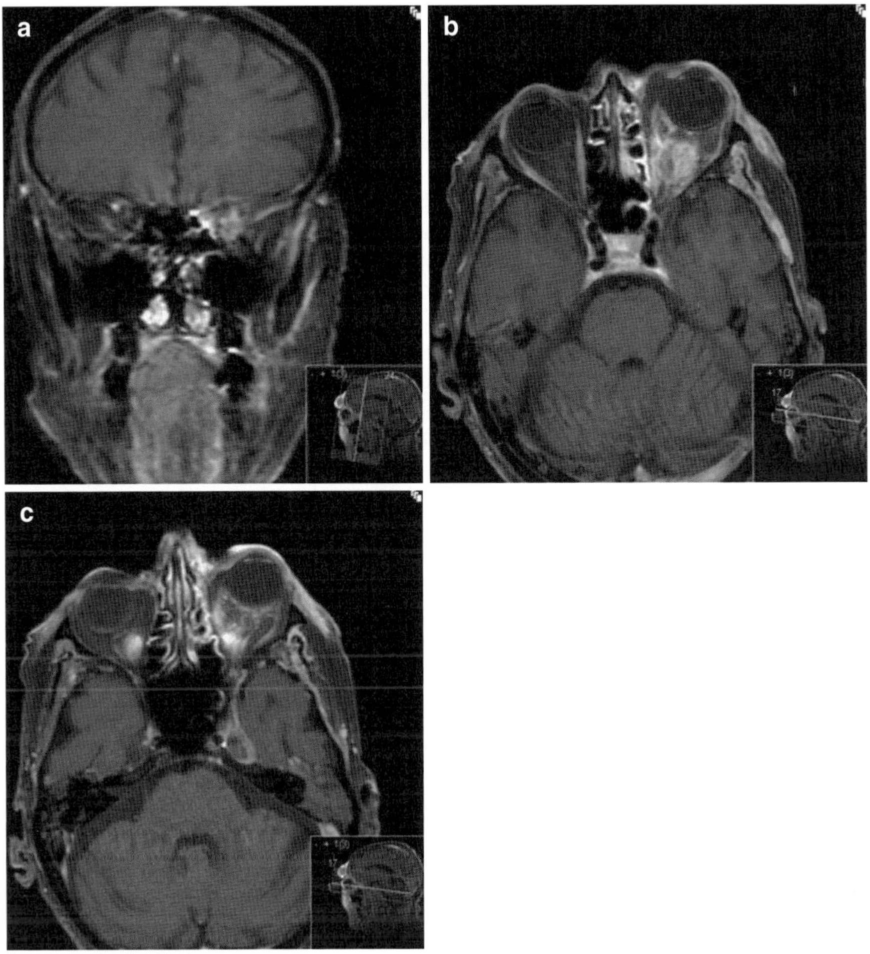

Fig. 4.1 T1-weighted gadolinium enhanced (**a**) coronal and (**b**, **c**) axial magnetic resonance imaging demonstrating enhancing tissue within the medial orbital wall extending back to the orbital apex along the path of the left supraorbital nerve, and into Meckel's cave

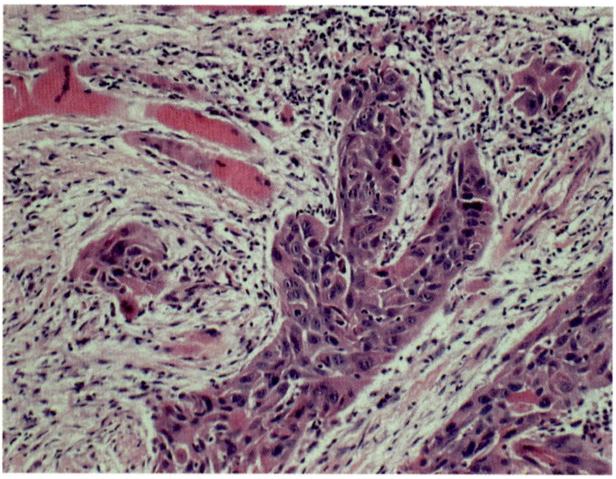

Fig. 4.2 Histopathology demonstrating nests of moderately differentiated squamous cell carcinoma cells infiltrating between muscle fibers (hematoxylin and eosin) (courtesy of Dr Nigel Kirkham, Consultant Histopathologist, Royal Free Hospital) (This figure is reproduced with permission from a previously published case report on the same patient in Koukkoulli et al. [6])

Discussion

Squamous cell carcinoma (SCC) accounts for 5–10 % of all periocular tumors. It is associated with increasing age, fair complexion, prolonged sun exposure, male gender (due to occupational sunlight exposure), chronically injured skin (ulcers and scars), certain genetic skin disorders (xeroderma pigmentosa, albinism), and immunosuppression following organ transplantation [1]. SCC causes local tissue destruction but may also spread via lymphatic, hematogenous and perineural routes.

Perineural invasion (PNI) into the orbit and intracranial cavity occurs along the routes of cranial nerves V and VII as a result of their extensive subcutaneous distribution. The frontal region is especially prone due to the rich supply provided by the supraorbital nerve. The incidence of PNI in periocular SCCs is 4–8 % and is associated with recurrent disease, poorly-differentiated histological features and lesions larger than 2 cm and deeper than 4 mm [1, 2].

PNI is asymptomatic in its early stages in 60–70 % of cases and is often not suspected until the orbit and cavernous sinus have been invaded. Perineural spread often cannot be visualized on neuroimaging and sensitivities have been reported to be as low as 76 %, for non-contrast MRI and CT [3]. MRI with contrast enhancement may show nerve enlargement, foraminal enlargement, obliteration of fat planes, pseudocystic masses and convexity of the lateral cavernous sinus wall [4].

In one series of 21 cases the majority were male, the forehead and brow were the most common primary sites for SCC with PNI and the lesion was often larger than 2 cm. The average time between primary excision to clinical presentation with PNI was 2 years. Many presented with reduced trigeminal sensation before other signs of orbital involvement arose. Once the tumor has spread to the orbital apex and beyond, treatment is palliative; the median duration from presentation of PNI to death secondary to disease in that series was 3 years [4]. Radiotherapy (as in this case) is given although there seems to be no clear evidence that it is helpful [5].

References

1. Limawararut V, Leibovitch I, Sullivan T, Selva D. Periocular squamous cell carcinoma. Clin Experiment Ophthalmol. 2007;35:174–85.
2. Esmaeli B, Ahmadi MA, Gillenwater AM, Faustina MM, Amato M. The role of supraorbital nerve biopsy in cutaneous malignancies of the periocular region. Ophthal Plast Reconstr Surg. 2003;19:282–6.
3. Bower JD, Sullivan TJ, Whitehead KJ. The management of perineural spread of squamous cell carcinoma to the ocular adnexae. Ophthal Plast Reconstr Surg. 2003;19:275–81.
4. McNab AA, Francs IC, Benger R, Crompton JL. Perineural spread of cutaneous squamous cell carcinoma via the orbit. Clinical features and outcome in 21 cases. Ophthalmology. 1997;104: 1457–62.
5. Waxweiler W, Sigmon J, Sheehan D. Adjunctive radiotherapy in the treatment of cutaneous squamous cell carcinoma with perineural invasion. J Surg Oncol. 2011;104:104–5.
6. Koukkoulli A, Koutroumanos N, Kidd D. Perineural spread of cutaneous squamous cell carcinoma manifesting as ophthalmoplegia. Neuro-ophthalmology 2015;39:144–6.

Case 5

History

This 45 year old lady noticed a drooping of her eyelids about 2 years before, and this appeared slowly to worsen. It was associated with an impairment of vision particularly when tired, when she found it hard to open the eyes widely enough. There was no double vision.

There was no muscular weakness and no other symptom, although of late her partner had noticed that her speech had changed a little. She found that she had to be careful when eating, and couldn't bolt her food or drink, although there was no choking or regurgitation.

There were no other or prior neurological symptoms, and she was otherwise well.

Examination

The anterior visual pathways were normal. The retinal examination and discs showed normal appearances. There was a bilateral symmetrical ptosis. Levator function was 6 mm on each side. There was a diminishment of upgaze on each side, and horizontal eye movements were normal. The saccadic velocities were reduced.

The face was not weak. Hearing was unimpaired. The bulbar muscles were strong but there was a slurring dysarthria. A 10 ml water swallow resulted in a wet voice quality for a time but there was no choking or coughing.

Neck flexion was weak but both proximal and distal limb muscles were strong.

D.P. Kidd, *Neuro-Ophthalmology*, DOI 10.1007/978-1-4471-2410-8_5

Clinical Evaluation

This lady presents with bilateral ptosis, an eye movement disorder without double vision, a change in voice and some difficulties with swallowing and chewing. The examination shows poor levator function (the normal is 15–20 mm) and slow saccadic velocities. The face is not weak but the neck flexors are. There are no other abnormal signs.

Myasthenia gravis would be associated with ptosis but commonly there are signs of neuromuscular blockade with a Cogan's twitch and fatigability, and the eye movement disorder is usually associated with diplopia. The face is very commonly involved in myasthenia.

A brain stem lesion such as an intrinsic glioma or lymphoma would be associated with long tract signs, and extra-axial tumors such as meningioma of the cerebellopontine angle or schwannoma of the VIIth or VIIIth nerves would not show symmetrical signs. Inflammatory lesions, particularly multiple sclerosis in its primary progressive form, would also not be so symmetrical and would be associated with long tract signs and ataxia.

An ocular myopathy would be more likely; the absence of diplopia and in particular the slow saccadic velocities would be in keeping with this. Chronic progressive external ophthalmoplegia would not be associated with bulbar involvement (see Case 7) and Kearns Sayre syndrome is associated with retinal pigmentation and cardiac conduction defects. Facio-scapulo-humeral muscular dystrophy and Dystrophia Myotonica are associated with a very prominent facial paralysis.

Imaging and electrophysiological investigations would be helpful.

Family History

Her mother's father had used ptosis props in later life. Her mother had developed ptosis in her 50s and later developed swallowing problems sufficiently severe to warrant the use of a PEG feeding tube. She had died at the age of 72 years with bronchopneumonia. Her mother's brother also had ptosis but the remainder of his family are well.

She has two brothers; one is well, the other has had ptosis surgery and recently has been to see a Neurologist with swallowing problems.

She has had no children.

Investigations

Biochemical screening including CK was normal. Acetyl choline receptor antibodies were negative. An EMG was not performed, but blood was sent to the Neurogenetics laboratory. This revealed a mutation in PABPN 1.

Discussion

Oculopharyngeal muscular dystrophy is an uncommon disease caused by alanine expansion mutations in the gene encoding poly (A)-binding protein nuclear 1 (PABPN 1) on chromosome 14q. This results in the accumulation of mutant PABPN 1 in the cell nucleus and the formation of insoluble aggregates [1, 2]. The prevalence in France is 1×10^5, but it is more common in French Canadians (100×10^5) and certain Jewish groups, in whom the prevalence is 1 per 600 [1]. It is to the most part autosomal dominant, with some families showing a recessive pattern of inheritance, and becomes fully penetrant by 70 years. Phenotypic anticipation does not occur.

Patients present most often in the fifth and sixth decades with bilateral ptosis, then dysarthria and increasing dysphagia. The serum CK is rarely raised, and the EMG shows myopathic potentials.

The pathological process is of degeneration and fibrosis in the affected muscles. Muscle biopsy reveals dystrophic features, with angulated fibers and fiber type variation, ragged red fibers and rimmed vacuoles (although these are not specific features and occur in other muscle disorders such as Inclusion Body myositis). A specific feature is the presence of intranuclear inclusions composed of tubular filaments of a size not seen in other muscle diseases.

The clinical features are as noted in this case, with an onset in the fifth or sixth decade of bilateral ptosis then swallowing problems about 10 years later. Later weakness of the proximal muscles and face may develop. A restriction of the extraocular muscles is common but complete external ophthalmoparesis is rare.

The swallowing disorder is different to that seen in neurogenic dysphagia; the fibrotic dystrophic pharyngeal muscles propel the bolus less efficiently towards the esophagus and the cricopharyngeus muscle fails to relax leading to a blocking effect at the pharyngo-esphageal junction. This results in a greater problem in dealing with solid food than liquids. It may be treated effectively for some time with cricopharyngeal myotomy or dilatation [1, 3], although it may recur later requiring repeated treatment. A recent trial of implantation of autologous myoblasts suggests a more prolonged effect [4].

References

1. Bais B. Oculopharyngeal muscular dystrophy. Handb Clin Neurol. 2011;101:181–92.
2. Trollet C, Gidaro T, Klein P, Butler-Browne G, Lacau St Guily J. Oculopharyngeal muscular dystrophy. GeneReviews(R) (internet) Seattle (WA), University of Washington 2014. 2014
3. Coiffier L, Perie S, Laforet P, Eymard B, St Guily JL. Long-term results of cricopharyngeal myotomy in oculopharyngeal muscular dystrophy. Otolaryngol Head Neck Surg. 2006;135: 218–22.
4. Perie S, Trollet C, Moully V, Vanneaux V, Mamchaoui K, Bouazza B, Marolleau JP, Lafroet P, Chapon F, Eymard B, Butler-Browne G, Larghero J, St Guily JL. Autologous myoblast transplantation for oculopharyngeal muscular dystrophy: a phase I/IIa study. Mol Ther. 2014;22: 219–25.

Case 6

History

This lady suffered a brief episode of double vision at the age of 36 years which settled spontaneously after 3 weeks. It recurred a year later and again resolved spontaneously, after 8 weeks. Two years later she developed a progressive worsening right sided ptosis and she was referred to her local Neurology department.

At that time screening blood tests were normal, an MRI scan of the brain was reported to be normal, and the CSF was acellular. No diagnosis was made, but the ptosis resolved spontaneously over 3 months.

Thereafter she remained well for 5 years, until she presented again, with a partial left sided ptosis. It came and went, then became complete and constant. She was referred to the Neuro-ophthalmology department.

Examination

There was a left sided complete ptosis without frontalis overaction. On the right side levator function was just within normal limits at 16 mm. There was limitation to upgaze on the left, with slight weakness of medial rectus on the same side. There were no other abnormal neurological signs.

D.P. Kidd, *Neuro-Ophthalmology*, DOI 10.1007/978-1-4471-2410-8_6

Clinical Evaluation

This was a complicated case initially; whilst a relapsing and remitting and in particular a spontaneously resolving problem with diplopia and ptosis must surely always be a neuro-muscular junction problem it is uncommon for such a complete ptosis to be so unilateral and furthermore that it should switch in an equally asymmetric way to the other side. The bilateral involvement, however, with temporal dispersion does make alternative causes, such as structural disorders at the orbital apex or cavernous sinus (tumors such as meningioma or pituitary adenoma and inflammatory lesions such as sarcoidosis and IgG4 disease) exceedingly unlikely.

An ocular myopathy, for example due to mitochondrial cytopathy, tends to be very symmetrical and diplopia is uncommon since the ophthalmoparesis is usually also very symmetrical. Oculopharyngeal muscular dystrophy and dystrophia myotonica may present late on with ptosis and diplopia but there are usually other neurological signs to discover. A family history is not always recognized in these disorders however.

Investigations

Screening blood investigations were normal. The CK was not raised. There were no acetylcholine or thyroid antibodies and she was not thyrotoxic. She did not have anti-MuSK antibodies.

Imaging of the orbits was undertaken; a regular axial brain scan does not show the orbital structures, orbital apex and cavernous sinus in sufficient detail. This was normal; the orbital muscles were of normal size. The midbrain was also seen to be normal.

An EMG showed normal compound muscle action potentials in the limbs, and no decrement on repetitive stimulation. Single fiber EMG showed abnormalities only in the orbicularis oculi on both sides, with jitter in two thirds of the muscles studies and blocking in half of those.

An MRI of the mediastinum showed no enlargement of the thymus gland.

Management

It was considered that Myasthenia Gravis was the most likely explanation and a trial of acetylcholinesterase inhibitors provoked a partial benefit. Her clinical features deteriorated and she developed bilateral ptosis and ophthalmoparesis, with a positive Cogan's twitch and the author felt more confident in recommending an escalation of treatment. She responded well to low dose (10 mg) prednisolone but quickly relapsed as the dose was reduced. She developed a rash to Azathioprine but responded well to Mycophenolate, with complete resolution of all abnormal signs on 750 mg bd. She has remained well since.

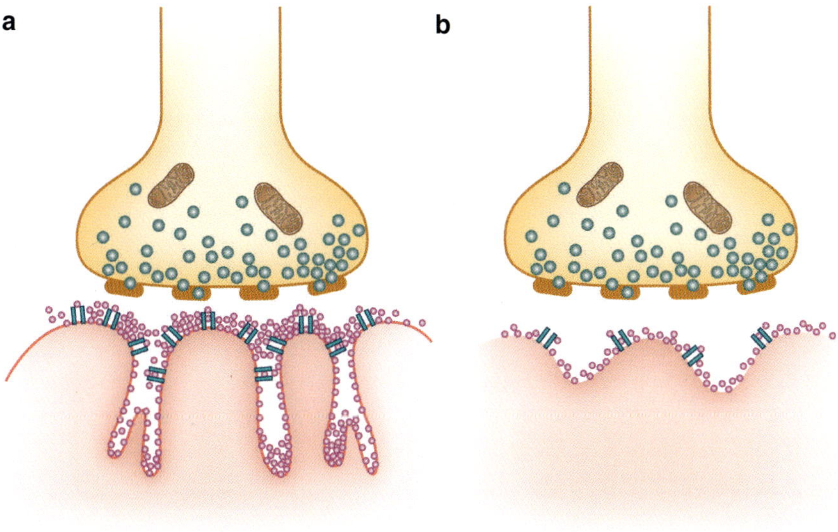

Fig. 6.1 Cartoon of the neuromuscular junction showing (**a**) normal appearances and (**b**) when acetylcholine receptor antibodies from and interfere with function

Discussion

Myasthenia Gravis is an autoimmune disease in which most (but not all) patients form antibodies against the alpha-1 subunit of the acetylcholine receptor. This leads to complement-mediated destruction of parts of the endplate so that the muscle fiber becomes less able to be stimulated by acetylcholine presented to it [1] (Fig. 6.1).

85 % of patients with generalized myasthenia and 50–60 % of those with ocular myasthenia possess acetylcholine receptor antibodies. The plasma concentration of antibodies does not correlate with disease severity. 10 % have muscle specific tyrosine kinase (MuSK) antibodies, leaving 5 % seronegative in the generalized form [2].

The prevalence of the disease is $14 - 20 \times 10^5$, more common in women in the second and third decades and more common in men in the seventh and eighth. The peak prevalence is in the seventh decade.

15 % have an associated thymoma, of whom the majority show anti-striated muscle antibodies. 70 % have thymic hyperplasia. Hyperplasia is more common in younger age groups.

The majority of patients present with ocular symptoms; those with the generalized form worsen to involve other muscle groups (the limbs and the bulbar muscles) within the first two years after symptom onset [3]. The ocular form, in which weakness of the extraocular muscles, levator and orbicularis oculi remains without generalization, is seen in around 15 % of cases. Electrophysiological abnormalities in the limbs are less common (but may be seen) and (as noted above) patients with the ocular form are more likely to be persistently seronegative.

Treatment is as noted above in this case; acetylcholinesterase inhibitors work by increasing the concentration of acetylcholine at the diseased endplate, so allowing a greater opportunity for stimulation of the endplate to occur. Corticosteroids and immune suppression work by altering the immune response. Intravenous immunoglobulin and apheresis are indicated in severe and treatment unresponsive cases. Thymectomy may abolish the disease in those with hyperplasia, or allow a substantial reduction in the requirement for treatment, whilst others are unaffected. Removal of thymoma is important but tends not to lead to changes in the severity of the associated neuromuscular disorder [4]. In the UK management guidelines have recently been published [5].

References

1. Vincent A. Autoantibodies in different forms of myasthenia gravis and in the Lambert-Eaton syndrome. Handb Clin Neurol. 2008;91:213–27.
2. Sommer N, Tackenberg B, Hohlfeld R. The immunopathogenesis of myasthenia gravis. Handb Clin Neurol. 2008;91:169–212.
3. Sanders DB, Massey JM. Clinical features of myasthenia gravis. Handb Clin Neurol. 2008;91:229–52.
4. Drachman DB. Therapy of myasthenia gravis. Handb Clin Neurol. 2008;91:253–72.
5. Sussman J, Farrugia ME, Maddison P, Hill M, Leite MI, Hilton-Jones D. Myasthenia Gravis: Association of British Neurologists' management guidelines. Pract Neurol. 2015;15:199–206.

Case 7

History

This lady first noticed a problem with her vision at the age of 46; she described a vertical separation worse when looking to the left but present in all directions of gaze. This had developed gradually and worsened, and only affected reading. It was very slight. Her optometrist was unable to correct the symptom with reading glasses and asked her GP to refer her to the Neurology department.

There was no variation and no accompanying neurological symptoms, specifically vestibular symptoms, muscle weakness, change in voice quality or difficulty swallowing.

Examination

The anterior visual pathways were normal. The ocular examination and the discs were also normal. There was no ptosis. The eye movements were full in the horizontal plane but restricted in upgaze, and there was a left over right hypertropia (the left eye was held higher than the right) (Appendix 3). The velocity of saccadic movements in all directions of gaze was reduced.

There were no other abnormal neurological signs.

D.P. Kidd, *Neuro-Ophthalmology*, DOI 10.1007/978-1-4471-2410-8_7

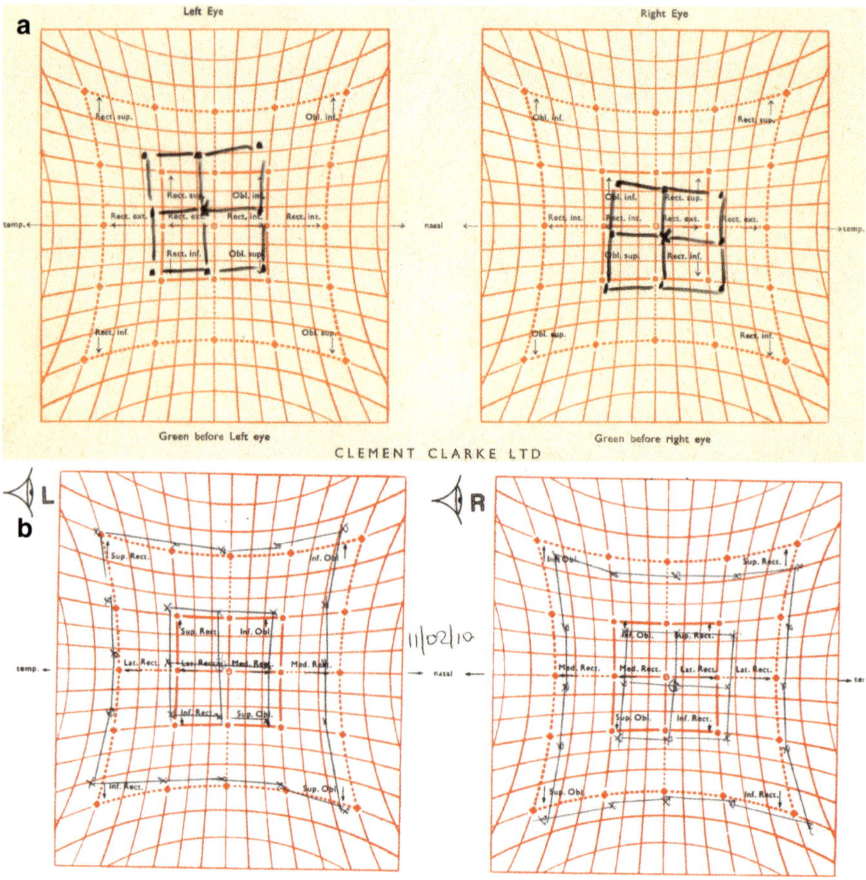

Fig. 7.1 Lees screen test chart showing restriction of eye movements in 1999 (**a**) and in 2010 (**b**)

Investigation and Management

She was assessed initially in the Neurology department and correctly both Myasthenia Gravis and thyroid orbitopathy were considered. Screening blood investigations were also normal and there were no antibodies against acetylcholine receptors nor thyroid tissue.

A 10 mg edrophonium ("tensilon") test was performed with no change in her vision.

In the ophthalmology department an orthoptic examination (Fig. 7.1a) showed a left over right hypertropia of 8 diopters in all directions of gaze for near which increased to 10 diopters in distance. A forced duction test suggested a restriction in eye movements rather than muscular weakness (Appendix 3).

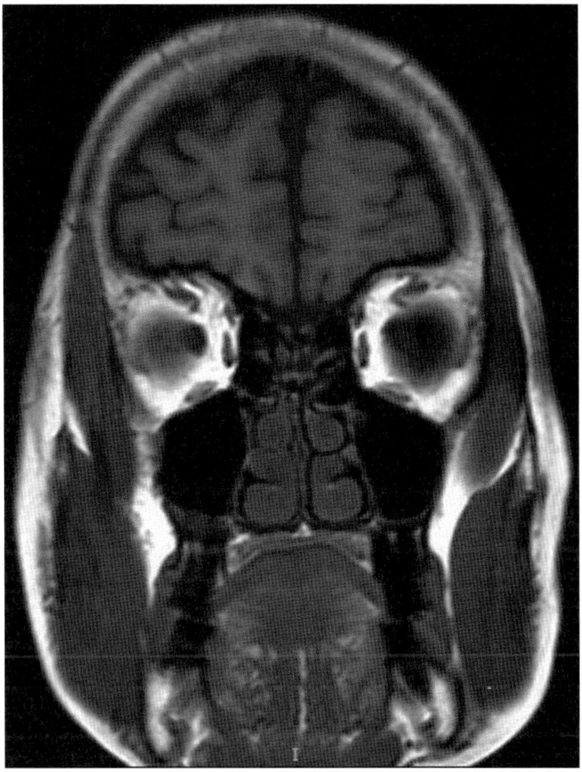

Fig. 7.2 MRI: coronal FATSAT image showing the rectus muscles symmetrically to be atrophied

An MRI scan of the orbits showed thinning of the extraocular muscles (Fig. 7.2).

She was referred to the Neuro-ophthalmology department. The investigations performed were reviewed and it was agreed that there was no evidence for thyroid orbitopathy, myasthenia or a brain stem lesion causing a gaze palsy. The examination findings were unchanged.

A diagnosis of ocular myopathy was made and it was explained that whilst further investigations were likely to lead to a confirmatory diagnosis it was unlikely that any meaningful form of treatment would follow. The patient opted to monitor the condition carefully, and she attended at yearly intervals thereafter, without any objective change in her condition (Fig. 7.1b).

Over the years her two sisters also came to the department with identical examination findings; one opted to undergo a muscle biopsy and this showed an excess of LDH positive, COX negative fibers in keeping with a mitochondrial cytopathy (Fig. 7.3). Genetic investigations did not identify a pathological mitochondrial DNA mutation or deletion.

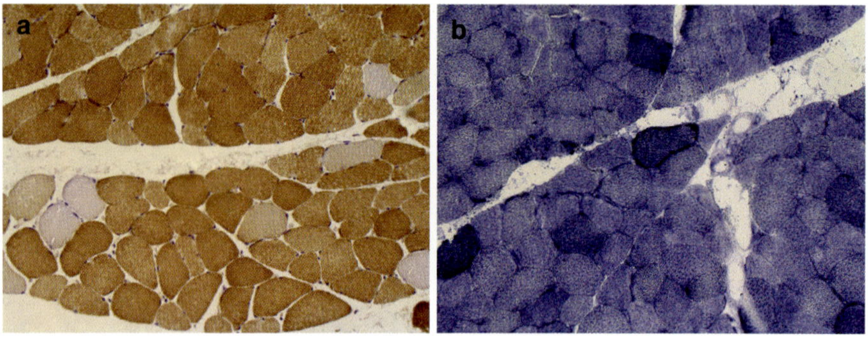

Fig. 7.3 Muscle biopsy of her sister: (**a**) staining for cytochrome oxidase shows several unstained fibers. Although occasional negative fibers may be seen in older patients as a consequence of normal aging, the frequency of negative fibers is beyond the level expected for the patient's age. (**b**) histochemical staining for succinate dehydrogenase activity shows scattered fibers with a darkly staining rim, indicating the accumulation of peripheral mitochondria. These fibers are referred to as 'ragged-red equivalents'. They are often seen in patients with mitochondrial disorders (Pathology images courtesy of Dr Malcolm Galloway, Consultant Neuropathologist, Institute of Neurology and the Royal Free Hospital, London, UK)

Discussion

Chronic progressive external ophthalmoplegia refers to a slowly progressive restriction of eye movements in all directions of gaze accompanied by ptosis. It is highly symmetrical, painless and rarely is associated with subjective double vision (because the ophthalmoparesis is symmetrical). The severity varies and if the eyes can move the velocity of saccadic movements is reduced, helping to differentiate it from myasthenia gravis and thyroid orbitopathy. It may be confused with other ocular myopathies such as oculopharyngeal muscular dystrophy, dystrophia myotonica, or MYH2-related myopathy. Miller Fisher syndrome may present in a similar way but subacutely with or without an internal ophthalmoparesis (paralysis of the sympathetic and parasympathetic supply to the ciliary body). The orbital muscles are seen to be atrophied [1] as seen here. This too is helpful is differentiating the disorder from a more subacute one such as thyroid orbitopathy, myasthenia gravis and Miller Fisher syndrome.

It is the most common clinical feature of neurological diseases related to inherited disorders of the respiratory chain. Whilst most patients go on to develop other neurological features such as neuropathy, ataxia, spasticity, myopathy and dystonia, some show an isolated CPEO, as in this family. What proportion of those with a mitochondrial disorder show the clinical phenotype of an isolated CPEO is not known, nor indeed what proportion have an identifiable mitochondrial or nuclear deletion or point mutation (AHV Schapira, personal communication). The association of CPEO with an early onset retinal pigmentation and cardiac conduction defects is termed Kearns-Sayre syndrome. The association of CPEO with gastrointestinal dysmotility, deafness and neuropathy is known as mitochondrial neurogastrointestinal encephalomyopathy (MNGIE).

Mitochondrial DNA mutations impair the workings of the respiratory chain, resulting in defective oxidative phosphorylation if present in sufficient proportion, leading to a reduction in energy supply. In addition there may be a resultant increase in production of free radicles, and finally defective mitochondrial function may allow early initiation of apoptosis [2]. It is associated with single mitochondrial deletions or point mutations which are usually sporadic, inherited mitochondrial RNA or protein coding genes, such as MT-TL1, or associated with nuclear-encoding genes which are involved in mitochondrial DNA replication, for example POLG, OPA-1 and SPG7 (reviewed in [3]), in which a maternally-derived family history is identified. However in around 50 % of cases no genetic defect has so far been identified, although in these cases a biopsy of skeletal muscle reveals clear evidence for mitochondrial disease, with a mosaic pattern of cytochrome s oxidase deficient fibers and ragged red fibers (caused by accumulation of sub-sarcolemnal accumulation of diseased mitochondria) [4]. Deletions in mitochondrial DNA within the muscle are usually seen.

Recently mutations in SRG-7, which is associated also with hereditary spastic paraparesis, have been shown to be associated with a form of CPEO associated with cerebellar ataxia [5].

References

1. Yu-Wai-Man C, Smith FE, Firbank MJ, Guthrie G, Guthrie S, Gorman GS, Taylor RW, Turnbull DM, Griffiths PG, Blamire AM, Chinnery PF, Yu-Wai-Man P. Extraocular muscle atrophy and central nervous system involvement in chronic progressive external ophthalmoplegia. PLoS One. 2013;8:e75048.
2. Schapira AHV. Mitochondrial diseases. Lancet. 2012;379:1825–34.
3. Horga A, Pitceathly RD, Blake JC, Woodward CE, Zapater P, Fratter C, Mudanohwo EE, Plant GT, Houlden H, Sweeney MG, Hanna MG, Reilly MM. Peripheral neuropathy predicts nuclear gene defect in patients with mitochondrial ophthalmoplegia. Brain. 2014;137:3200–12.
4. Petty RK, Harding AE, Morgan-Hughes JA. The clinical aspects of mitochondrial myopathy. Brain. 1986;109:915–38.
5. Pfeffer G, Gorman GS, Griffin H, Kurzawa-Akanbi M, Blakely EL, Wilson I, Sitarz K, Moore D, Murphy JL, Alston CL, Pyle A, Coxhead J, Payne B, Gorrie GH, Longman C, Hadjivassiliou M, McConville J, Dick D, Imam I, Hilton D, Norwood F, Baker MR, Jaiser SR, Yu-Wai-Man P, Farrell M, McCarthy A, Lynch T, McFarland R, Schaefer AM, Turnbull DM, Horvath R, Taylor RW, Chinnery PF. Mutations in the SPG7 gene cause chronic progressive external ophthalmoplegia through disordered mitochondrial DNA maintenance. Brain. 2014;137:1323–36.

Part II
The Nerve

Case 8

History

This 26 year old lady developed a mild 'flu-like illness around Christmas time; there was fever, aches and pains in the joints, myalgia, cough and then a headache. As the symptoms improved 48 hours later she noticed blurred vision in both eyes. This worsened over a further day and she noticed a patch of missing vision in the central visual field causing difficulty with reading and seeing people's faces. There was no pain. There had been no prior neurological symptoms. She presented to the emergency department and was briefly admitted for investigations.

Examination

The systemic examination was normal.

The visual acuities were 6/9 N10 on the right 6/6 N6 on the left. Color vision was slow but within normal limits. There was no pupillary asymmetry. The discs and ocular media were normal. The visual fields confirmed the presence of bilateral central scotomas (Fig. 8.1).

The remainder of the neurological examination was normal.

D.P. Kidd, *Neuro-Ophthalmology*, DOI 10.1007/978-1-4471-2410-8_8

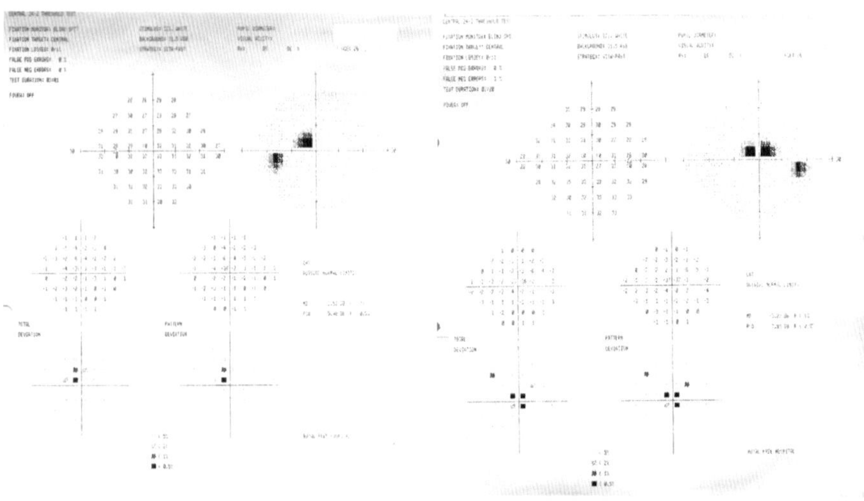

Fig. 8.1 Humphrey visual field showing bilateral small central scotomata

Evaluation

This young lady has presented with bilateral visual symptoms and signs of involvement of the optic nerve on both sides. The visual fields show bilateral involvement of the nerve (*ie* involvement of both sides of the midline on both sides) and so a symmetrical involvement by a disease process of both occipital poles would be unlikely.

An acute demyelinating optic neuropathy is possible; the absence of pain is against it (90 % of cases have pain at onset), and whilst bilateral cases occur in up to 30 % of published series (reviewed in [1]) it is much more common for the clinical signs to be very asymmetrical. Table 8.1 shows a list of possible causes of a subacute bilateral optic neuropathy; after structural causes have been outruled by imaging, inflammatory and infectious causes should be considered next, and nutritional, metabolic and inherited causes may be considered in further enquiry by history.

Investigations are warranted, looking for uncommon causes.

Investigations

Full blood count and ESR were normal. The CRP was 45. Biochemical screening was normal. Serological tests for ANA, ENA, ANCA, phospholipid and aquaporin-4 were normal. The serum ACE was not raised. A chest X-ray was normal. Viral screening studies showed an IgM response to H1N1 in keeping with the so-called swine 'flu infection.

An MRI scan of the brain was normal.

Table 8.1 Causes of bilateral subacute optic neuropathy

Inflammatory:	Demyelinating disease
	Sarcoidosis
	Post-infectious immune activation
	Neuromyelitis Optica
	Anti-MOG (myelin-oligodendrocyte glycoprotein) associated optic neuritis
	CRION (chronic relapsing inflammatory optic neuropathy)
	Connective tissue disease *e.g.* SLE, Sjogren's syndrome
	Behçet's syndrome
Infection:	Tuberculosis
	Bartonella Henselai
	Borrelia Burgdorferi
	Syphilis
	Viral diseases including HIV
Vascular:	Anterior and posterior ischemic optic neuropathy
	Vasculitis: giant cell arteritis, polyarteritis nodosa, Churg-Strauss syndrome, granulomatosis with polyangiitis
Metabolic:	Tobacco-alcohol amblyopia
	Methanol, solvents
	Ethambutol, chemotherapy agents
	B12 deficiency
	Endemic nutritional deficiencies
Space-occupying lesions:	Giant carotid aneurysms
	Mucocoeles of the paranasal sinuses
	Choristomas and cysts of the parasellar region
	Meningiomas and schwannomas of the parasellar region
Inherited disorders:	Leber's hereditary optic neuropathy

She was improving spontaneously and so no treatment was recommended; over 18 months her fields improved. Despite a small residual scotoma she found her vision to be unimpaired.

Discussion

Optic neuritis associated with viral infections is well recognized [2]. It is more common in children and more often bilateral than unilateral. A viral prodrome within the previous 3 weeks then visual loss and pain is the most common clinical syndrome. The clinical characteristics are indistinguishable from a demyelinating optic neuritis. Other neurological symptoms may arise if the disorder affects other parts of the nervous system, causing acute disseminated encephalomyelitis (ADEM); if the brain is unaffected (by ADEM) the MRI is normal. The spinal fluid tends to be active with a raised protein and a lymphocytosis. Recovery is good in most cases, and there is no evidence that steroids enhance this recovery [3].

Neuroretinitis may be seen, and a concurrent uveitis, retinitis and retinal vasculitis may also arise [2].

There is only one other published report of optic neuritis following H1N1 infection [4], but vaccinating against the illness has been associated with acute disseminated encephalomyelitis and optic neuritis [5, 6].

References

1. Kidd DP, Plant GT. Optic neuritis. In: Kidd DP, Biousse V, Newman NJ, editors. Neuro-ophthalmology. Philadelphia: Butterworth Heinemann Elsevier; 2008. p. 140–1.
2. Brazis PW, Miller NR. Viruses (except retroviruses) and viral diseases. In: Miller NR, Newman NJ, editors. Walsh and Hoyt's clinical neuro-ophthalmology. Philadelphia: Lippincott Williams & Wilkins; 2005. p. 3115–322.
3. Farris BK, Pickard DJ. Bilateral post-infectious optic neuritis and intravenous corticosteroid therapy in children. Ophthalmology. 1990;97:339–45.
4. Lai CC, Chang YS, Li ML, Chang CM, Huang FC, Tseng SH. Acute anterior uveitis and optic neuritis as ocular complications of influenza A infection in an 11 year old boy. J Pediatr Ophthalmol Strabismus. 2011;6:48.
5. Lapphra K, Huh L, Scheifele DW. Adverse neurologic reactions after both doses of pandemic H1N1 influenza vaccine with optic neuritis and demyelination. Pediatr Infect Dis. 2011;30:84–6.
6. Fuji K, Suyama M, Chiba K, Okunushi T, Oikawa J, Kohno Y. Acute disseminated encephalomyelitis following 2009 H1N1 influenza vaccine. Pediatr Int. 2012;54:539–41.

Case 9

History

This man was found to have poor vision in childhood. Investigations were performed and no cause for the visual loss was found. A successful amateur boxer, he applied at 21 for a professional license but was refused since his acuities were found to be 6/12.

He was referred at the age of 33 following a field examination by his optometrist. He had noted that his vision slowly had deteriorated over many years.

There were no headaches, other or prior neurological symptoms, and no symptoms on systematic enquiry. There was no known family history of neurological or ophthalmic disease.

Examination

The central visual acuity was 6/24 N8 in both eyes. There was a red – green color blindness which was symmetrical. The visual fields showed incomplete centrocaecal scotomas (Fig. 9.1). The ocular media were clear and the retinae normal. The discs showed a bilateral temporal pallor without excavation (Fig. 9.2). The remainder of the neurological examination was normal.

D.P. Kidd, *Neuro-Ophthalmology*, DOI 10.1007/978-1-4471-2410-8_9

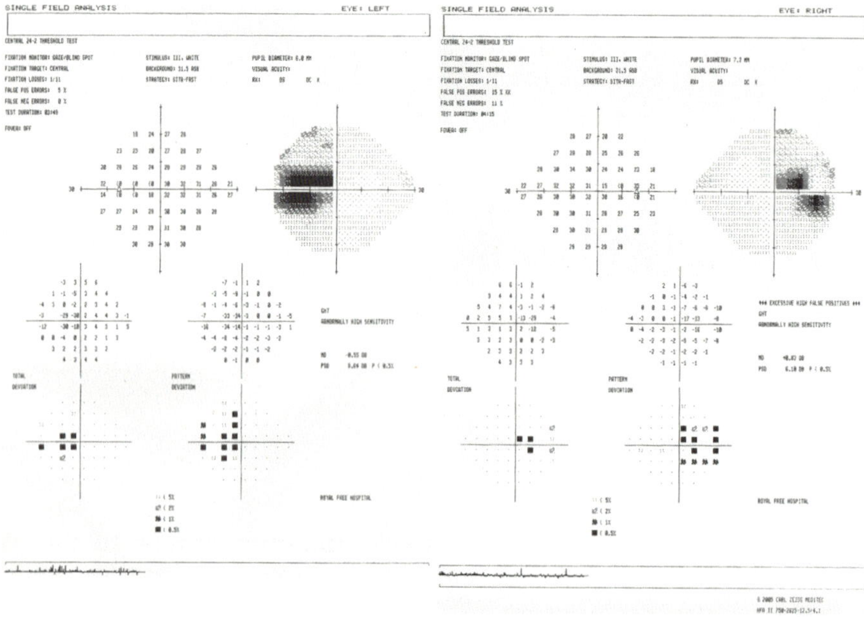

Fig. 9.1 Humphrey automated visual filed showing bilateral centrocaecal scotomas

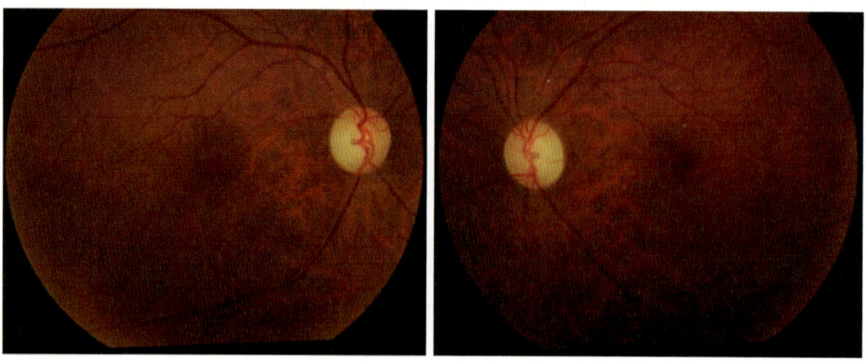

Fig. 9.2 Fundus photograph showing symmetrical bilateral disc pallor

Investigation

Full blood count and screening biochemical tests were normal. Serological tests showed no evidence for an underlying vasculitis, connective tissue disease or Sarcoidosis.

MRI scan of orbits showed rather slender optic nerves but no intrinsic lesion or enhancement, no compressive mass and no lesion within the brain (Fig. 9.3).

A spinal fluid examination showed no abnormalities. Oligoclonal bands were absent.

Electrophysiological tests of optic nerve and retinal function revealed an undetectable pattern reversal VEP and markedly subnormal amplitude flash VEPs. Pattern electroretinograms showed profound loss of the N95 peak and a shortening of P50 latency. The full field ERG was normal on each side.

An optical coherence tomographic (OCT) examination of the discs revealed a profound loss of retinal nerve fiber layer thickness (Fig. 9.4).

Genetic tests for mutation in the mitochondrial genome were negative for Leber's hereditary optic neuropathy. However tests did reveal a mutation in the OPA-1 gene at exon 6: c.649C>T.

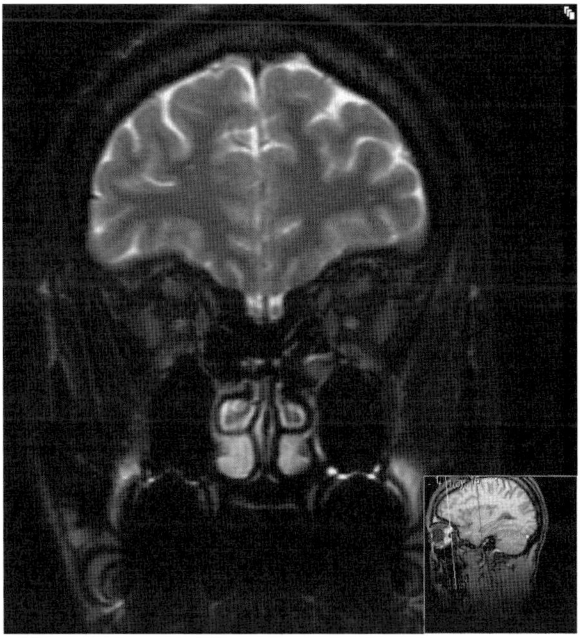

Fig. 9.3 T2 weighted coronal MRI showing that both optic nerves are slender

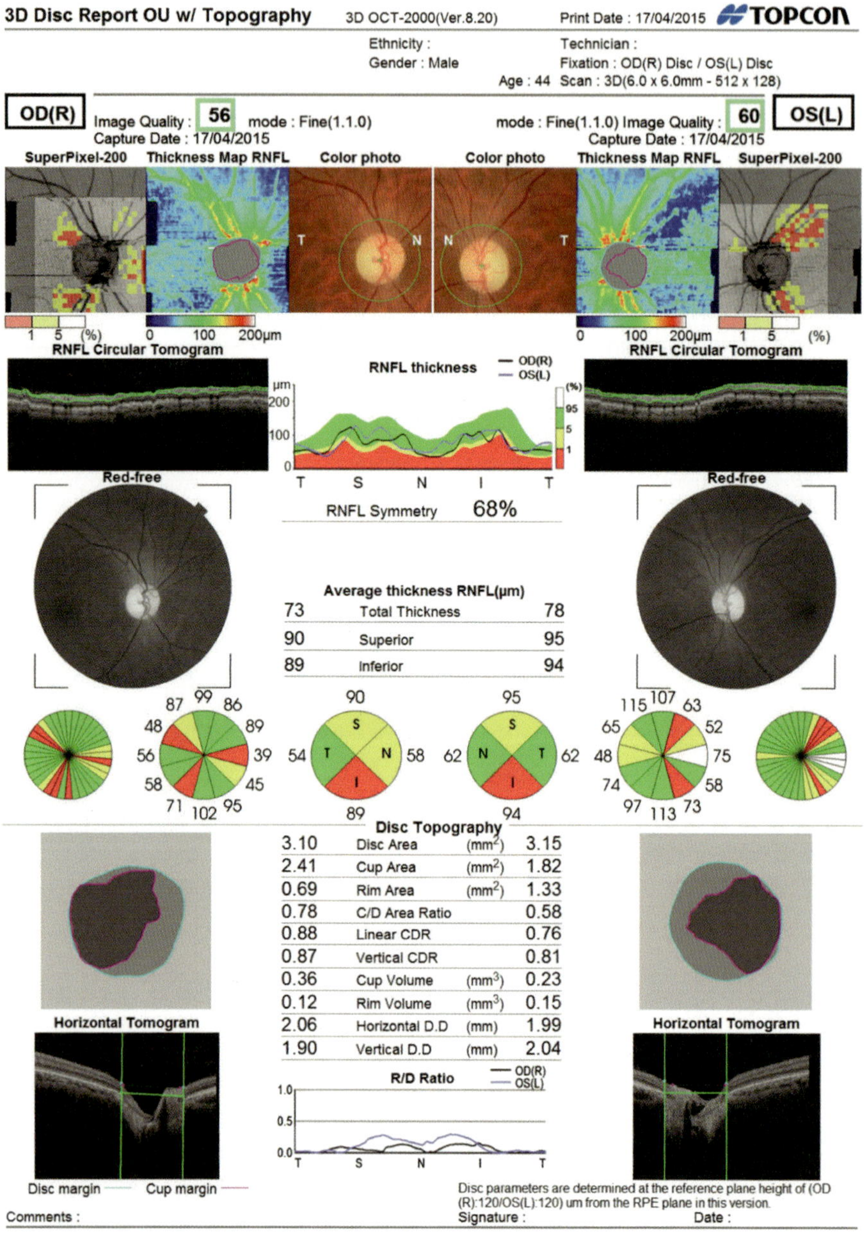

Fig. 9.4 Optical coherence tomogram (OCT) showing reduction in the thickness of the retinal nerve fiber layer (RNFL) on both sides

Clinical Evaluation

This man presented with a slowly progressive visual loss possibly from childhood, without any family history of a similar disorder. The examination findings are in keeping with an optic neuropathy; there is loss of central acuity and color vision (although congenital color blindness does occur in 8 % of men), the visual field defect is in keeping with an optic neuropathy and in particular, because it is centrocaecal, the papillomacular bundle. Finally there is temporal pallor of the optic disc, again in keeping with involvement of the papillomacular bundle. An OCT showed a reduction in the thickness of the retinal nerve fiber layer. Visual evoked potentials were abnormal, and there was a specific reduction in the N95 peak of the ERG, in keeping with a loss of retinal ganglion cell function in addition to an optic neuropathy.

Imaging showed no evidence for a compressive or inflammatory cause, blood and CSF investigation failed to identify a systemic or local inflammation or infection. A nutritional amblyopia would not evolve so slowly. An inherited disorder, therefore, was considered the most likely, and dominant optic atrophy the most likely of these.

Discussion

The history and examination findings are typical for dominant optic atrophy. The disorder is common, with a prevalence of 1 in 35,000 [1]. The penetrance and clinical severity varies amongst affected family members. Characteristically the disorder is noticed in the second decade of life and gradually deteriorates. In most families the visual loss reaches a plateau in late middle age, and it is uncommon for the acuity to become worse than 6/60 over a lifetime [1, 2].

The fields usually show central or centrocaecal loss, bitemporal defects are sometimes also seen. The discs are uniformly or temporally pale, and the retinal nerve fiber layer thickness is reduced, even in the very early stages, and in particular within the region of the papillomacular bundle [3, 4]. The retinae are normal. The pupillary responses are normal because the melanopsin ganglion cells in the photoreceptor layer are not involved [5].

The genetic abnormalities are widespread, with many different single base pair substitution mutations within the OPA-1 gene, and also missense mutations, deletions and insertions. The result is that the OPA-1 protein is reduced and abnormal, leading to oxidative stress and retinal ganglion cell death.

No treatment has been shown to be helpful.

References

1. Man PYW, Griffiths PG, Burke A, Sellar PW, Clarke MP, Gnanaraj L, Ah Kine D, Hudson G, Szermin G, Taylor RW, Horvath R, Chinnery PJ. The prevalence and natural history of dominant optic atrophy due to OPA-1 mutations. Ophthalmology. 2010;117:1538–46.
2. Lenaers G, Hamel CP, Lelettre C, Amati-Bonneau P, Procaccio V, Bonneau P, Milea D. Dominant optic atrophy. Orphanet J Rare Dis. 2012;7:46. epub July 9 2012.
3. Berninger TA, Jaeger W, Krastel H. Electrophysiology and colour perimetry in dominant infantile optic atrophy. Br J Ophthalmol. 1991;75:49–52.
4. Milea D, Sander B, Wegener M, Jensen H, Kjer B, Jorgensen TM. Axonal loss occurs early in dominant optic atrophy. Acta Ophthalmol. 2010;88:342–6.
5. Man PYW, Bailie M, Atawan A, Chinnery PF, Griffiths PG. Pattern of retinal ganglion cell loss in dominant optic atrophy due to OPA-1 mutations. Eye (Lond). 2011;25:596–602.

Case 10

History

This 61 year nursing Sister presented with sudden onset visual loss in the right eye. It lasted 10 seconds then resolved in entirety. Later that day she developed an incomplete reduction in vision on the left side which remained. She attended the ophthalmic emergency clinic in her own hospital.

There had been headache for the previous 2 months, which had increased. She had noticed aches and pains around the shoulders and an odd feeling in her jaw on the left when chewing, which resolved with rest.

Her past medical history had been unremarkable and she took no regular medications.

Examination

The central acuities were 6/5 on the right and 6/9 on the left. Color vision and pupillary responses had not been measured. The ocular media and discs were described as normal.

D.P. Kidd, *Neuro-Ophthalmology*, DOI 10.1007/978-1-4471-2410-8_10

Investigation

Her ESR was 115, CRP 134 and platelets 513. The white cell count was normal, and hemoglobin was 9 g/dl with normal red cell indices. Renal and liver functions were normal.

Evaluation

This lady presents with two episodes of amaurosis fugax over the course of a day. Patients with carotid stenosis often present with an escalating series of such symptoms, but virtually always (because carotid stenosis is more often asymmetric) on the same side. She ostensibly has no risk factors for the development of early atheromatous disease and so alternative explanations do need to be considered. Furthermore the condition has affected each side.

Amaurosis fugax is a transient monocular visual loss which is abrupt and which recovers within 30 minutes (although most commonly it only lasts 5 minutes or less). Patients may experience a total loss of visual field, but most note a curtain drawing phenomenon either vertically or horizontally, with an incomplete loss. Sometimes the affected field is colored green or blue. Rarely speckles or scintillations are observed. In the North American symptomatic carotid endarterectomy trial [1] half reported a sudden painless and complete loss of vision and a quarter an altitudinal curtain effect. The presence of pain is uncommon in carotid atheromatous disease.

Pain is common in carotid dissection (see Case 29), vasculitis and in migraine, although the pain is subacute and the timing is different; furthermore the visual disorder is more commonly (although not always) associated with positive phenomena such as scintillations and teichopsia. Acute angle closure glaucoma, in which repeated and self-limiting episodes of visual loss and ocular pain often with nausea may simulate migrainous neuralgia or cluster headache. On closer enquiry these patients may find that the attacks are brought on by exposure to low levels of background illumination (the author had a patient who only had attacks at night or at the movies).

Hemorrhage into a pituitary adenoma (pituitary apoplexy) would be associated with a more constant visual loss and ophthalmoparesis. Infections from the sinuses or an infective meningitis should also be considered, but again involvement of the ocular motor nerves would be likely.

In this case there are other symptoms which are extremely important; a constitutional disorder which had evolved over weeks, specific myalgic pains and latterly a feeling of tightness in the masseter muscles when eating and talking. This is jaw claudication. There is muscle ischemia as well as ocular ischemia. A vasculitic cause would be highly likely in this case.

Management

She was prescribed prednisolone 60 mg per day and referred to the Royal Free Hospital. Her headaches and aches and pains resolved entirely within 24 h of taking steroids. On the following day, however, she awoke with worsening vision on the left side and was admitted through the emergency department.

Examination

The central acuities were 6/9 on the right and there was no perception of light on the left. Color vision was present on the right side. There was an afferent pupillary defect on the left. Each disc was swollen left greater than right; there were disc hemorrhages on the left side. The left superficial temporal artery was non-pulsatile and was tender to palpate.

Further Evaluation and Management

This lady presents with a rather rapid onset systemic disorder with headaches and aches and pains then bilateral visual loss which was initially transient, then constant and worsening. It is notable that her vision deteriorated further despite having started steroids and noting that the headache and constitutional symptoms were improving.

The constellation of headache, malaise, aches and pains, and jaw claudication culminating in the development of optic neuropathy is very typical of Giant Cell arteritis. It is disappointing but well recognized that despite a prompt diagnosis and treatment, the condition may continue to evolve. Others cases have for example lost all vision in one eye then gone on within days to lose vision on the other despite treatment [2].

The differential diagnosis includes non-arteritic anterior ischemic optic neuropathy, and vasculitis of another type, for example ANCA positive vasculitis, Churg-Strauss syndrome and polyarteritis nodosa. Inflammatory disorders such as a demyelinating optic neuritis (which is bilateral in 30 % of cases) and granulomatous optic neuropathy should also be considered, but would not have such an abrupt onset.

She underwent a left superficial temporal artery biopsy (Fig. 10.1) and she was treated with 1 g intravenous methylprednisolone per day for three days, then oral prednisolone at 80 mg per day. Her vision did not deteriorate further, indeed an enlargement of her field on the left occurred sufficient to attain an acuity of finger counting. Her disc swelling resolved and the systemic symptoms did not recur. She was treated with a reducing dose of steroids over the following three years.

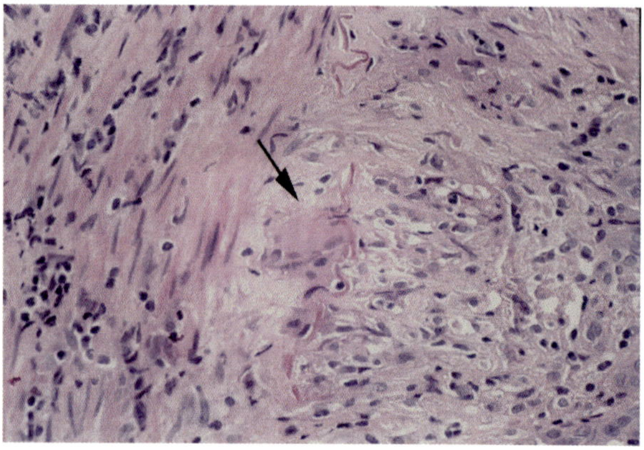

Fig. 10.1 H & E stained section of the left superficial temporal artery showing a giant cell (*arrow*) and disruption of the internal elastic lamina. On the left there is a mononuclear inflammatory cell infiltrate, on the right the thickened intima (Courtesy of Prof Tamas Revesz, Department of Neuropathology, Institute of Neurology)

Discussion

Giant cell arteritis is an autoinflammatory disease which never affects people under the age of 50 years. It is more common in women (3:1) and more common in those with Caucasian heritage than African. There is an association with HLA DR4. A granulomatous inflammation develops within the walls of medium and large arteries. The granulomas are composed of activated macrophages and CD4 T cells. The vascular endothelium becomes inflamed leading to hyperplasia of the intimal layer and vessel occlusion occurs [2].

The disease affects the aortic arch and its branches, leading to ischemic disorders of the brain, the structures of the head and neck, and the upper limbs. Stroke may arise, and even coronary occlusion, and the aorta may dissect or rupture. Uptake of FDG tracer within the walls of large vessels such as the aorta and the carotids may be seen on CT/PET scans (Fig. 10.2).

The ocular and neuro-ophthalmic complications are the most common and widely known [2, 3]. Ischemic disorders of the choroid, branch retinal arterioles and the central retinal artery, in which the retinal will appear white, with sparing of the macula (the cherry red spot) and retinal edema will develop. The most common disorder however is the development of anterior ischemic optic neuropathy, due to occlusion of the posterior ciliary arteries. The disc is swollen and pale, and there may be cotton wool spots and flame shaped intraretinal hemorrhages in the peripapillary region. Visual loss is often profound, and, as in this case, there if often a preceding history of brief ipsi- or contralateral transient visual loss in the recent past. A posterior ischemic optic neuropathy may arise, in which the disc is not seen to be swollen, and, when other arteries are involved, a chiasmal syndrome or tractopathy may be seen, with a bitemporal or homonymous hemianopia. Diplopia may arise when the vessels supplying the IIIrd, IVth and VIth nerves are affected. Oculomotor paresis is the most common, and tends to be pupil-sparing [3].

Treatment is with high dose corticosteroids (1 mg/kg or above), and as in this case, prompt institution of treatment is no guarantee that further visual loss may

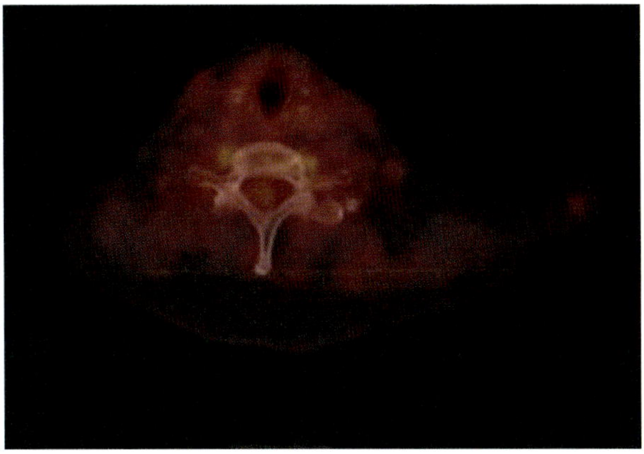

Fig. 10.2 CT PET scan of another patient with giant cell arteritis showing uptake within the carotid arteries on both sides

arise. There appears not to be any difference between oral and intravenous steroids. Those who are steroid unresponsive or high doses are required to suppress the disease may need immunosuppressive therapies, although these adjunctive agents proffer no greater effect on disease control [4]. It is disappointing that biological agents against TNFα have not shown benefit in placebo controlled trials [5, 6].

If the ESR is raised this investigation may be used as a monitor of disease control. Treatment is normally required for 18–24 months but some relapse upon steroid withdrawal after many months of apparent quiescence on very low doses of steroids, so great care must be taken to ensure that the disease has been brought under satisfactory control.

References

1. Barnett HJ, Taylor DW, Eliasziw M, Fox AJ, Ferguson GG, Haynes RB, Rankin RN, Clagett GP, Hachinski VC, Sackett DL, Thorpe KE, Meldrum HE, Spence JD. Benefit of carotid endarterectomy in patients with symptomatic moderate or severe stenosis. North American Symptomatic Carotid Endarterectomy Trial Collaborators. N Engl J Med. 1998;339:1415–25.
2. Weyand CM, Liao TJ, Goronzy JJ. The immunopathology of giant cell arteritis. J Neuroophthalmol. 2012;32:259–65.
3. Galetta SL. Vasculitis. In: Miller NR, Newman NJ, editors. Walsh and Hoyt's clinical neuro-ophthalmology. 6th ed. Philadelphia: Lippincot Williams and Wilkins; 2005. p. 2347–65.
4. Yates M, Loke YK, Watts RA, MacGregor AJ. Prednisolone combined with adjunctive immunosuppression is not superior to prednisolone alone in terms of efficacy and safety in giant cell arteritis: meta-analysis. Clin Rheumatol. 2014;33:227–36.
5. Hoffman GS, Cid MC, Rendt-Zagar KE, Merkel PA, Weyand CM, Stone JH, Salvarani C, Xu W, Visvanathan S, Rahman MU, Infliximab-GCA Study Group. Infliximab for maintenance of glucocorticosteroid-induced remission of giant cell arteritis: a randomized trial. Ann Intern Med. 2007;146:621–30.
6. Seror R, Baron G, Hachulla E, Debandt M, Larroche C, Puéchal X, Maurier F, de Wazieres B, Quéméneur T, Ravaud P, Mariette X. Adalimumab for steroid sparing in patients with giant-cell arteritis: results of a multicentre randomised controlled trial. Ann Rheum Dis. 2014;73: 2074–81.

Case 11

History

This 28 year old lady developed pain around the left eye which spread to form a periorbital ache which worsened over 2 days. As she developed visual blurring the pain began to recede, but she noted sharp stabbing pain when she looked up and to the left side. The right side was normal and there were no other symptoms. There had not been any previous neurological symptom.

She was assessed in her local ophthalmic department and saw a Neurologist there too who diagnosed optic neuritis. She was referred to the Royal Free Hospital.

Examination

By then she saw 6/6 in both eyes with normal color vision but there was a mild left sided relative afferent pupillary defect and the left field showed a mild central loss (Fig. 11.1a). The optic discs were normal. There were no other abnormal neurological signs.

D.P. Kidd, *Neuro-Ophthalmology*, DOI 10.1007/978-1-4471-2410-8_11

Evaluation

The history was typical of a left sided demyelinating type optic neuritis and since she was recovering spontaneously no treatment was recommended. A series of blood investigations was performed and a discussion about the pros and cons of imaging took place. It was explained that it would be helpful to rule out alternative causes for the disorder such as structural disorders and infections, but that the risk of identifying any of these would be low. The relationship between optic neuritis

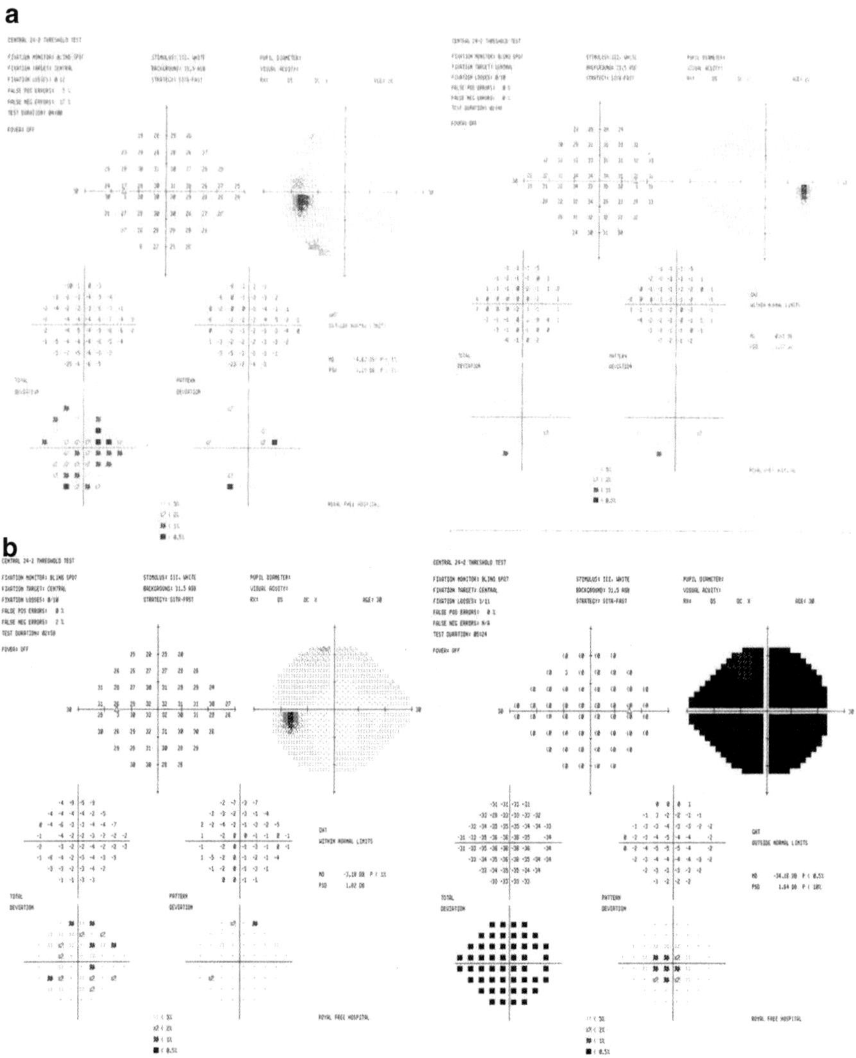

Fig. 11.1 (**a**) Humphrey visual field during recovery from the first episode of optic neuritis, and (**b**) at presentation of and (**c**) during recovery from the second episode

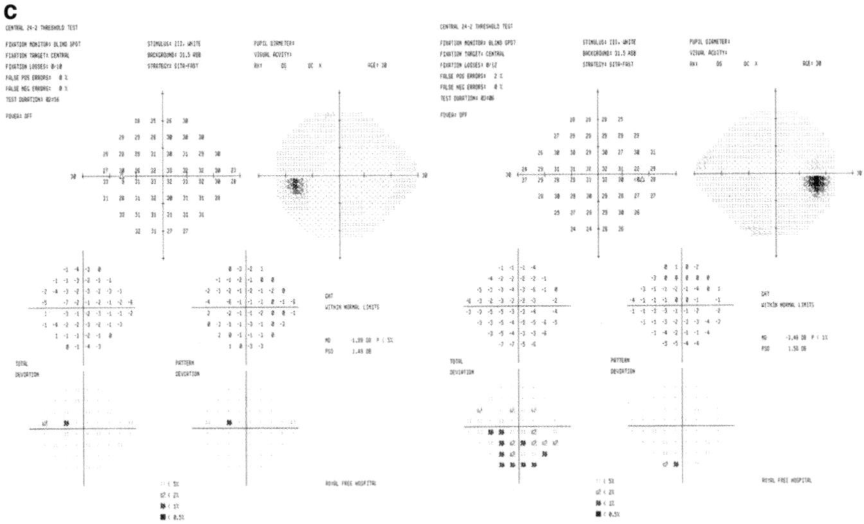

Fig. 11.1 (continued)

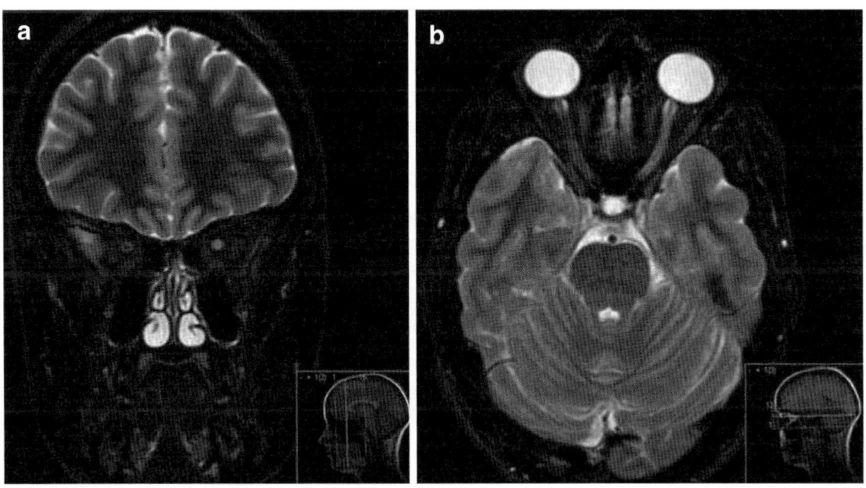

Fig. 11.2 MRI: coronal (**a**) and axial (**b**) T2 weighted scans showing a high signal lesion within the left optic nerve

and multiple sclerosis was discussed, in particular the relationship between this and the number of white matter lesions seen on the scan together with the fact that were a number of white matter lesions to be seen there was no clear way of identifying if and when a second attack would arise.

She opted to undergo the MRI scan, which showed a high signal lesion within the optic nerve and none elsewhere (Fig. 11.2a, b).

Since the blood investigations were normal it was recommended that she be allowed to recover and that she be monitored in the Neuro-ophthalmology clinic.

When she attended again 6 weeks later the neuro-ophthalmic examination was normal aside from a mild temporal pallor of the left optic disc. She had noted a mild Uhtoff's phenomenon when in the gym but no other symptoms.

She was well 6 months later, and again 6 months after that, but a month later returned with rather prominent pain in the right eye which developed and worsened over 5 days, then a subacute visual loss on the right side.

Examination

She saw hand movement perception on the right, 6/6 on the left (Fig. 11.1b). Color vision was absent on the right and there was an afferent pupillary defect on the same side. The disc was swollen (Fig. 11.3), and the retinae were normal.

Evaluation

This young lady presents with a second, contralateral, optic neuropathy with symptoms and signs strongly suggestive of an inflammatory disorder. Previous investigations did not identify a definite relationship between the original disorder and multiple sclerosis, but it had been discussed as the most likely etiological association. Imaging and blood investigations were repeated.

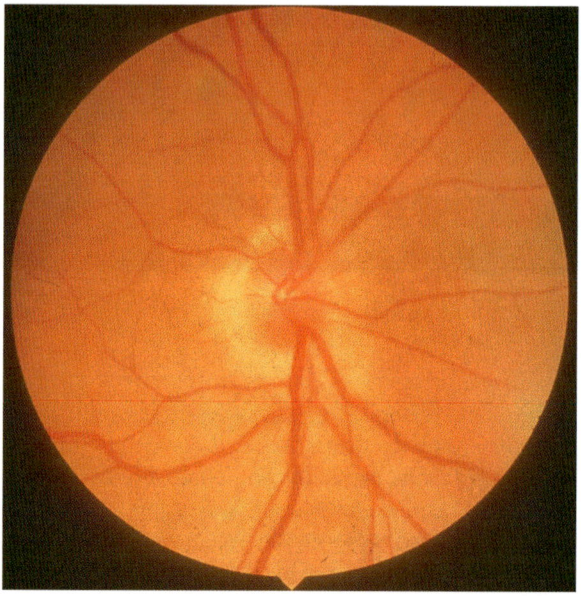

Fig. 11.3 Optic disc photo showing mild disc edema

ESR, biochemical screening, serum ACE, ANA, ENA, anti-phospholipid and aquaporin-4 antibodies were normal or negative.

A second MRI scan of the orbits revealed a high signal lesion on the right with a continuance of the previous lesion on the left (Fig. 11.4a, b). There was mild enhancement following administration of Gadolinium (Fig. 11.4c). There remained no lesions within the brain.

Her anti-MOG antibodies returned and were raised.

Again she improved spontaneously (Fig. 11.1c) and no treatment was recommended. She will be observed and immunosuppression will be recommended should there be a third event.

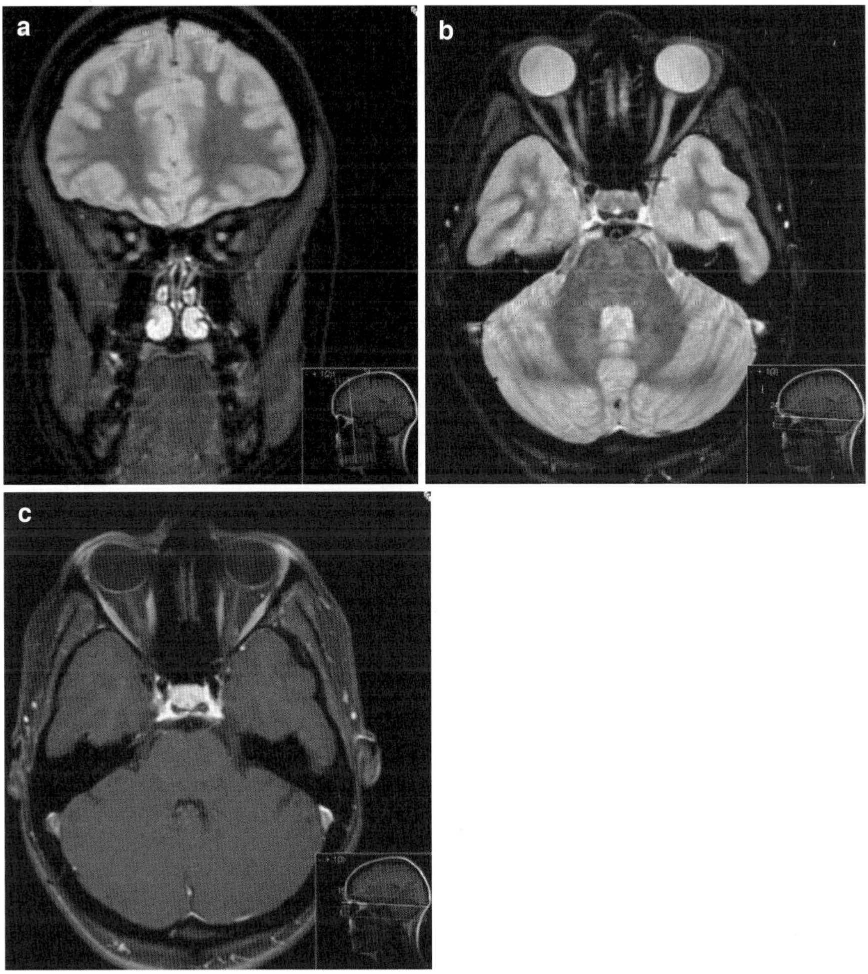

Fig. 11.4 MRI: coronal (**a**) and axial (**b**) T2 weighted scan of the optic nerves showing high signal on both sides, and (**c**) axial T1 weighted scan following administration of contrast showing minor enhancement of the right optic nerve

Discussion

Optic Neuritis

Optic neuritis is a disorder of the young (mean age 32 years) and two thirds are female. The incidence in Sweden was 1.46×10^5 person years [1]. This case describes the typical clinical features of a demyelinating optic neuritis [2, 3]. The pain, and in particular the pain on eye movements, is characteristic, affecting 90 % of patients; it commonly settles as the visual scotoma develops. 30 % see phosphenes or photopsias. 35 % have disc swelling and 3 % vitreous cells. The prevalence of an intermediate uveitis either before or during optic neuritis [4] is very low. The visual acuity diminishes to a nadir over 1–7 days, remains for a short time then begins quickly to recover. The mean nadir in the Optic Neuritis Treatment Trial [2] was 20/80 (6/24) but varied from 20/20 (6/6) to no perception of light. A substantial return of acuity occurs within 2 weeks, and 75 % have regained a normal visual acuity after 6 months. Residual symptoms are common however; loss of stereopsis and contrast sensitivity, minor field defects and washed-out color acuity correlate with axonal loss in the retinal nerve fiber layer [5].

Relationship with Multiple Sclerosis

In a 20 year prospective study of patients with clinically isolated demyelinating syndromes (CIS) about 64 % of patients developed clinically definite multiple sclerosis [6]. There was a relationship throughout the study between the number of MRI brain lesions seen at onset and the risk of developing MS; 21 % of those with a normal MRI at baseline *vs* 82 % of those whose scan was abnormal. So too was there are relationship between disability at 20 years and number of MRI lesions seen at baseline; 45 % of those with 10 or more lesions had difficulty walking or were wheelchair bound, whereas only 6 % of those with normal MRI had become disabled to the same degree [6]. 42 % of the cohort had developed the secondary progressive disease course. Importantly it was seen that those who went on to develop a progressive disease showed a greater accrual of lesion volume per year than those with a more mild disease course.

In a larger cohort of 1015 Spanish patients followed prospectively for a mean of 81 months 299 (30 %) had normal MRI at baseline, of whom 7 % developed clinically definite MS during the study period. 72 % of those with abnormal brain MRI developed MS during the same period. There was a clear relationship between lesion load at baseline together with the presence of CSF oligoclonal bands and the development of disability over time [7]. It was also noted that prescribing disease modifying treatments prior to the onset of the second attack failed to alter the risk of developing disablement. Patients with optic neuritis as their CIS had a greater chance of escaping disablement (other studies which have also shown this are cited in [7]).

Anti-MOG and Optic Neuritis

Myelin-oligodendrocyte glycoprotein is expressed by oligodendrocytes. It has been shown to induce demyelination in experimental models [8, 9] and has been found increasingly over the past decade to be associated with demyelinating disorders, particularly in children, in whom 46 % of one study [10] of consecutive patients under the age of 16 with optic neuritis in Austria were found to be seropositive. Pediatric patients with a wide range of inflammatory neurological disorders such as ADEM, Neuromyelitis Optica and relapsing optic neuritis have been found to be associated with anti-MOG antibodies [11].

More recently it has been found that a proportion of aquaporin-4 seronegative Neuromyelitis Optica patients have anti-MOG antibodies [12, 13], and that these patients may have a more steroid-responsive disease and a less severe outcome. A study of NMO spectrum disorder aquaporin-4 seronegative patients from Australia has demonstrated a clear relationship between anti-MOG antibodies and bilateral optic neuropathy in such patients, not seen in those with longitudinally extensive transverse myelitis and without optic neuritis [14]. These patients had good visual outcomes, demonstrated a rapid steroid responsiveness, and a tendency to have recurrent disease.

This subgroup of patients seem to have a more severe disease severity but a greater degree of recovery, and it was noted in one study [13] that the associated MRI lesions resolved in entirety with recovery. It appears that the antibody titer reduces over time, although few become seronegative. There is no evidence base on the most effective treatment, nor its duration; most have been treated with steroids and immunosuppression, and plasma exchange or IVIg [12].

A series of 51 patients with isolated or recurrent optic neuritis without imaging evidence for a risk of development of MS revealed that 10 had anti-MOG, 6 had aquaporin-4 antibodies and 7 had antibodies to Glycine receptor α1 subunit [15]. The 10 patients with anti-MOG had a better visual outcome than those with aquaporin 4 antibodies. Five had a monophasic disorder and seemingly had had no treatment, whilst 5 had a recurrent optic neuritis, of whom 3 had received no long term treatment and 2 azathioprine. Three others with both anti-MOG and anti GlyR antibodies had relapsing optic neuropathies of whom one was receiving treatment (with methotrexate).

References

1. Jin YP, Pedro-Cuesta J, Soderstrom M, Link H. Incidence of optic neuritis in Stockholm, Sweden 1990–1995. Arch Neurol. 1999;56:975–80.
2. Optic neuritis study group. The clinical profile of optic neuritis; experience of the optic neuritis study group. Arch Ophthalmol. 1991;109:1673–8.
3. Toosy AT, Mason DF, Miller DH. Optic neuritis. Lancet Neurol. 2014;13:83–99.
4. Biousse V, Trichet C, Bloch-Michel E, Roullet E. Multiple sclerosis associated with uveitis in two large clinic-based series. Neurology. 1999;52:179–81.

5. Trip SA, Schlottmann PG, Jones SJ, Altmann DR, Garway-Heath DF, Thompson AJ, Plant GT, Miller DH. Retinal nerve fibre layer axonal loss and visual dysfunction in optic neuritis. Ann Neurol. 2005;58:383–91.
6. Fisniku LK, Brex PA, Altmann DR, Miskiel KA, Benton CE, Lanyon R, Thompson AJ, Miller DH. Disability and T2 MRI lesions: a 20-year follow up of patients with relapse onset of multiple sclerosis. Brain. 2008;131:8080–817.
7. Tintore M, Rovira À, Río J, Otero-Romero S, Arrambide G, Tur C, Comabella M, Nos, Arévalo MJ, Negrotto L, Galán I, Vidal-Jordana A, Castilló J, Palavra F, Simon E, Mitjana R, Auger C, Sastre-Garriga J, Montalban X. Defining high, medium and low impact prognostic factors for developing multiple sclerosis. Brain. 2015;135:1863–1874.
8. Schleusener HJ, Sobel RA, Linington C, Weiner HL. A monoclonal antibody against a myelin oligodendrocyte glycoprotein induces relapses and demyelination in central nervous system auto-immune disease. J Immunol. 1987;139:808–17.
9. Reindl M, Di Pauli F, Rostasy K, Berger T. The spectrum of MOG autoantibody-associated demyelinating diseases. Nat Rev Neurol. 2013;9:455–61.
10. Rostasy K, Mader S, Schanda K, et al. Anti-myelin oligodendrocyte glycoprotein antibodies in pediatric patients with optic neuritis. Arch Neurol. 2012;69:752–6.
11. Brilot F, Dale RC, Selter RC, et al. Antibodies to myelin-oligodendrocyte glycoprotein in children with inflammatory demyelinating central nervous system disease. Ann Neurol. 2009;66:833–42.
12. Kitley J, Woodhall M, Waters P, Leite MI, Devenney E, Craig J, Palace J, Vincent A. Myelin-oligodendrocyte glycoprotein antibodies in adults with a neuromyelitis optica phenotype. Neurology. 2012;79:1273–7.
13. Kitley J, Waters P, Woodhall M, Leite MI, Murchison A, George J, Kuker W, Chandrate S, Vincent A, Palace J. Neuromyelitis optica spectrum disorders with aquaporin-4 and myelin-oligodendrocyte glycoprotein antibodies: a comparative study. JAMA Neurol. 2014;71:276–83.
14. Ramanathan S, Reddel SW, Henderson A, Parratt JD, Barnett M, Gatt PN, Merheb V, Kumaran RY, Pathmanandavel K, Sinmaz N, Ghadiri M, Yiannikas C, Vucic S, Stewart G, Bleasel AF, Booth D, Fung VS, Dale RC, Brilot F. Antibodies to myelin-oligodendrocyte glycoprotein in bilateral and recurrent optic neuritis. Neurol Neuroimmunol Neuroinflamm. 2014;1, e40.
15. Martinez-Hernandez E, Sepulveda M, Rostasy K, Hoftberger R, Grauss F, Harvey RJ, Saiz A, Dalmau J. Antibodies to aquaporin 4, Myelin-Oligodendrocyre Glycoprotein, and the Glycine receptor alpha1 subunit in patients with isolated optic neuritis. JAMA Neurol. 2015;72:187–193.

Case 12

History

This 25 year old lady developed a subacute blurring of vision in the right eye at 35 weeks into her first pregnancy. This gradually worsened. There was no pain and no other symptom. There had been no prior neurological symptoms. There had been no complication of pregnancy and her blood pressure was normal. There was no proteinuria.

Examination

The central visual acuity was 6/9 N6 on the right with reduced color vision. The vision was normal on the left. There was a central visual field defect on the right side (Fig. 12.1a). There was a prominent relative afferent pupillary defect. The ocular media were clear and the retinae normal. The right disc was diffusely swollen (Fig. 12.2). The retinal vessels were normal. The eye movements were unimpaired and the trigeminal sensation normal. There were no other abnormal neurological signs.

D.P. Kidd, *Neuro-Ophthalmology*, DOI 10.1007/978-1-4471-2410-8_12

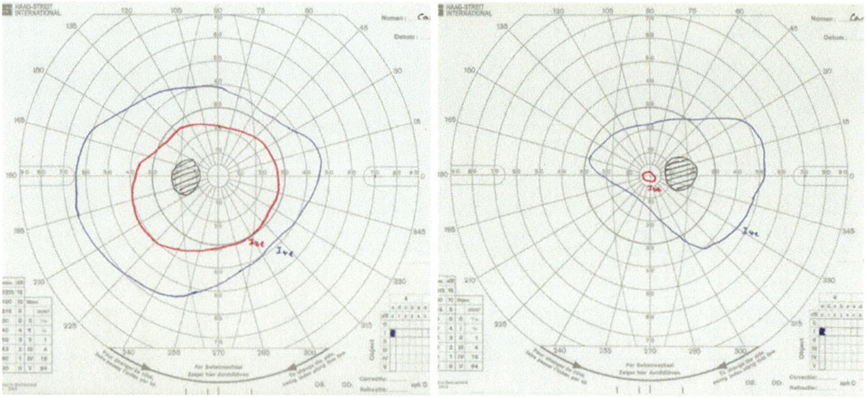

Fig. 12.1 Goldman fields at presentation

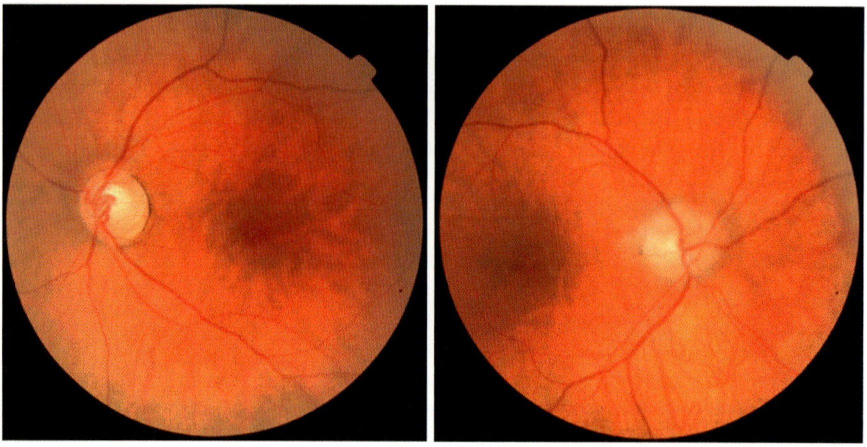

Fig. 12.2 Fundus photograph showing optic disc swelling on the right

Evaluation

Visual loss in pregnancy requires urgent investigations; pituitary adenomas and meningiomas may all present at this age and can enlarge substantially during pregnancy. Infections and inflammatory disease also need to be considered. An uncommon inflammatory disorder of the pituitary, lymphocytic hypophysitis (see Case 28), is more common in the third trimester of pregnancy than at any other time. Posterior reversible leucoencephalopathy syndrome (PRES; see Case 43) occurs with pre-eclampsia. Vascular disorders, particularly venous sinus thrombosis, and including stroke also need to be considered.

In this case there were clear signs of an optic neuropathy on the right side and the disc was swollen, so a disorder involving the nerve itself rather than a compressive disorder along the anterior visual pathway would be more likely. Imaging should be undertaken.

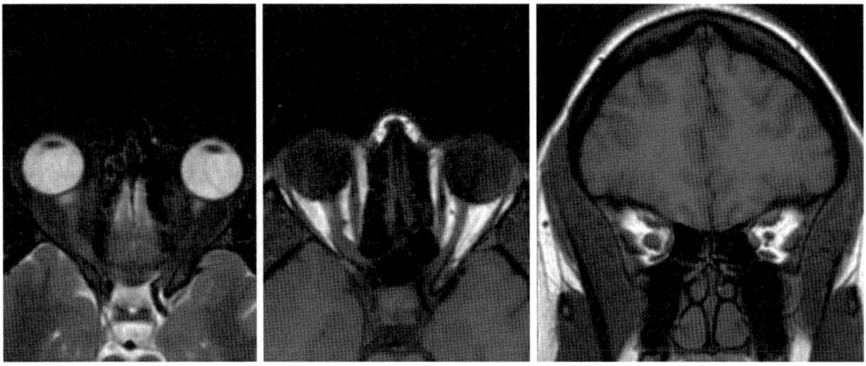

Fig. 12.3 MRI scan of orbits showing enlargement of the optic nerve – sheath complex on the right side

Management

An MRI scan of the orbits (Fig. 12.3) showed an enlargement of the optic nerve – sheath complex on the right side. Gadolinium is not given in pregnancy so it could not be ascertained whether or not the lesion enhanced.

It was considered to be either an optic nerve sheath meningioma or an optic perineuritis. After a series of blood investigation revealed no evidence for an underlying infection or inflammatory disorder the patient was allowed to continue to term and the vision watched carefully. She gave birth to a healthy girl at term three weeks later. Post-partum a spinal fluid examination was undertaken which was normal. Her vision improved spontaneously and returned to 6/6 with slightly reduced color vision and a normal field (Fig. 12.1b). The pupillary defect persisted.

Imaging was undertaken at yearly intervals and no change was observed. She underwent a second pregnancy three years later with a less dramatic visual change which improved incompletely post-partum. Thereafter the field constricted slightly although the scan showed no changes. It was recommended that she undergo radiotherapy and she received 50.4 Gy in 28 fractions using the Rapid Arc IMRT technique. She has remained well since, with stable visual function.

Discussion

Primary optic nerve sheath meningiomas (ONSM) are uncommon, comprising only 2 % of all meningiomas diagnosed [1, 2]. They are much less common than secondary meningiomas, which have spread in through the optic canal. In adulthood they are more common in women than men, and are only rarely bilateral. Around 10 % are seen in childhood, when they are more commonly bilateral. There is a close association with neurofibromatosis type 2.

The tissue spreads around the optic nerve through the subarachnoid space, interfering with axoplasmic transport and reducing blood supply.

95 % of adult ONSM are unilateral. They present most commonly in the fifth decade with a progressive painless impairment of vision. The signs are of an optic neuropathy; if the lesion is large enough there may be proptosis and diplopia. Transient obscuration of vision may occur and may be induced by eye movement if intraorbital pressure is high. Most have disc swelling without exudate or hemorrhage, and the pathognomonic retino-choroidal shunt vessels are seen only very late on, usually associated with optic disc atrophy. These develop when the nerve has become ischemic, and are opened collateral vessels from the choroidal circulation.

On imaging ONSM may show a fusiform, globular or tubular pattern (the most common) of mass effect, and the lesion enhances following administration of gadolinium. In tubular meningiomas a tram track effect may be seen, in which the enhanced meningioma contrasts with the lower signal arising from the nerve itself. On non-contrast CT scans longstanding lesions may be calcified. *Pneumosinus dilatans*, in which the posterior ethmoid and sphenoid sinuses are enlarged and aerated, may be seen. Since expression of somatostatin is elevated in meningioma, modern radioactive tracers such as 68-Ga-DOTA-TATE can be used to increase diagnostic certainty [3] (and to plan treatment or monitor recurrence).

Treatment

The ONSM shares the same pial blood supply as the nerve itself, so any surgical form of treatment will inevitably disrupt whatever remaining vision there is. Over the past 20 years there has been a great deal of progress in defining the mode and dose of radiotherapy which works best. On the one hand there is the effectiveness of therapy, and on the other the risk of delayed radiotherapy-associated complications including visual loss due to endarteritis and retinopathy, dry eyes, pituitary failure and temporal lobe atrophy. Conformal radiotherapy techniques such as intensity-modulated radiotherapy, stereotactic fractionated radiotherapy, radiosurgery and proton beam therapy all seem to work well with a low incidence of adverse effects and a high degree of visual stabilization. One recent review states that single fraction radiosurgery appears to have the best results [2].

References

1. Miller NR. Primary and secondary tumors of the optic nerve and its sheath. In: Kidd D, Biousse V, Newman NJ, editors. Neuro-ophthalmology. Philadelphia: Butterworth Heinemann Elsevier; 2008. p. 215–23.
2. Shapey J, Sabin HI, Danesh-Meyer HV, Kaye AH. Diagnosis and management of optic nerve sheath meningiomas. J Clin Neurosci. 2013;20:1045–56.
3. Klingensfein A, Haug AR, Miller C, Hintschich C. Ga-68-DOTA-TATE PET/CT for discrimination of tumors of the optic pathway. Orbit. 2015;34:16–22.

Case 13

History

This lady presented at the age of 44 with a slow onset ingravescent disturbance of vision on the right side. She noted that a band of opaqueness had developed over the central vision and deteriorated over the course of 3 months. There was a more sudden deterioration latterly and she had lost all vision in the right eye.

A year previously she had undergone hematological investigations for a low platelet and neutrophil count. A bone marrow biopsy revealed normal cellularity. A diagnosis of ITP was made and her blood indices improved on low dose prednisolone. She was otherwise well and noted no other symptoms on systematic enquiry.

Examination

There was no perception of light on the right. The central acuities were normal on the left. There was an afferent pupillary defect. The right disc was hyperemic and mildly swollen. The left was normal. The ocular media were clear.

There were no other abnormal neurological signs and the systemic examination was normal.

D.P. Kidd, *Neuro-Ophthalmology*, DOI 10.1007/978-1-4471-2410-8_13

Evaluation

This lady presents with a progressive painless optic neuropathy which accelerated and became severe. The clinical features were those of an optic neuropathy and there were no other signs. A progressive painless optic neuropathy could be caused by any pathological process; a 3 month history is more in keeping with a structural lesion such as meningioma or pituitary adenoma, but an inflammatory or infective disorder arises from or adjacent to the paranasal sinuses could also cause it. It would be most unlike a demyelinating optic neuritis. Metastatic lesions would have a more rapid disease course and would be likely to be painful. Vascular lesions would have a rapid onset, except for a giant aneurysm causing compression at the orbital apex. Most of the compressive lesions should be associated with other clinical signs referable to the orbital apex or the cavernous sinus. So an isolated optic neuropathy is most likely. Imaging or the orbits and chiasm is warranted, and blood investigations will investigate the possibility of a systemic inflammatory or infective disorder.

Investigations

The ESR and CRP were normal. The platelet count was 105, the neutrophil count was normal. Biochemical screening was normal aside from a speckled pattern ANA. ENA and ANCA were normal. There was no anticardiolipin antibody. The serum ACE was elevated at 63.

An MRI scan of the orbits without contrast enhancement revealed swelling and hyperintensity of the right optic nerve. There were no brain lesions.

The CSF was under normal pressure; the protein was 0.3 g/dl and acellular. The sugar was 3.4/6.6 mmol/dl. Oligoclonal bands were negative.

A Gallium scan (Fig. 13.1) showed uptake in the lacrimal glands, the mediastinal glands and the lungs. A CT scan of the thorax confirmed mediastinal and hilar lymphadenopathy. Biopsy of one of the mediastinal glands at mediastinoscopy revealed non-caseating granulomatous infiltration.

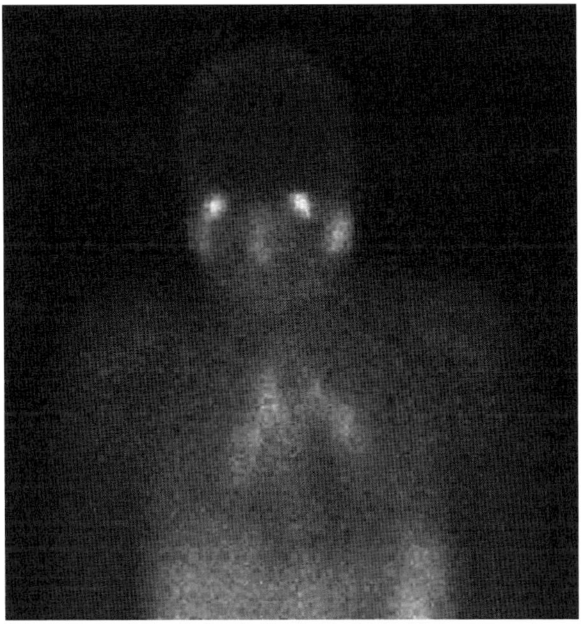

Fig. 13.1 Gallium-67 scintigram showing uptake of tracer within the lacrimal and parotid glands, and the mediastinal glands and lungs

Treatment

Her steroids were increased to 60 mg per day and her vision improved. Within 3 months she had regained a normal central acuity and color vision. The field was improving, and had returned to normal after 6 months. Her steroids were reduced and stopped, and although her ACE was intermittently modestly raised, she remained well.

Six years later she presented again with a recurrence of her optic neuropathy, on the other side, with a reduction in acuity to 6/60. She was treated with intravenous then oral steroids. Imaging showed clear signs of an optic neuritis with enhancement (Fig. 13.2). Her fields normalized over 6 months and an immunosuppressive agent was started. She has been well since then on azathioprine 150 mg per day, and off steroids.

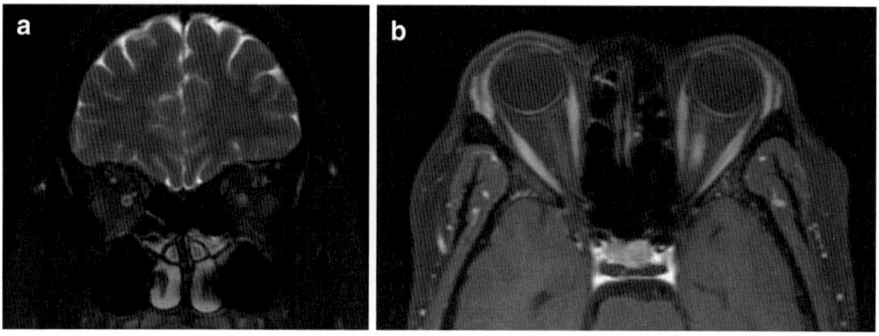

Fig. 13.2 MRI (**a**) coronal STIR image showing high signal within the left optic nerve, and (**b**) axial T1 weighted scan following injection of gadolinium showing a long region of enhancement of the left optic nerve

Discussion

Optic neuropathy in sarcoidosis is uncommon; in a recent series of 52 cases 80 % presented with a subacute optic neuropathy resembling optic neuritis, a more slowly progressive optic neuropathy occurred in the remainder. 30 % were bilateral. Concurrent intra ocular inflammation was seen in 36 %. Pain arose in only 27 % of cases. MRI findings showed optic nerve involvement in 75 % of cases, with more widespread adjacent inflammation in 30 % [1].

In general, therefore it is not usually possible to differentiate between optic neuritis related to sarcoidosis and a demyelinating optic neuritis; the diminishment in vision is often more slow, and often more severe, and a spontaneous improvement within 2–3 weeks is less frequent, and pain is less frequent but so too may all these features arise in a demyelinating optic neuritis due to multiple sclerosis or to Neuromyelitis Optica. The presence of an associated intraocular inflammation is cited by many as the main clue, but this arose in only 36 % of the series noted above. A high index of suspicion, and a careful monitoring as the disorder is investigated is important; it is not sufficient to diagnose optic neuritis and reassure the patient that she will improve.

Thrombocytopenia is uncommon in sarcoidosis, considered to occur in 2 % of cases, and is found in patients with a more severe disease course. The etiology may be immune-based platelet destruction (as in this case), due to bone marrow replacement by disease, or associated with hypersplenism [2].

References

1. Kidd DP, Burton BJ, Plant GT, Graham EM. Optic neuropathy associated with systemic sarcoidosis. Neurol Neuroimmunol Neuroinflam. 2016;3:e270.
2. Mahévas M, Chiche L, Uzunhan Y, Khellaf M, Morin AS, Le Guenno G, Péronne V, Affo L, Lidove O, Boutboul D, Dion G, Ducroix JP, Papo T, Pacheco Y, Schleinitz N, Michel M, Godeau B, Valeyre D. Association of sarcoidosis and immune thrombocytopenia: presentation and outcome in a series of 20 patients. Medicine (Baltimore). 2011;90:269–78.

Case 14

History

This 39 year old lady developed a progressively worsening problem with vision in the left eye. She attended her local hospital ophthalmology department where they found her left disc to be swollen. Brain imaging was normal. During investigation the vision in the right eye began to deteriorate. There was no pain and no other visual symptom. There was no pain on eye movement. There had been no previous neurological symptom and she was otherwise well, taking no regular medication. There were no systemic symptoms, and there had been no illness prior to the onset of the visual disorder.

She was referred to the Royal Free Hospital, admitted and underwent a series of investigations.

Examination

On admission the visual acuities were PL and NPL. Color vision was absent and the pupillary reflexes were sluggish. Both discs were swollen. The ocular media were clear and examination of the retinae unremarkable. The remainder of the neurological examination was normal. There were no systemic signs.

D.P. Kidd, *Neuro-Ophthalmology*, DOI 10.1007/978-1-4471-2410-8_14

Evaluation

This is a very urgent problem. She presents with an escalating and sequential visual loss. There is no color vision but the acuities are not sufficient to see the plates, and the pupils are symmetrical and sluggish. This is not necessarily an optic neuritis, therefore; intracranial hypertension due to a venous sinus thrombosis or to the so-called Idiopathic Intracranial Hypertension disorder more common in young women with high BMI may present with an evolving papilloedema which begins on one side then the other may cause this but the fields would be constricted and a central scotoma would not arise, and it would be likely in such a severe case that the papilloedema would be associated with retinal hemorrhage; a disorder of the posterior circulation could cause asymmetric visual loss which spreads to both sides; a tumor, ischemic disease or PRES (see Case 43) may present thus but would not be associated with sequential disc edema. A mass lesion of the anterior visual pathway for example at the chiasm would not be associated with disc swelling, and again the fields would show abnormalities commensurate with a chiasmal disorder. So the visual fields in this circumstance are extremely important.

These showed a central scotoma in the seeing eye (Fig. 14.1), which would make an optic neuropathy likely; the presence of sequential disc edema would corroborate this.

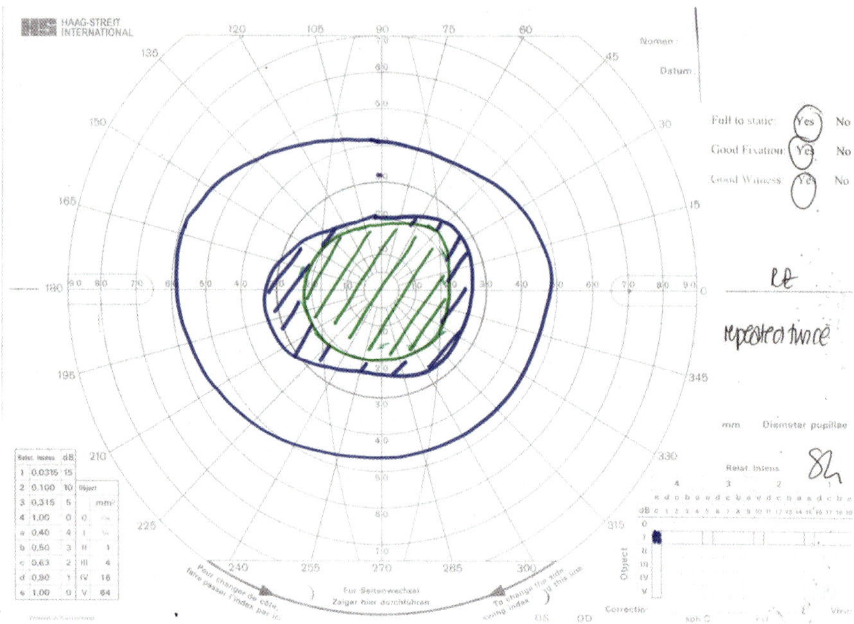

Fig. 14.1 Goldman visual field showing a central visual field defect on the right

Investigations

Screening blood tests were all normal, in particular there was no ANA, anticardiolipin antibody or ENA, ANCA was negative and there were no aquaporin 4 antibodies.

The MRI scan of orbits revealed swelling of the optic nerves on both sides associated with enhancement following injection of contrast (Figs. 14.2 and 14.3).

The CSF was under normal pressure; protein was 0.3 g/dl, the specimen was acellular, oligoclonal bands were negative.

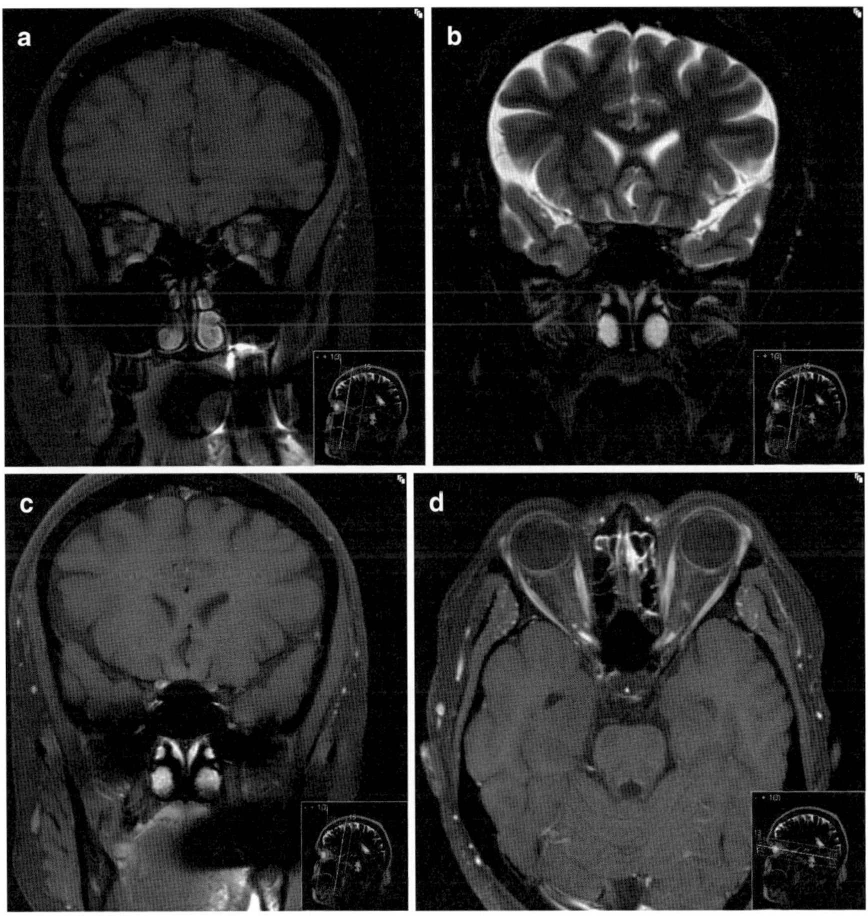

Fig. 14.2 T2 weighted (**a**) coronal MRI showing high signal in both nerves and T1 weighted coronal and axial scans following administration of contrast, with swelling of the optic nerve – sheath complex within the posterior aspect of the orbit (**b**), enhancement of the right nerve (**c**) and enhancement of both nerves within the optic canals (**d**). There are no other abnormalities, in particular white matter lesions within the brain

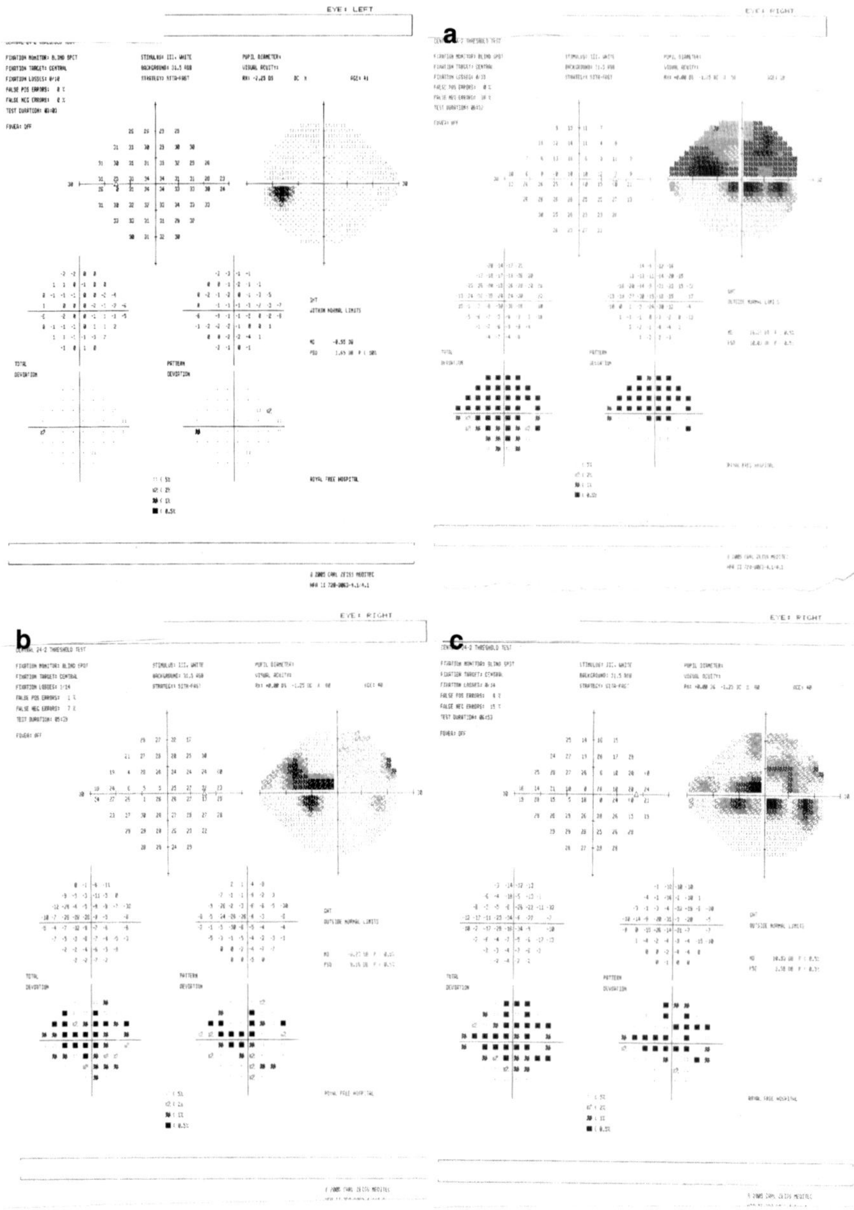

Fig. 14.3 Series of Humphrey visual fields which fluctuated then improved on the right as treatment increased

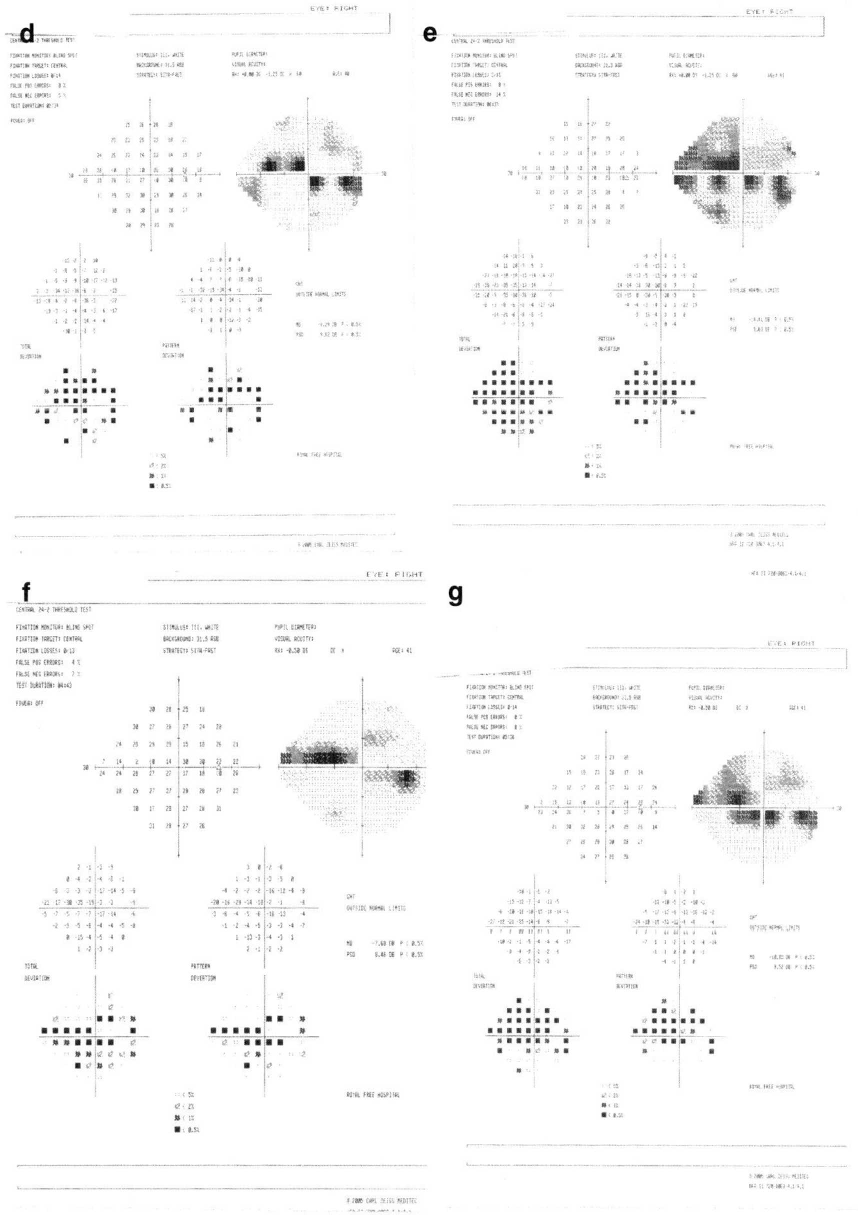

Fig. 14.3 (continued)

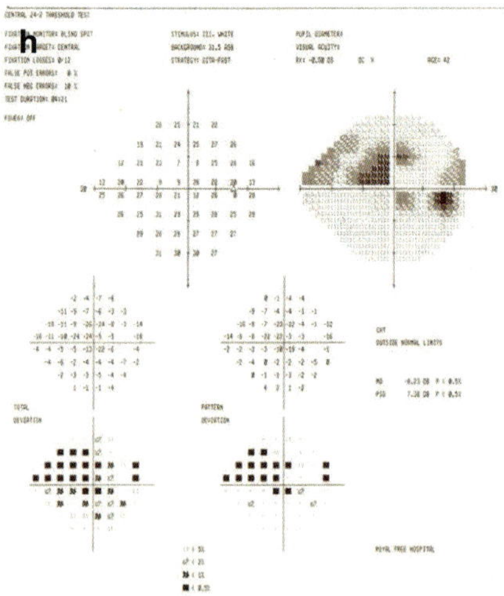

Fig. 14.3 (continued)

Management

A granulomatous optic neuropathy was postulated and she was treated with high dose oral steroids. She made a rapid improvement, regaining central acuities of 6/36 and 6/9 over the course of the following month, but relapsed in both eyes as the dose of steroids was reduced to 40 mg. Her vision improved again on 100 mg of prednisolone to 6/24 and 6/6. Methotrexate was added and increased slowly. The optic disc swelling resolved.

On 10 mg Methotrexate and 5 mg prednisolone her right visual acuity again deteriorated and settled with increases of both drugs. One further relapse occurred but she has been stable on 17.5 mg methotrexate per week and prednisolone 10 mg per day. Her acuities are 6/9 and 6/5. The left disc is normal, the right shows temporal pallor.

Discussion

This patient has a relapsing, steroid responsive optic neuritis in keeping with chronic relapsing inflammatory optic neuropathy (CRION) [1, 2]. This is a diagnosis made after exclusion of alternative explanations, particularly multiple sclerosis, in which bilateral optic neuritis may arise in around 30 % of cases, Neuromyelitis Optica, the syndrome known as auto-immune optic neuropathy [3] which shares clinical features and steroid-responsiveness but which is associated with anti-nuclear antibodies, SLE itself (although a chiasmitis is more commonly cited in the literature), sarcoidosis (see Case 13) and then vasculitic disorders such as Churg-Strauss syndrome and polyarteritis nodosa. Giant cell arteritis does not occur at such a young age.

Devic's syndrome related to aquaporin-4 antibodies, associated with anti-Ro and –La antibodies in Sjogren's syndrome, and to anti-phospholipid antibodies, tends not to cause a steroid responsive relapsing disorder, and the outcome even following prompt treatment is usually not as good (see Case 19). Bilateral steroid responsive optic neuropathy is also associated with the presence of anti- myelin-oligodendrocyte glycoprotein (MOG) antibodies (see Case 11), which were assessed following treatment in this case, and found to be negative.

Infective disorders such as sinus mucocoele, tuberculosis, Lyme disease and viral infections would provoke a monophasic illness. Similarly (but important to consider in this case) is toxic amblyopia which may present with synchronous or sequential optic neuropathy with central scotoma.

Sequential optic neuropathy with disc swelling is seen in Leber's hereditary optic neuropathy, and whilst it may improve spontaneously, does not respond to steroids. Enhancement of the nerves has however been reported (see Case 17).

The clinical syndrome described above is typical for the disorder CRION; steroid responsiveness is gratifyingly rapid but so too is relapse if steroids are reduced too quickly, and those who do always require high dose immunosuppression with Azathioprine, Methotrexate or Mycophenolate. Imaging of the brain is normal, that of the optic nerves reveals lesions on both sides, often (although not always) with enhancement. The CSF is acellular but the protein may be raised, and oligoclonal bands are not seen. Systemic antibodies including aquaporin-4 and myelin-oligodendrocyte glycoprotein (MOG) are absent in most cases [4].

References

1. Kidd D, Burton B, Plant GT, Graham EM. Chronic relapsing inflammatory optic neuropathy (CRION). Brain. 2003;126:276–84.
2. Petzold A, Plant GT. Chronic relapsing inflammatory optic neuropathy: a systematic review of 122 cases published. J Neurol. 2014;261:17–26.
3. Kupersmith MJ, Burde RM, Warren FA, Klingele TG, Frohman LP, Mitnick H. Auto-immune optic neuropathy: evaluation and treatment. J Neurol Neurosurg Psychiatry. 1988;51:1381–6.
4. Petzold A, Pittock S, Lennon V, Magiore C, Weinshenker BG, Plant GT. Neuro-myelitis optica IgG (aquaporin-4) autoantibodies in immune mediated optic neuritis. J Neurol Neurosurg Psychiatry. 2010;81:109–11.

Case 15

History

This 50 year lady was referred to her local ophthalmic department by her Optometrist when she presented with a month long progressive painless reduction in vision on the right side. There was no pain on eye movement, and no phosphenes. They found a reduction in vision to 6/18 and a swollen optic disc. She was referred in turn to a Neurologist who arranged a brain MRI which showed an abnormality of the optic nerve on the right, but no other lesion. He gave her a course or oral steroids and referred her to the Royal Free Hospital Neuro-ophthalmology unit.

Her past medical history was unremarkable and she took no regular medication. There were no other symptoms on systematic enquiry.

Examination

The central acuity was counting fingers in the right eye. The color vision was absent and there was a relative afferent pupillary defect. The acuities on the left were normal. The right disc was seen to be swollen. No retinal or choroidal lesion was seen. There was no proptosis and the eye movements were normal. Trigeminal sensation was normal and there were no other abnormal neurological signs.

D.P. Kidd, *Neuro-Ophthalmology*, DOI 10.1007/978-1-4471-2410-8_15

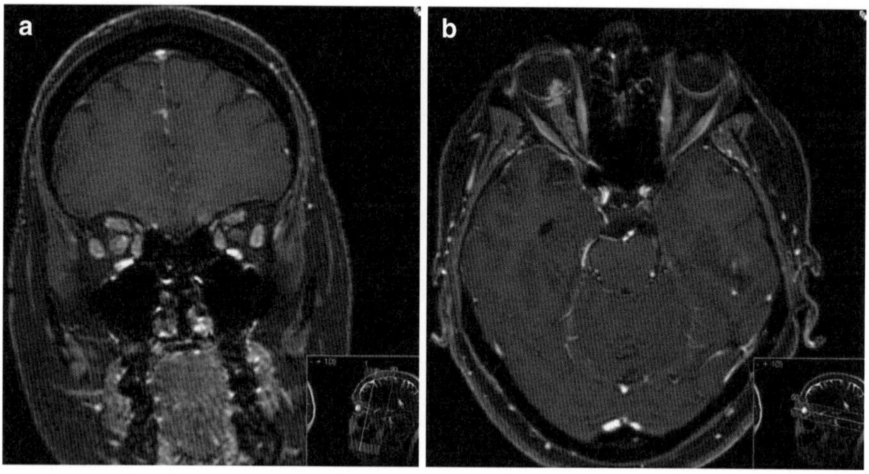

Fig. 15.1 MRI of orbits showing high signal within the right optic nerve – sheath complex extending from the bulbar segment through the optic canal to the chiasm. There is patchy enhancement

Evaluation

There were clear signs of an optic neuropathy, with a reduction in central acuity, a loss of ipsilateral color vision and a relative afferent pupillary defect. The affected disc was seen to be swollen.

The history is not at all typical for a demyelinating optic neuritis; the absence of pain, and the undoubted slowly evolving loss of vision would be most unlike this (see Case 11 for comparison). The MRI was reviewed (Fig. 15.1). This showed an enlargement of the optic nerve-sheath complex on the right with enhancement not of the nerve but of the sheath itself. It extends from the globe to the optic canal.

The Neuro-radiological differential diagnosis was of an inflammatory disorder or infiltration. It was felt not to be meningioma.

Investigations

Screening blood investigations revealed a normal blood count; the ESR was 20, the CRP 12. Renal function was normal but the liver function showed a modest rise in transaminases. The serum calcium was raised at 2.70. ANA, ANCA, rheumatoid factor and TPHR were negative. The serum ACE was normal. The protein electrophoresis revealed a slight monoclonal band; IgG was raised and the lamda light chains elevated. The lamda: kappa ratio was normal at 0.22. A full viral screen was normal aside from evidence for a previous infection with EBV. Borrelia, Bartonella, Cryptococcus and toxoplasma serologies were negative.

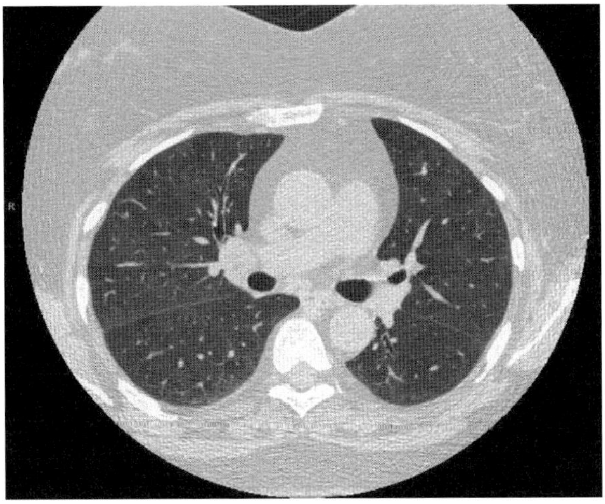

Fig. 15.2 Chest CT: there is a diffuse ground glass appearance throughout the lungs without fibrosis

The MRI scan (Fig. 15.1) showed high signal within the right optic nerve, with thickening and enhancement of the optic nerve sheath. This suggested that the pathological process was within the optic nerve sheath and not the nerve itself.

The CSF was under normal pressure and clear. The protein was 0.4 g/dl, there were six white cells and there were matched oligoclonal bands. The CSF/blood sugars were 3.1/7.4.

A chest X-ray showed a patchy ground glass appearance and a high resolution CT scan of the thorax revealed small mediastinal nodes but no hilar lymphadenopathy, and the ground glass parenchymal changes seen on the chest X-ray (Fig. 15.2).

A mantoux test was negative at 10 units. Quantiferon was negative.

A trans-bronchial biopsy of the lung was normal. The bronchoalveolar lavage revealed lymphocytes and alveolar macrophages. A trans-jugular liver biopsy revealed steatosis and no inflammation or fibrosis. A bone marrow aspiration and trephine biopsy revealed normal haemopoetic tissue, no plasma cell dyscrasia and no lymphoma.

An α1-anti-trypsin level was normal.

It was clear that this lady had a systemic disorder and it was frustrating that a wide series of investigations had failed to allow us to differentiate between an inflammatory, an infective or a neoplastic disease. Her vision deteriorated to counting fingers then hand movements. The respiratory abnormalities, the raised calcium and the monoclonal gammopathy are all in keeping with sarcoidosis but so too in malignant disease and lymphoma, and indeed in tuberculosis.

A PET/CT scan was undertaken; this showed numerous active lymph nodes within the neck, axilla, mediastinal and abdomen (Fig. 15.3).

A biopsy was then undertaken of the cervical node and showed granulomatous infiltration in keeping with sarcoidosis (Fig. 15.4).

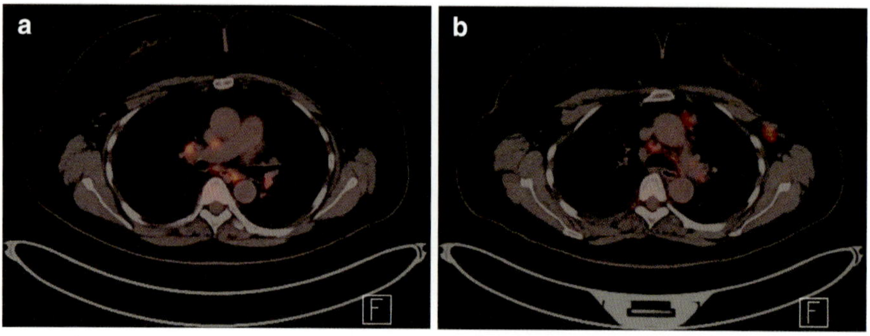

Fig. 15.3 CT PET scan showing uptake of FDG tracer in the cervical lymph nodes on both sides, the left axilla and the upper mediastinum. There were also nodes within the abdomen

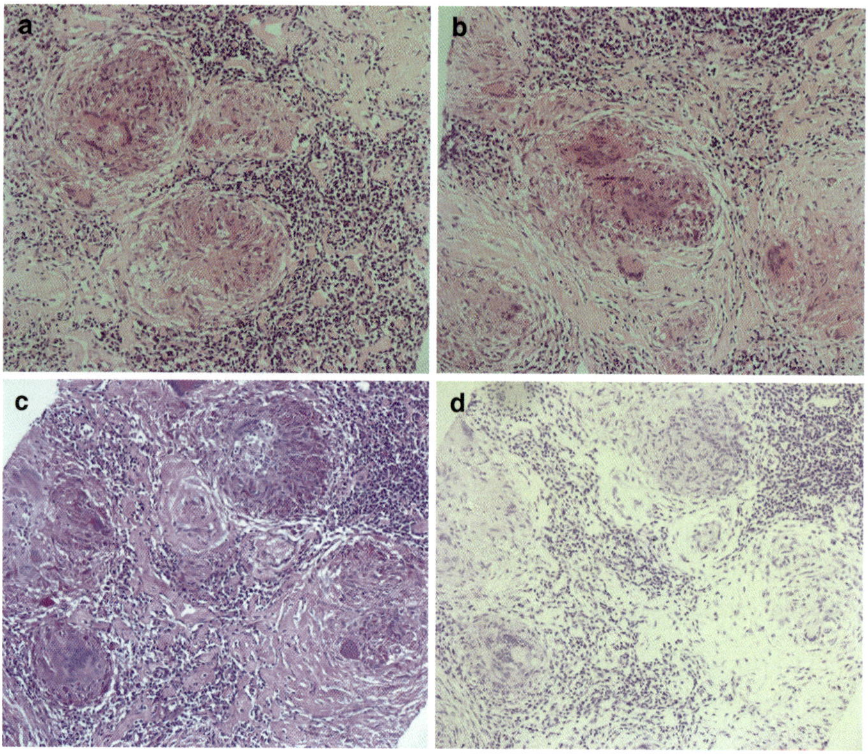

Fig. 15.4 Histology: There are numerous well formed epithelioid granulomas and Langhan's giant cells (**a**, **b**; H&E, ×400 magnification); (**c**) PAS stained slide showing no evidence of fungal infection; (**d**) ZN stained slide showing no evidence of Acid-fast bacilli. The features are of a chronic granulomatous lymphadenitis (Courtesy of Prof Peter Isaacson, Department of Celluar Pathology, Royal Free Hospital)

Treatment and Progress

She was treated with intravenous methyl prednisolone and oral prednisolone at 60 mg per day. There was an immediate albeit gentle response and over 3 weeks the visual acuity improved to 6/36. The steroids were reduced and the acuity worsened, but improved with further steroids and intravenous cyclophosphamide. Her systemic symptoms abated and she had been well on low dose oral steroids and weekly methotrexate. Her latest acuity is 6/24 with a constricted field.

Discussion

Optic perineuritis is in modern terms a diagnosis made using MRI; the pattern of enhancement is different to that seen in optic neuritis, in which the nerve enhances in the same region as the high signal lesion. In perineuritis the optic nerve-sheath complex enhances and is often seen as a tramline rather similar to that seen in optic nerve sheath meningioma on axial images, and as a doughnut on coronal scans [1]. There is high signal within the nerve, but the enhancement tends to be outside.

There are in addition several important clinical differences; in general the patients are older, the visual loss is more progressive than subacute and pain is more long-lasting. The field defect is less often central and frequently a peripheral constriction.

It is associated with inflammatory disorders including sarcoidosis, granulomatosis with polyangiitis and rheumatoid arthritis, and infections such as tuberculosis and syphilis. It has been seen to be associated with viral-mediated meningoencephalitis, usually in children. In these cases the literature suggests that there are usually other features which can be found to make the diagnosis, as in this case. In granulomatosis with polyangiitis the ESR will be raised and the ANCA found (either pANCA or cANCA), and in tuberculosis and syphilis there will similarly be other features on blood and radiological investigations. The condition may be mild, presenting with pain and little visual change, the diagnosis being made on imaging after the disc or discs are seen to be swollen. Those associated with viral infections are usually children in whom a lymphocytic pleocytosis is found in the CSF.

Those in whom no such cause is identified are deemed to have the idiopathic form, which was studied in [1]; pain is a prominent symptom and the visual loss proceeds over weeks rather than days. The disc is swollen but the ocular examination is otherwise normal. Most cases show a rapid and pleasing response to steroids although there may be relapse were the dose reduced too quickly. All but two of their 14 cases recovered well with treatment. One of their cases (who had been steroid unresponsive and had deteriorated to no light perception) underwent an optic sheath biopsy which showed marked thickening of the sheath and expansion of the pial septae and a chronic lymphocytic infiltration with fibrosis.

Reference

1. Purvin V, Kawasaki A, Jacobson DM. Optic perineuritis: clinical and radiographic features. Arch Ophthalmol. 2001;119:1299–306.

Case 16

History

This 43 year old lady had no symptoms but her optometrist at a routine check identified a visual field defect on the left side. She was referred to her GP and then to the Royal Free Hospital for evaluation.

Examination

The central acuities, color vision and pupillary responses were normal. The fields (Fig. 16.1) were abnormal; either a bilateral arcuate defect left greater than right, or an upper bitemporal quadtrantic defect. The discs were normal. The ocular examination was normal save for the identification of nodules on the iris on both sides (Fig. 16.2).

Further examination of the skin revealed several large café au lait patches and some axillary freckling.

D.P. Kidd, *Neuro-Ophthalmology*, DOI 10.1007/978-1-4471-2410-8_16

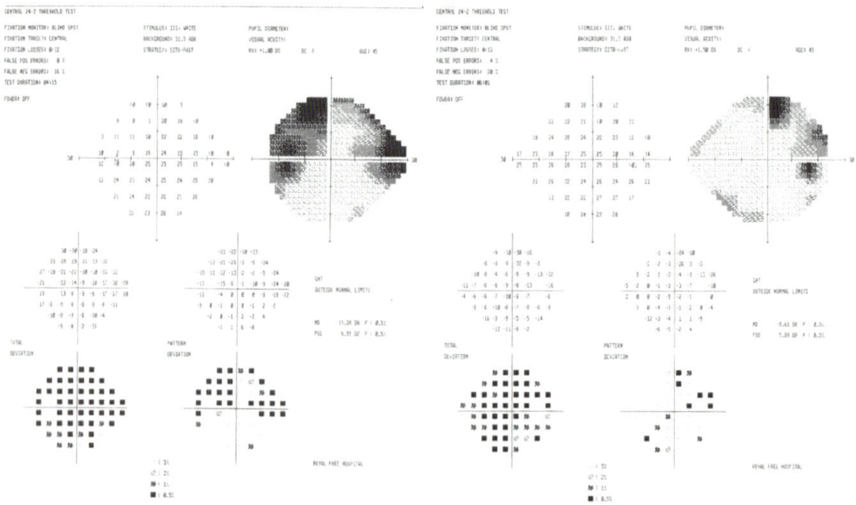

Fig. 16.1 Humphrey visual field showing an upper temporal abnormality on the both sides. The field defect obeys the vertical midline, which would make a neurological field defect much more likely than one due to retinal disease or glaucoma. Thus imaging is important in this case

Fig. 16.2 Lisch nodules on the iris

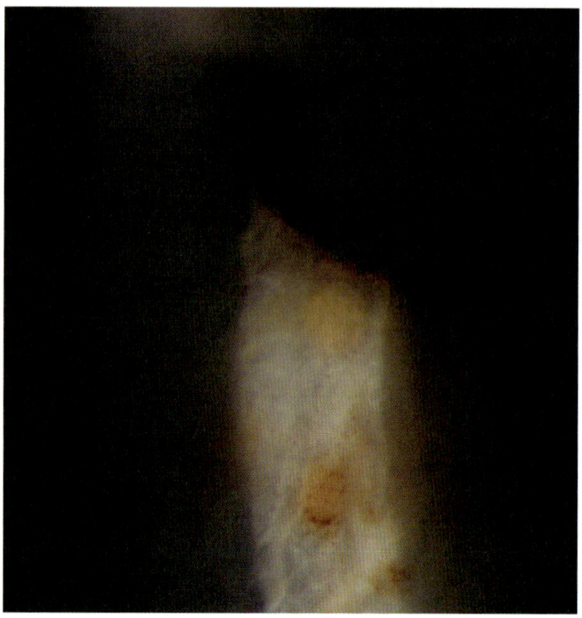

Evaluation

You never know what kind of interesting case is going to walk in through the door next. This lady, seemingly well, whose optometrist was concerned about a visual field defect walks in assuming that the Doctor she sees is going to be reassuring, until the ocular examination reveals a clue which leads to an examination of the skin which leads to the diagnosis.

The neuro-ophthalmic exam was within normal limits save for the abnormal visual field, but the presence of the iris nodules together with the skin lesions led to the MRI scan shown in Fig. 16.3.

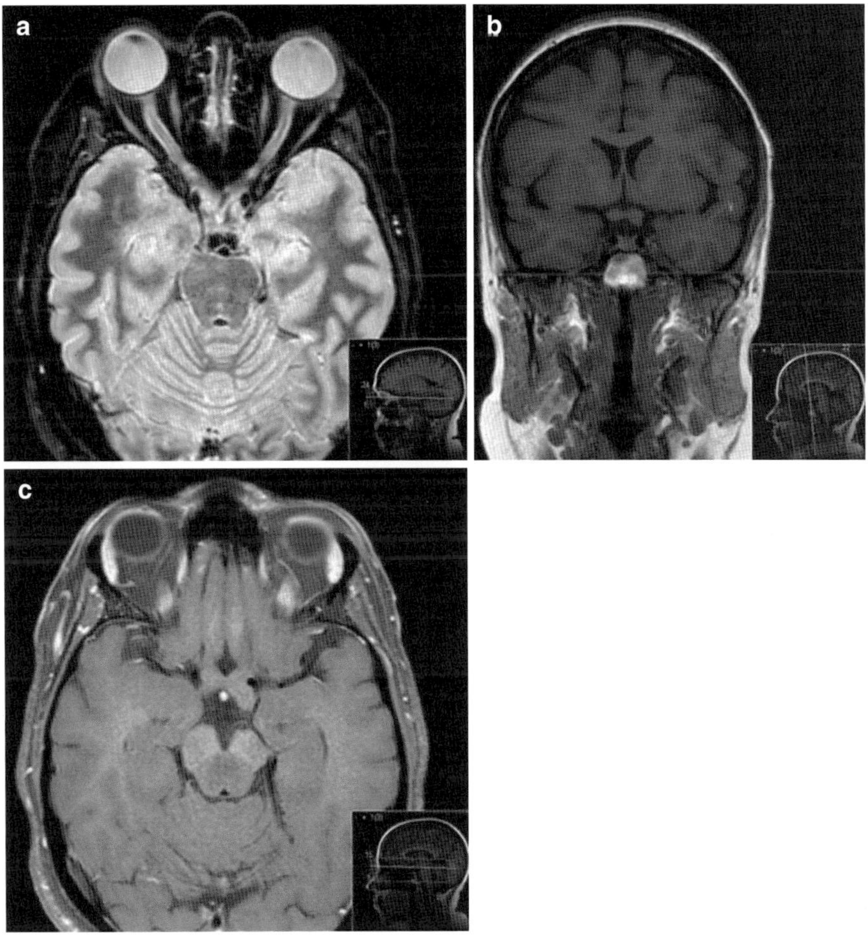

Fig. 16.3 MRI: (**a**) T2 weighted axial MRI showing enlargement of the right optic nerve extending back to and involving the chiasm and left optic tract, (**b**) coronal T1 weighted scan and (**c**) T1 weighted scan following administration of contrast, showing no enhancement of the asymmetric chiasmal enlargement

Investigations

Screening blood investigations were normal

An MRI scan of the orbits and chiasm revealed enlargement of the right optic nerve, chiasm and both optic tracts (Fig. 16.3) without enhancement.

She was referred to the Neurogenetics clinic of the hospital where genetic testing confirmed that she had Neurofibromatosis type 1.

Discussion

The MRI features are those of a low grade glioma of the chiasm. There is no enhancement, as there would be were the lesion to be high grade, and the absence of any significant disturbance of the function of the anterior visual pathway proves that the lesion, although striking on the scan, allows normal conduction through it.

Optic nerve gliomas are uncommon neoplasms which comprise over half of optic nerve primary tumors. They are most common below the age of 10 years, and the natural history of one of considerable variation, from rapidly progressive visual loss to seeming spontaneous regression of the lesion without treatment [1]. Thirty percent have neurofibromatosis type 1 [2].

In a recent series of 445 patients only 89 were aged over 20 years [3]. Of those 131 who had had biopsies 96 % of patients less than age 20 showed low tumor grade, whereas 66 % of those between 20 and 50 were low grade and only 22 % of those above the age of 50. Malignant gliomas of the anterior visual pathway are not related to neurofibromatosis, present in old age with a very rapidly progressive visual disorder with chiasmal enlargement and enhancement, and spread forwards into the nerves on both sides and backwards into the hypothalamus [2].

Twenty percent of children with NF1 have optic nerve gliomas, and most who have them have NF1. Only half of those with optic nerve gliomas will have a symptomatic visual loss; those who do present with visual loss, nystagmus, proptosis and strabismus. Since most are diagnosed with NF1 in childhood, brain scans are undertaken regularly in order to identify intracranial complications of the disease, and gliomas are identified even when asymptomatic [1].

Most childhood optic nerve gliomas are pilocytic astrocytomas; others are pilomyxoid and fibrillary (diffuse) astrocytomas, which may have greater mitotic rates. Malignant glioma is very uncommon in childhood, particularly those associated with NF1 [1, 4].

Treatment is given only to those with a documented tumor progression, some 30–50 % of cases, and chemotherapy is given nowadays; radiotherapy was formerly given, but is associated with a high risk of adverse effects. Surgery is rarely performed since it induces visual loss and does not influence outcome [4].

Following chemotherapy a quarter improve, a quarter deteriorate and the remainder stay the same [5].

Neurofibromatosis 1

It is an autosomal dominant disorder with an incidence of 1 in 2500. Half of the cases have new mutations and so no family history [6]. The gene is located on chromosome 17q11.2, and the protein neurofibromin controls cell growth and proliferation; inactivating mutations result in stimulation of RAS signaling leading to the development of RAS-linked neoplasia [7].

In the peripheral nerves neurofibromas occur in all cases, plexiform neurofibromas in 60 % and malignant nerve sheath tumors in 5 %. Within the brain optic pathway glioma occurs in 15–20 %; gliomas in the brain or spinal cord in 3 % and dysembryoplastic neuroepithelial tumors in 5 %. aquaduct stenosis and Arnold Chiari malformations are seen rarely.

In the eye Lisch nodules are seen in the iris in 95 % of cases, and choroidal nodules in 99 %. Lisch nodules are dome shaped lesions of the iris, composed of pigmented cells, fibroblasts and mast cells, similar to neurofibromas.

There is a higher incidence of low IQ, epilepsy, cerebrovascular disease and multiple sclerosis than in the general population. The peripheral nerve sheath tumors may transform into sarcomas. In addition, patients with NF1 show a higher incidence of gastrointestinal stromal tumors, somatostatinomas, pheochromocytomas, leukemias and breast cancer [6–8].

So this lady with Neurofibromatosis 1 presents with a mild field defect which has not deteriorated and so has in all likelihood been present since her optic nerve gli oma developed in early childhood and which has not (and presumably will not in the future) progressed to any significant degree. It is being monitored and no treatment is planned.

Table 16.1 Clinical diagnostic criteria for NF-1

Patients must have two or more of the following in order to fulfill the clinical criteria:
A first degree relative with NF1
Six or more *café au lait* patches
Axillary or groin freckling
Two or more Lisch nodules
Optic pathway glioma
Two or more cutaneous or subcutaneous neurofibromas
One plexiform neurofibroma
Bony dysplasia

References

1. Avery RA, Fisher MJ, Liu GT. Optic pathway gliomas. J Neuroophthalmol. 2011;31:269–78.
2. Dutton JJ. Gliomas of the anterior visual pathway. Surv Ophthalmol. 1994;38:427–52.
3. Mishra MV, Andrews DW, Glass J, Evans JJ, Dicker AP, Shen X, Lawrence YR. Characterization and outcomes of optic nerve gliomas: a population-based analysis. J Neurooncol. 2012;107:591–7.
4. Fried I, Tabori U, Tihan T, Reginald A, Bouffet E. Optic pathway gliomas: a review. CNS Oncol. 2013;2:143–59.
5. Fisher MJ, Loguidice M, Gutmann DH, Listernick R, Ferner RE, Ullrich NJ, Packer RJ, Tabori U, Hoffman RO, Ardern-Holmes SL, Hummel TR, Hargrave DR, Bouffet E, Charrow J, Bilaniuk LT, Balcer LJ, Liu GT. Visual outcomes in children with neurofibromatosis type 1-associated optic pathway glioma following chemotherapy: a multicenter retrospective analysis. Neuro Oncol. 2012;14:790–7.
6. Ferner RE, Gutmann DH. Neurofibromatosis type 1 (NF1): diagnosis and management. Handb Clin Neurol. 2013;115:939–55.
7. Niemeyer CM. RAS diseases in children. Haematologica. 2014;99:1653–62.
8. Madanikia SA, Bergner A, Ye X, Blakeley JO. Increased incidence of breast cancer in women with NF1. Am J Med Genet. 2012;158A:3056–60.

Case 17

History

This 20 year old lady presented with a mild central visual loss which she first noticed in the right eye when putting on make-up. This worsened over a couple of days and was not painful. She attended the ophthalmic emergency department of her local hospital and was found to have reduced acuities in both eyes and swollen optic discs. There were no other or prior neurological symptoms and no symptoms were identified on systematic enquiry. Her past medical history was unremarkable and she took no regular treatment.

A series of investigations was performed and she received treatment with intravenous corticosteroids without benefit. Her vision stabilized but did not improve. She was referred to the Neuro-ophthalmology Unit of the Royal Free Hospital.

Examination

She saw 6/36 N18 right, 6/12 N8 left. The color vision was absent. The pupillary responses were unimpaired and symmetrical. Each disc was slightly swollen (Fig. 17.1). The ocular examination was normal, in particular there was no uveitis or retinal lesion. The fields showed asymmetric centrocecal scotomata (Fig. 17.2). The eye movements were normal and there were no other abnormal neurological signs.

D.P. Kidd, *Neuro-Ophthalmology*, DOI 10.1007/978-1-4471-2410-8_17

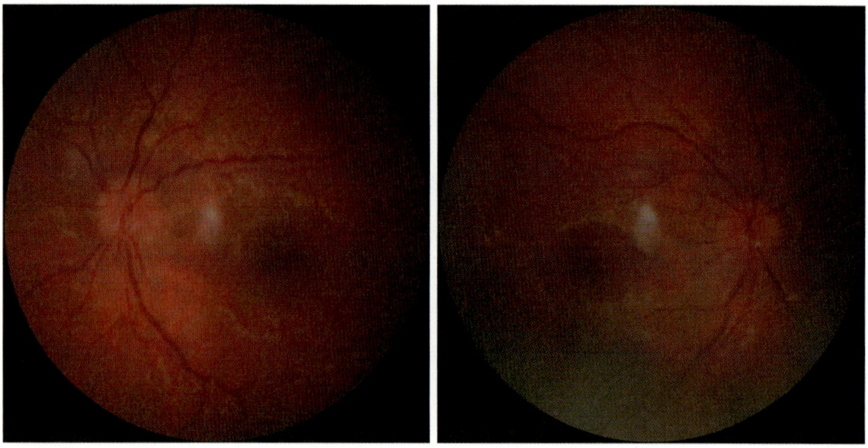

Fig. 17.1 Disc photographs showing mild edema around the disc; the peripapillary retina is more swollen than the disc itself

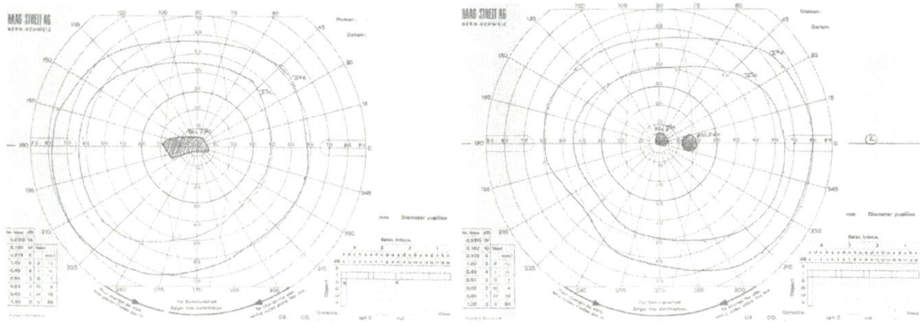

Fig. 17.2 Goldman visual field showing a central scotoma on the *right*, centrocecal on the *left*

Evaluation

This is a young lady with a painless optic neuropathy which probably developed and progressed simultaneously, although it is difficult to be certain since she had not noted a problem with the left, less severely affected eye. Bilateral synchronous optic neuritis of a demyelinating cause is uncommon and it is most uncommon for there to be no eye pain. Other causes of optic neuritis in which bilateral involvement is more common, including sarcoidosis, SLE, CRION, that associated with aquaporin-4 and anti-MOG antibodies and parainfectious optic neuritis should all be considered (see Case 11). A demyelinating cause should be associated with abnormalities on brain MRI (although not always) and systemic inflammatory disorders would be associated with clues in the blood and serological tests. A chiasmal disorder due for example to a pituitary adenoma would be unlikely with this particular pattern of visual field defect, and bilateral papilloedema due for example to idiopathic intracranial hypertension would not be associated with a central scotoma and loss of color vision.

It is difficult to say whether or not the absence of a pupillary abnormality is significant; when each nerve is affected the degree of conduction block may be similar even if the acuities are not, and so the relative defect which can often be seen in unilateral optic neuropathy may not be apparent.

Investigations

The blood count and biochemical screens were normal. ANA, ENA and ANCA were negative. ESR, ACE, vitamin B1 and B12 was within normal limits. Serological tests for Borrelia, Brucella (she lived in a rural community) and Bartonella were negative. An aquaporin-4 antibody titer was normal.

An MRI scan of the orbits was normal. A visual evoked potential was normal.

The fluorescein angiogram showed no leakage at the disc nor from the vessels (Fig. 17.3).

A spinal fluid examination showed normal pressure; protein and sugar levels were within normal limits. There were no lymphocytes and no oligoclonal bands.

Genetic testing for Leber's hereditary optic neuropathy revealed a mutation at thc 11778 rcgion.

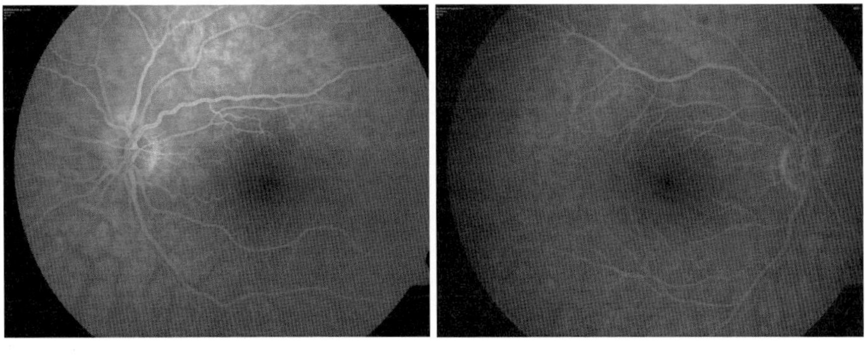

Fig. 17.3 Fluorescein angiogram showing no disc leakage at 4 min

Discussion

Whilst there is a chance that her optic neuropathy was not related to the genetic disorder and she was simply carrying the gene, we felt that having ruled out inflammatory and structural causes and having already ascertained that she had not responded to treatment with intravenous steroids, it was reasonable to associate the two. The clinical syndrome is in keeping with it, and on follow up her vision has not changed since. She was treated with Idebenone, a derivative of co-enzyme Q-10.

Leber's Hereditary Optic Neuropathy

Three point mutations in the mitochondrial genome account for 90 % of cases of Leber's hereditary optic neuropathy [1]. That located at position 11778 account for 70 % of cases, and those at positions 14484 and 3460 account for around 14 % each, although these proportions vary in different populations. These mutations are found only in families with LHON. The genetic defect has a low rate of penetrance; around 50 % of men with the mutation will present with optic neuropathy and only 10 % of females. The risk is greatest in the third decade (the median age of onset is 20 years in men and older in females), so the risk reduces with age. A family history of diagnosed optic neuropathy is absent in around 40 % of cases. The risk of visual loss in asymptomatic carriers of any of the three pathogenic mutations is 46 % in men and 11 % in women. Males become affected five times more commonly than females, most often in the second and third decades, although it has been seen in children and also in late age. Ninety-five percent of those affected will have become clinically manifest by the sixth decade [1]. Environmental triggers are important; cigarette smoking seems to have an important link, with 93 % of affected men being smokers in a retrospective study, and drugs, in particular antibiotics such as Ethambutol and Erythromycin and anti-retroviral drugs have shown a close link to the development of visual loss in those with mutations.

The majority presents with a subacute painless unilateral optic neuropathy. In 25 % the visual loss is bilateral and synchronous [2, 3]. The acuity drop varies; some still see 6/6 (20/20) whilst others lose all sight in the eye. The majority reduces to 6/60 (20/200) or counting fingers. Color vision is lost in the affected eye, but in contrast to inflammatory optic neuropathies the pupillary response is not delayed (because the melanopsin ganglion cells in the photoreceptor layer are not involved [4, 5]). The field defect varies, but the common defect is a central or centrocecal scotoma (Fig. 17.2), which was seen in 87 % of one series [3]. This increases in size and density over days after onset of symptoms and often becomes absolute i.e. there is no light perception within the defect.

The chambers of the eye are quiet, but the disc often shows characteristic appearances: a circumpapillary telangiectatic microangiopathy, in which there is capillary dilatation within the disc, and sometimes vascular engorgement in the retinal vessels. There is swelling not of the disc but of the retina immediately around the disc, and (for the same reason) an absence of leakage of fluorescein from the disc at angiography. These signs may arise during acute visual loss, but also later in the other presymptomatic eye, and in unaffected carrying relatives. Other abnormalities may also be seen, for example a general disc swelling, macular edema and retinal hemorrhage. In 20 % of cases the disc is normal.

In the vast majority of cases the other eye becomes affected within a year, normally within 8 weeks; persisting unilateral involvement is exceedingly rare. Over time visual improvement may arise; this may be modest, for example islands of vision appearing within the central scotoma, but may be appreciable. Those with the 14484 mutation are most likely to improve and those with the 11778 least likely. This improvement often begins slowly a year after symptom onset but has been seen to occur many years after a constant severe visual impairment [6].

References

1. Man PYW, Griffiths PG, Hudson G, Chinnery PF. Inherited mitochondrial optic neuropathies. J Med Genet. 2009;46:145–58.
2. Nikoskelainen EK. Clinical picture of LHON. Clin Neurosci. 1994;2:115–20.
3. Riordan-Eva P, Sanders MD, Govan GG, Sweeney MG, DaCosta J, Harding AE. The clinical features of Leber's hereditary optic neuropathy defined by the presence of pathogenic mitochondrial DNA mutations. Brain. 1995;118:319–37.
4. Kawasaki A, Herbst K, Sander B, Milea D. Selective wavelength pupillometry in Leber hereditary optic neuropathy. Clin Experiment Ophthalmol. 2010;38:322–4.
5. LaMorgia C, Ross-Cisneros FN, Sadun AA, Hannibal J, Munarini A, Mantovani V. Melanopsin retinal ganglion cells are resistant to neurodegeneration in mitochondrial optic neuropathies. Brain. 2010;133:2426–38.
6. Man PYW, Griffiths PG, Chinnery PF. Mitochondrial optic neuropathies – disease mechanisms and therapeutic strategies. Prog Retin Eye Res. 2011;30:81–114.

Case 18

History

This 66 year old man had a long history of lumbar spondylitis disease and had undergone successful surgery in 2007 for a cauda equina compression at L5/S1, with resolution of symptoms. In 2012 sciatic pain recurred with claudicant symptoms on walking, leading to a feeling of iced water running down his leg at L4 and L5 on the right side. Reinvestigation led to the identification of a further lumbar canal stenosis at L3/L4, and it was decided that he should undergo a decompressive laminectomy. This duly took place under the care of the spinal neurosurgeons and at surgery nothing untoward was seen to occur; there was for example no excessive blood loss and the anesthetist reported no cardiovascular instability.

Nonetheless upon waking in the recovery room he noted a marked and painless visual impairment.

He was not known to have ischemic heart disease but was hypertensive. There was no history of hypercholesterolemia or diabetes. He was a non-smoker. There was a family history of ischemic heart disease but not of stroke. His past medical history was otherwise unremarkable.

Examination

He saw hand movements on the right and 6/24 on the left, and no color vision. There was a right relative afferent pupillary defect. Neither disc was swollen and the ocular examination was normal.

There was no measurable field on the right and the left showed an inferior altitudinal defect and a superior arcuate defect (Fig. 18.1). The eye movements were normal and there were no other new abnormal neurological signs

D.P. Kidd, *Neuro-Ophthalmology*, DOI 10.1007/978-1-4471-2410-8_18

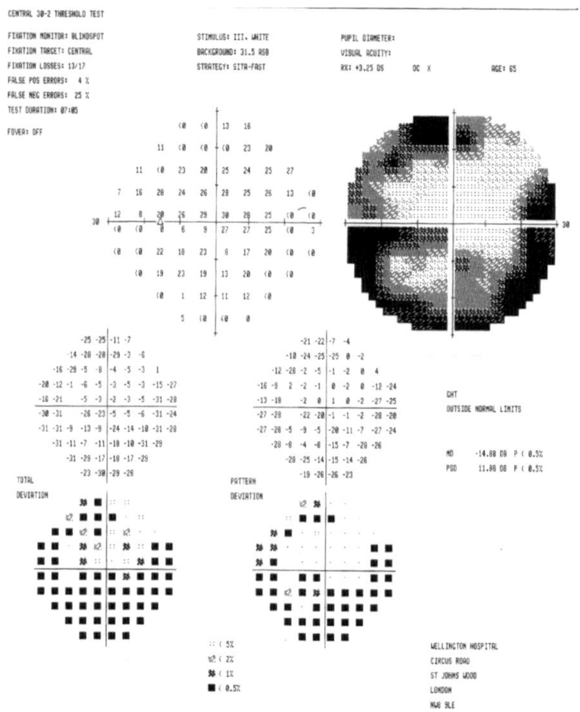

Fig. 18.1 Humphrey visual field on the *left* showing inferior altitudinal and superior arcuate field defects

Evaluation

This was an alarming post-operative emergency in which bilateral optic neuropathies had arisen during anesthesia and surgery. Nothing seemingly untoward had arisen during or after surgery, and so an ischemic disorder of the occipital cortex would be unlikely, although still needs to be considered since the only clear sign of an optic neuropathy is the relative afferent pupillary defect. An ocular disorder such as bilateral retinal detachment would have been seen at the time of the post-operative ocular examination. An unassociated disorder of the anterior visual pathway needs to be considered; for example a pituitary adenoma with hemorrhage, meningioma, and aneurysm. Imaging is warranted, and urgently.

Investigation

Post-operative blood tests were normal; the hematocrit was not abnormally high. Biochemical screening was normal. An MRI scan of the orbits was normal.

Management

A diagnosis of posterior ischemic optic neuropathy (PION) was made. No treatment is available and the patient was monitored. Over the following 3 months the discs became noticeably pale, right greater than left, and no meaningful improvement in vision arose. He was registered with a certificate of visual improvement.

Discussion

In a review of 72 cases seen in two Neuro-ophthalmology centers in the US over 20 a year period Sadda et al. [1] defined posterior ischemic optic neuropathy to be:

1. An acute deficit in visual acuity, visual field or both
2. An ipsilateral relative afferent pupillary defect
3. Documented absence of optic disc swelling or peripapillary hemorrhage at the time of the visual loss
4. Exclusion of compressive, inflammatory or other optic nerve disorder (for example disc drusen or glaucoma).

There were 34 men and 38 women of mean age 62 (18–88) years. Six were subsequently found to have arteritis, for example Giant Cell arteritis. Of the remainder, 28 suffered visual loss after surgery and 38 with no preceding event. Risk factors for atheromatous disease (hypertension, diabetes, ischemic heart disease, smoking etc.) were identified in 87 %. Twenty-six cases were bilateral, particularly in the arteritic group and following surgery. Only 21 % of cases in the non-surgical, non-arteritic group were bilateral. Visual loss was less severe in this group compared with the other two, and recovery of vision more likely to occur. Overall half the patients were left with acuities less than 20/200 (6/60).

Twenty-eight developed PION after surgical procedure. Half of these was associated with spinal surgery; the patients were younger than the other groups, were less likely to have vascular risk factors (those with PION following other surgery, for example cardiac or abdominal surgery had the same prevalence of risk factors as the other non-arteritic group). Fifty-four percent were bilateral.

The blood supply to the optic nerve is complex (Fig. 18.2); that to the anterior part is derived from a pial plexus served by branches from the ophthalmic artery and the central retinal artery. That to the disc is supplied by a more rich network supplied by branches of the short posterior ciliary arteries, choroidal feeder vessels and pial vessels from the ophthalmic artery. The posterior part of the nerve however is supplied only by the pial capillary plexus which surrounds it, with poor penetrance into the nerve itself, with the result the central part of the nerve posteriorly has a relatively poor arterial supply. This would render this part of the nerve at risk of ischemia during periods of low perfusion pressure, for example during blood loss.

The American Society of Anaesthesiology post-operative visual loss registry studied through multivariate analysis 80 cases of visual loss following spinal surgery

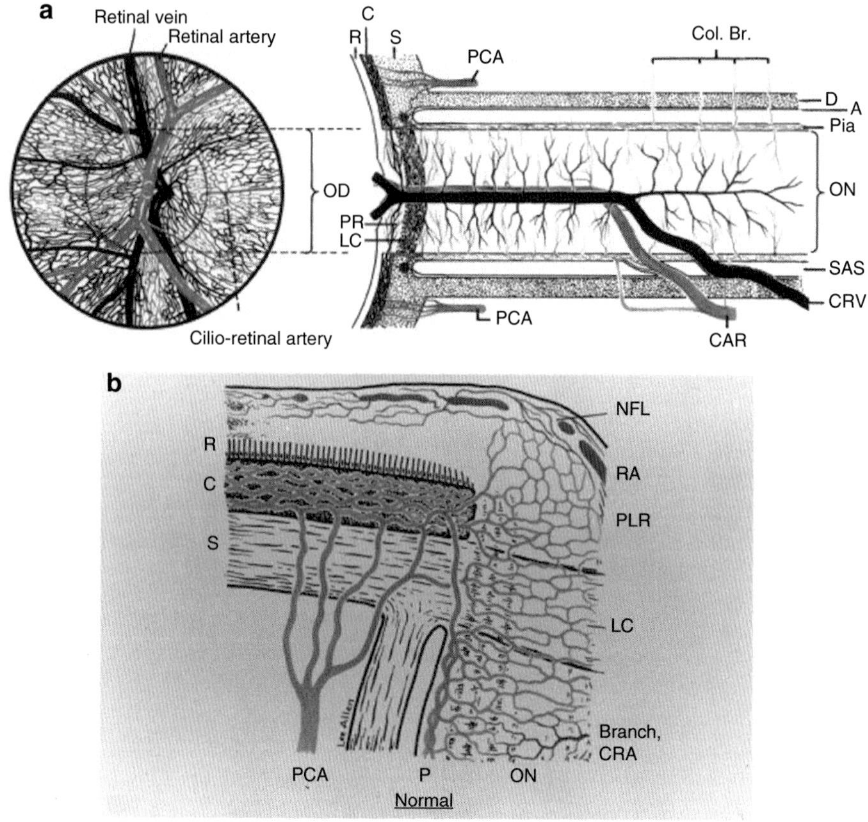

Fig. 18.2 The blood supply to the optic nerve (Reprinted with permission of Elsevier from Hayreh [2]). *A* arachnoid, *C* choroid, *D* dura, *LC* lamina cribrosa, *PR* prelaminar region, *R* retina, *S* sclera, *Pia* pia arachnoid, *ON* optic nerve, *SAS* subarachnoid space, *NFL* surface nerve fiber layer of the disc, *CRA* central retinal artery, *ICA* internal carotid artery, *CRV* central retinal vein, *PCA* posterior ciliary artery, *OA* ophthalmic artery

[3] and identified male sex, obesity, estimated blood loss and use of colloid as blood volume replacement as risk factors, as well as duration of anesthesia. There is much discussion in the literature on the use of head frames and their compressive effect on intraocular pressure, venous stasis as the head is held below the heart, but no conclusions have been drawn.

A study of the incidence of visual loss in a cohort of all 4.7 million spinal surgical procedures carried out in the US between 1993 and 2002 revealed an incidence of 0.094 %; risk factors included ages less than 18 and greater than 40, vascular risk factors and anemia [4]. A further study of 5.6 million surgical procedures in the US over a 10 year period revealed an incidence of 8.64/10000 after cardiac surgery and 3.09/10000 after spinal fusion [5]. This included all forms of visual loss including cortical blindness which is common after cardiac surgery in children.

References

1. Sadda SR, Nee N, Miller NR, Biousse V, Newman NJ, Kouzis A. Clinical spectrum of posterior ischemic optic neuropathy. Am J Ophthalmol. 2001;132:743–50.
2. Hayreh SS. The blood supply of the optic nerve head and the evaluation of it – myth and reality. Prog Retin Eye Res. 2001;20:563–93.
3. Postoperative visual loss study group. Risk factors associated with ischemic optic neuropathy after spinal fusion surgery. Anesthesiology. 2012;116:15–24.
4. Patil CG, Lad EM, Lad SP, Ho C, Boakye M. Visual loss after spine surgery: a population-based study. Spine. 2008;33:1491–6.
5. Shen Y, Drum M, Roth S. The prevalence of perioperative visual loss in the United States: a 10 year study from 1996 to 2005 of spinal, orthopaedic, cardiac and general surgery. Anesth Analg. 2009;109:1534–45.

Case 19

History

This 35 year old lady was admitted for investigation of a subacute painless visual loss on the right side. It had begun a week previously and had progressively deteriorated to no perception of light. There were no phosphenes and no pain on eye movement. The left eye was normal and her vision previously had been good.

There was a significant past neurological history of severe quadriplegia whose cause was diagnosed as neurosarcoidosis 9 years before. On further investigation it was found that she had had a subacute severe weakness and sensory loss affecting all four limbs; MRI had shown a longitudinally extensive cervico-thoracic spinal cord lesion, and the CSF had shown a raised protein and some white cells. There were matched oligoclonal bands. There had been no evidence for systemic sarcoidosis. The condition relapsed several times over the ensuing 5 years, was temporarily responsive to steroids, but with the accrual of an increasing quadriparesis. Her condition had seemingly been stable for the previous 4 years; after rehabilitation she managed well with a wheelchair and adaptations to her home. She had ventilatory support at night with a BiPAP system. There had been no other neurological symptoms in the intervening period although there had been problems with bladder function, culminating in the implantation of a suprapubic catheter.

She took no regular treatment and was otherwise well. There was no family history of neurological disease.

Examination

The left acuities were normal. There was no perception of light on the right. There was an afferent pupillary defect. The ocular examination was unremarkable and the disc was initially normal in appearance.

There was a very severe spastic quadriparesis with only slight movement in the right arm, and tendon contractures. The higher cortical functions were normal.

The systemic examination was normal.

D.P. Kidd, *Neuro-Ophthalmology*, DOI 10.1007/978-1-4471-2410-8_19

Evaluation

This young lady presents with a clear history and examination findings of a unilateral optic neuropathy and is obvious that the previous disorder should be considered part of the new problem. This disorder was a relapsing transverse myelitis. Sarcoidosis may well cause the clinical syndrome, so too would SLE, Sjogren's syndrome, anti-phospholipid antibody syndrome and paraneoplastic disorders. Infections such as HIV, HTLV-1, tuberculosis, Brucella, borrelia and syphilis. The clinical features are of Neuromyelitis Optica; the diagnostic criteria are noted in the Table 19.1.

Table 19.1 NMOSD diagnostic criteria for adult patients

Diagnostic criteria for NMOSD with AQP4-IgG
1. At least one core clinical characteristic
2. Positive test for AQP4-IgG using best available detection method (cell based assay strongly recommended)
3. Exclusion of alternative diagnosis
Diagnostic criteria for NMOSD without AQP4-IgG or NMOSD with unknown AQP4-IgG status
1. At least 2 core clinical characteristics occurring as a result of one or more clinical attacks and meeting all of the following requirements:
(a) At least one core clinical characteristic must be optic neuritis, acute myelitis with LETM, or area postrema syndrome
(b) Dissemination in space (two or more different core clinical characteristics)
(c) Fulfillment of additional MRI requirements, as applicable
2. Negative tests for AQP4-IgG using best available detection method, or testing unavailable
3. Exclusion of alternative diagnosis
Core clinical characteristics
1. Optic neuritis
2. Acute myelitis
3. Area postrema syndrome: episode of otherwise unexplained hiccups or nausea and vomiting
4. Acute brain stem syndrome
5. Symptomatic narcolepsy or acute diencephalic clinical syndrome with NMOSD-typical diencephalic MRI lesions
6. Symptomatic cerebral syndrome with NMOSD-typical brain lesions
Additional MRI requirements for NMOSD without APQ4-IgG and NMOSD with unknown AQ4-IgG status
1. Acute optic neuritis: requires brain MRI showing (a) normal findings or only non-specific white matter lesions or (b) optic nerve MRI with T2-hyperintense lesion or T1-weighted gadolinium-enhancing lesion extending over >1/2 optic nerve length or involving chiasm
2. Acute myelitis: requires associated intramedullary MRI lesion extending over ≥ 3 contiguous segments (LETM) or ≥ 3 contiguous segments of focal spinal cord atrophy in patients with history compatible with acute myelitis
3. Area postrema syndrome: requires associated dorsal medulla/area postrema lesions
4. Acute brainstem syndrome: requires associated periependymal brainstem lesions

Reproduced with permission from [2]

Investigations

Screening blood investigations were normal. Serum ACE, ANA, ENA, anti-phospholipid antibodies were all normal.

MRI scan of the orbits showed high signal within a swollen right optic nerve (Fig. 19.1) and severe atrophy of the whole spinal cord (Fig. 19.2). Previous scans were obtained and showed a severe longitudinally extensive myelitis some years before (Fig. 19.3).

Aquaporin-4 antibodies were found to be positive.

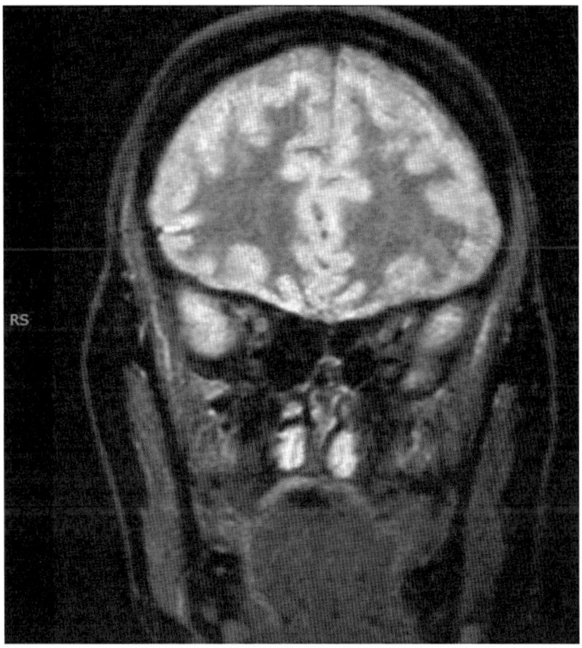

Fig. 19.1 T2 FATSAT coronal MRI showing swelling of and high signal within the right optic nerve

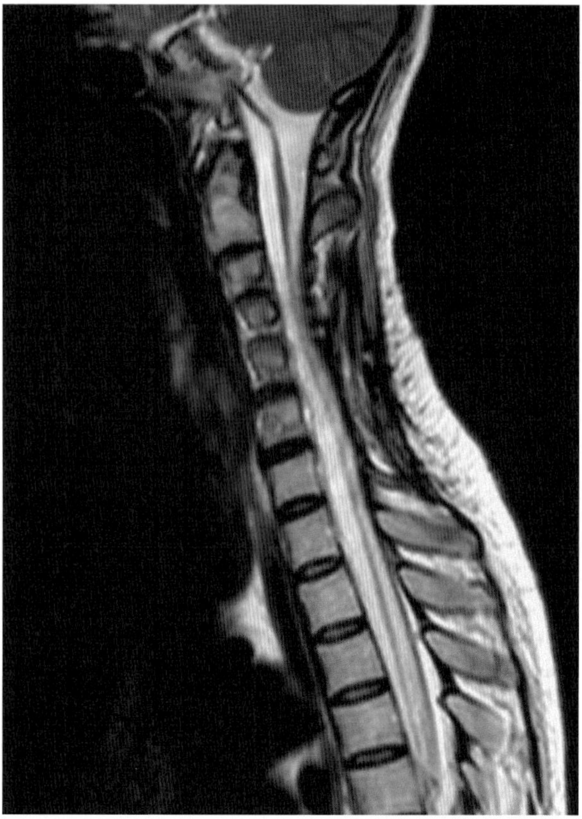

Fig. 19.2 T2 weighted sagittal MRI showing a very striking atrophy of the cord from lower medulla to the mid thoracic region

Management

She was treated with 5 g intravenous methylprednisolone, and plasma exchange for 5 days, then underwent treatment with Rituximab 2000 mg. Her vision improved to 6/18 and the disc became pale but not atrophic. The signs of the cord lesion did not alter.

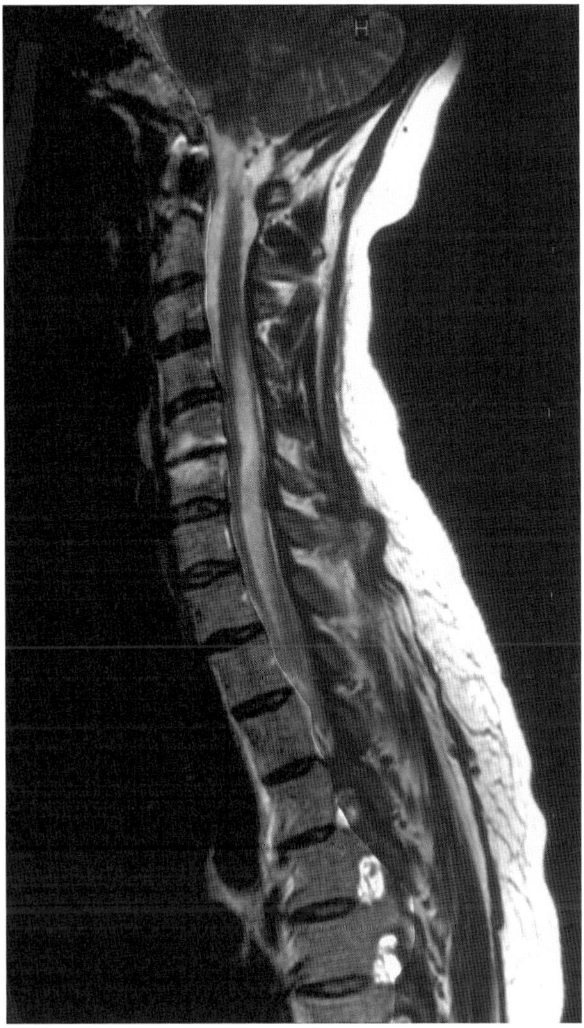

Fig. 19.3 T2 weighted sagittal MRI of the cervical spinal cord showing a longitudinally extensive swelling with high signal from 7 years before

Discussion

Neuromyelitis Optica

Neuromyelitis Optica (NMO) is an uncommon inflammatory disorder of the central nervous system very distinct from multiple sclerosis. The classical features are of a severe transverse myelitis and bilateral optic neuropathy.

The prevalence varies amongst different genetic groups, being more common in south East Asian populations (in which it accounts for around 40 % of all demyelinating disease, *vs* 1–2 % of Caucasians) and, in the US, African Americans, who account for one third of all cases. The prevalence is estimated to be 0.3–4.4 × 10^5 [1]. There is a wider age range of involvement, including a higher incidence in children (10 % of all cases in the US), and the median age is older than in multiple sclerosis; 39 years. The disorder affects females some nine times more than men.

The target antigen is the aquaporin-4 antibody; aquaporin-4 is a water channel expressed in astrocytic end feet at the blood–brain barrier, particularly at nodes of Ranvier and synapses, and the supra-optic and paraventricular nuclei of the hypothalamus, and the gray matter around the ventricles (the subfornical organ, the lamina terminalis and the area postrema).

Aquaporin-4 antibodies are present in 90 % of cases of NMO spectrum disorders, and their presence implies a high risk of relapsing disease, to the extent that long term immunosuppression is advocated upon their identification [1]. A proportion of those without aquaporin-4 antibodies have MOG antibodies.

Around 50 % have antinuclear antibodies and many others have Sjogren's syndrome associated antibodies and rheumatoid factor. Thirty-five percent have neural-specific auto-antibodies such as acetylcholine receptor, voltage gated potassium and CRMP-5 antibodies, which may not be associated with symptoms of those diseases [1]. However there is also a high prevalence of coexisting auto-immune disease, such as diabetes, thyroid disease, pernicious anemia, coeliac disease, polymyositis and connective tissue diseases. It may also be associated with malignant disease, particularly in the elderly, as a paraneoplastic phenomenon.

The CSF is active with lymphocytes, neutrophils and eosinophils. The protein is raised. IL-6 levels are elevated. The prevalence of oligoclonal bands is 30 %.

The myelitis is a longitudinally extensive lesion occupying more than three vertebral segments on MRI. Previously it was considered that the brain was unaffected, but there is now accumulating evidence that up to 60 % have brain lesions and these are periventricular and basal in position, corresponding to the prevalence of aquaporin-4 channel density noted above. Hypothalamic dysfunction including diabetes insipidus may occur, and a syndrome of nausea and persistent hiccups related to involvement of the area postrema has been seen (cited in [1, 2]).

Involvement of the optic nerve is no longer a prerequisite for the diagnosis (see Table 19.1), but is a very common clinical manifestation. Factors suggestive of NMO-associated optic neuritis include simultaneous bilateral involvement, chiasmal involvement, poor nadir acuity and an altitudinal field defect [2]. In one series of 30 patients [3] 28 were female and 23 had had optic neuritis. This was retrobulbar in all but 4. Four presented with a bilateral synchronous optic neuritis. All had relapsing disease with a mean of 2.7 attacks per patient. The median time to severe monocular and binocular visual loss was 2 and 13 years respectively.

In general the nadir acuity is less than in an MS-associated optic neuritis, and the improvement less complete [4]. MRI shows a longer lesion and one more likely to be posteriorly placed, even to spread back into the chiasm and tract. OCT demonstrates a proportionately greater loss of retinal nerve fiber layer thickness than that seen after an MS-associated optic neuritis [5].

With modern treatment the prognosis for visual loss has substantially improved, with fewer nor progressing to severe visual loss than before.

The pathogenesis is the release of antibodies to aquaporin-4 which bind to astrocytes and thereby induce a severe immune cascade leading to neutrophil, lymphocyte and macrophage activation, a complement mediated cytotoxicity leading to damage and death of astrocytes, oligodendrocytes and axons. The pathological appearances are of an immune activation with perivascular demyelination, loss of astrocytes and axons, and tissue necrosis which affects both gray and white matter structures.

Treatment since the identification of aquaporin-4 antibodies and the removal of this patient group from multiple sclerosis has improved enormously; steroids remain helpful initially but aggressive immunosuppression and plasma exchange are now the accepted therapies; immunosuppression with azathioprine, mycophenolate and methotrexate and early use of rituximab augments recovery, reduces tissue destruction and lowers relapse frequency. Experimental monoclonal antibody treatments with eculizumab and toculizumab may also provoke greater benefits [1]. Treatment for multiple sclerosis such as interferon β may make patients worse [6].

References

1. Pittock SJ, Lucchinetti CF. Neuromyelitis optica and the evolving spectrum of autoimmune aquaporin-4 channelopathies: a decade later. Ann N Y Acad Sci. 2016;1366:20–39.
2. Wingerchuk DM, Banwell B, Bennett JL, Cabre P, Carroll W, Chitnis T, de Seze J, Fujihara K, Greenberg B, Jacob A, Jarius S, Lana-Peixoto M, Levy M, Simon JH, Tenembaum S, Traboulsee AL, Waters P, Wellik KE, Weinshenker BG, International Panel for NMO Diagnosis. International consensus diagnostic criteria for neuromyelitis optica spectrum disorders. Neurology. 2015;85:177–89.
3. Merle H, Olindo S, Bonnan M, Donnio A, Richer R, Smadja D, Cabre P. Natural history of the visual impairment of relapsing neuromyelitis optica. Ophthalmology. 2007;114:810–5.
4. Levin MH, Bennett JL, Verkman AS. Optic neuritis in neuromyelitis optica. Prog Retin Eye Res. 2013;36:159–71.
5. Merle H, Olindo S, Donnio A, Richer R, Smadja D, Cabre P. Retinal peripapillary nerve fiber layer thickness in neuromyelitis optica. Invest Ophthalmol Vis Sci. 2008;49:4412–7.
6. Palace J, Leite MI, Nairne A, Vincent A. Interferon beta treatment in neuromyelitis optica: increase in relapses and aquaporin 4 antibody titers. Arch Neurol. 2010;67:1016–7.

Case 20

History

This 26 year old lady presented to her local hospital as an emergency with an escalating history of feeling unwell with headache and blurred vision. The headache had begun suddenly but without precipitant, and was generalized. There were no migrainous features although it felt pulsating. As the headache increased it showed an increase in intensity with Valsalva maneuver such as coughing or straining. The vision was normal but as she stood up from sitting there would be a diminution of vision for 10 seconds or so before it improved again. It felt like a dark cloud passed briefly across her vision on both sides.

There was increasing lassitude, a feeling of fever with sweating at night, generalized aches and pains and prominent fatigue. There were no flu-like symptoms. Latterly she had developed swelling and duskiness of the legs, and finally painful raised red lesions on the shins. On further enquiry she admitted to having suffered from recurrent bouts of oral ulceration since her early teens, and then painful genital ulcers.

She was otherwise well with no past medical history and took no treatment. There was no family history of neurological disease.

Examination

On admission she saw 6/5 N5 with normal color vision. The visual fields were not formally tested. The ocular examination revealed bilateral papilloedema. The anterior chambers were normal and no abnormality was detected within the retina.

The systemic examination revealed her to be unwell although afebrile. There were tender raised red skin lesions on the shins and there was a dusky hue to the skin of the legs, with pitting edema. There were several 1 cm sized tender ulcers in the soft palate and tonsil, and two within the labial mucosa of the vulva.

She was referred to the Royal Free Hospital.

D.P. Kidd, *Neuro-Ophthalmology*, DOI 10.1007/978-1-4471-2410-8_20

Evaluation

This is a severe and evolving systemic disorder with headache, optic disc swelling initially with unaffected vision but then with unilateral visual loss.

1. The neuro-ophthalmic disorder
   Her vision is normal but her discs are swollen; this would make a bilateral inflammation of the optic nerves most unlikely since inevitably optic nerve function would be reduced. In the presence of a systemic vascular disorder causing ischemia on occasion the disc may swell without the development of an ischemic optic neuropathy initially, but usually only for a short time.

   The transient visual change she describes is known as visual obscuration; this is related to papilloedema (see discussion of Case 34). She is young and female, but not overweight; this would make idiopathic intracranial hypertension an unlikely cause, since the prevalence of IIH increases 20 fold in young women who are obese. The syndrome of IIH can be caused by drug ingestion, for example vitamin A (including retinoic acid), tetracycline, lithium, amiodarone, ciprofloxacin, phenytoin and progesterone, and metabolic disorders such as Addison's disease, hypothyroidism, hypoparathyroidism and renal failure.
2. The systemic disorder
   She is clearly unwell and becoming worse. Infection, inflammation and vasculitis should all be considered first, then neoplastic disorders; at her age lymphoreticular disorders would be more common than epithelial malignancy. Of the infective causes of a meningeal disorder with systemic features HIV should be considered, herpesvirus infections (particularly EBV and HHV 6 and 7), tuberculosis, syphilis, Bartonella Henselai (cat scratch disease), Borrelia Burgdorferi (Lyme disease), Tropherimi Whipplei (Whipple's disease).

   The presence of orogenital ulceration is important here, particularly the fact that the lesions had been recurrent and of long standing. Immunological disorders such as immunodeficiency and allergy such as Stevens-Johnson syndrome, and sarcoidosis and Behçet's syndrome, connective tissue diseases such as Rheumatoid arthritis, Sjogren's syndrome and systemic lupus erythematosus, and B27 associated diseases such as Reiter's syndrome, may all cause these symptoms, as may inflammatory bowel disease such as Crohn's disease or ulcerative colitis, and Coeliac disease.

   Vasculitis at her age would involve consideration of Takayasu's arteritis (more common in women but with arterial problems), polyarteritis nodosa (more common in men and associated with hepatitis B but again more associated with arterial problems), cryoglobulinemia (associated with hepatitis C), polyangiitis with granulomatosis (associated with sinus and meningeal disease and renal failure) and Churg Strauss syndrome (associated with eosinophilia and asthma).

Investigations

The ESR was 80 and the CRP 156. Biochemical screening was normal and the FBC within normal limits. ANA, ENA, ANCA, anticardiolipin and endomysial antibodies were all negative. Serological investigations into HIV, hepatitis B and C, EBV and HHV6 were all negative. A CT scan of the chest abdomen and pelvis showed normal organs but a widespread bilateral thrombosis of the iliac veins.

The MRI scan of brain showed no parenchymal disorder but clear evidence for a thrombosis of the entirety of the superior sagittal sinus (Figs. 20.1a and 20.2). There was clear evidence for raised pressure in that the optic nerve sheaths were patulous (Fig. 20.1b).

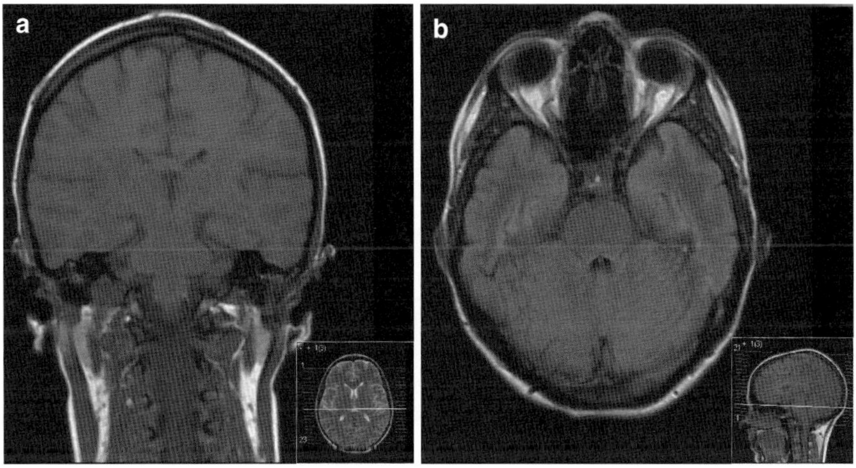

Fig. 20.1 Coronal T1 weighted MRI (**a**) showing no flow within the superior sagittal sinus and (**b**) T2 weighted axial MRI showing patulousness of the optic nerve sheaths on both sides, but without an empty sella (implying that the pressure is raised but has only recently become so)

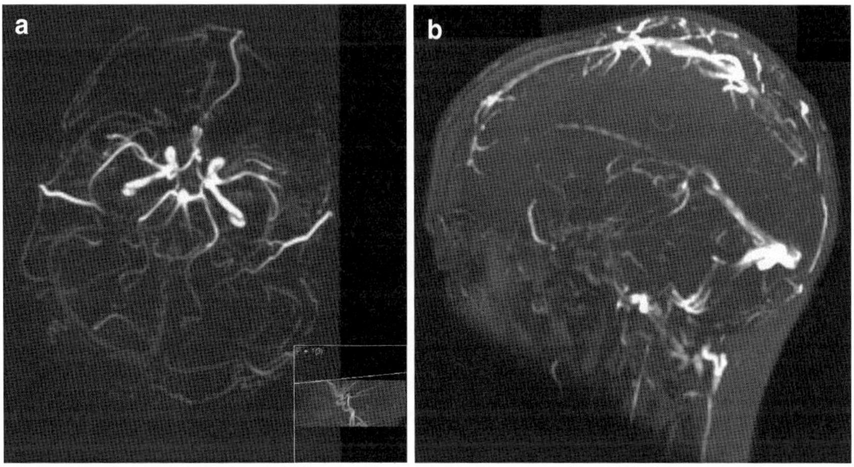

Fig. 20.2 MR venogram showing an absence of flow within the superior sagittal sinus

The CSF was under high pressure >40 cm CSF, but the constituents were normal. The sugar differential was 3.2/5.4 and culture and PCR examinations were negative for infection.

Evaluation

The presence of longstanding episodic orogenital ulceration, skin lesions, erythema nodosum and thrombosis of the iliac veins and the superior sagittal sinus would make Behçet's syndrome the most likely cause for this severe disorder.

She was treated with intravenous megadose steroids, subcutaneous heparin and her visual fields monitored carefully. Her CSF pressure did not settle and the fields became constricted, and so a lumboperitoneal shunt was implanted in order to reduce pressure quickly. Her fields stabilized then slowly enlarged. Her papilloedema resolved.

She is on oral prednisolone and azathioprine and a slow steroid wean is underway, watching to see if or when her systemic disease reactivates.

Papilloedema

The disc swells as a result of axoplasmic stasis; raised pressure prevents the return of axoplasm, so that it collects at the optic nerve head. It takes 1–5 days for this to take place. The first sign of papilloedema is a swelling on the nasal side in a C shape. The temporal side remains clear. Then the swelling spreads to the temporal side and the cup becomes less distinct. As it evolves the cup becomes obscured altogether and there is an obvious swelling of the retinal nerve fiber layer. The disc looks pink and the vessels on the disc surface become obscured.

The presence of papilloedema does not interfere with vision, unless the cause also interferes with optic nerve function. However with sustained and severe raised intracranial pressure optic nerve function fails, due to ischemic complications at the disc itself (references in Case 34); small arcuate defects are seen, and nasal steps, and sometimes nasal scotomata. The presence of a restriction in peripheral field gives an assessment of how severe the pressure is. If the pressure is not dealt with the disc becomes pale – consecutive optic atrophy. An atrophic nerve cannot become swollen (because there is no axon and hence no axoplasm).

Pseudopapilloedema

Frequently discs appear to be swollen when they are not; in hypermetropia the discs are small and therefore crowded and hyperemic, optic disc drusen are common and can even be associated with transient visual obscuration, and some discs are tilted so that one side lies within the retina whilst the other protrudes away from it.

Drusen appear as bumps on the surface of the discs, although they may be buried within it. The disc is elevated, the cup is usually absent and the disc would not be hyperemic, nor would the capillaries be dilated. Drusen can be seen on CT since they are often calcified, and with orbital ultrasound.

Discussion

Behçet's Syndrome

Behçet's syndrome is an uncommon autoinflammatory disease in which oral and genital ulceration occurs, accompanied by skin lesions, arthritis, gastrointestinal involvement and a sight threatening retinal vasculitis and uveitis may arise [1]. It is much more common in Turkey than in any other country, but the prevalence is greater in the so-called Silk Road countries extending on either side of the Mediterranean Sea through the Middle East to Japan [2]. There is a clear association with HLA B51 which in Turkey is present in 70 % of patients *vs* 14 % of controls and in European patients much lower – perhaps 20 %. It confers a greater risk of ulceration, skin, vascular and ocular involvement, but not neurological complications [3].

Ocular involvement occurs in 70 % of patients and if untreated leads inevitably to severe damage. A non-granulomatous anterior and posterior uveitis develops, and retinal vasculitis leads to vessel occlusion and an ischemic, glaucomatous eye with macular scarring [4].

Involvement of the nervous system occurs in 5–10 % of cases. 80 % of cases develop an inflammatory meningoencephalitis, of whom half have brain stem lesions, although all other parts of the nervous system may be affected. A progressive disease course is unusual; the majority have single lesions (since treatment with immunosuppression prevents relapse) whilst a third have a more aggressive relapsing remitting disease requiring high dose immunosuppression and treatment with biological agents [5].

Vascular Involvement in Behçet's Syndrome

Of 5970 patients attending the Behçet's syndrome clinic of the University of Istanbul 882 (14.7 %) had had vascular involvement [6]. Only 10 % were women, and median time after diagnosis was 1.4 years (0–4.9 years). 87 % had lower limb DVT (13 also had concurrent upper limb DVT), 9 % and 8 % had superior and inferior vena cava thrombosis respectively, 2.4 % had Budd Chiari syndrome. 10 % had peripheral arterial thrombosis, 6 % had pulmonary artery thrombosis, and 4 % had venous sinus thrombosis. Around half those with venous sinus thrombosis also had DVT or pulmonary artery thrombosis or both.

Another systematic review of venous sinus thrombosis in Behçet's syndrome [7] showed that around half had superior sagittal sinus thrombosis and a third had transverse and sigmoid sinus thrombosis. A minority had cavernous sinus involvement, cortical vein and jugular vein thrombosis. In general the prognosis is good, unless optic neuropathy or cerebral hemorrhage occurs, and recurrence is uncommon. Patients are treated with steroids and immune suppression; there is an as yet unanswered debate about whether or not anticoagulation is required, since the pathogenesis of the vascular thrombosis is inflammation of the endothelium, and there appears to be no evidence for activation of pro-thrombotic factors such as protein C and S, yet at present I do recommend treatment with anticoagulation as well as immunosuppressive therapy.

References

1. Yazici H, Fresko I, Yurdakul S. Behçet's syndrome: disease manifestations, management and advances in treatment. Nat Clin Pract Rheumatol. 2007;3:148–55.
2. Verity DH, Marr JE, Ohno S, Wallace GR, Stanford MR. Behçet's disease, the Silk Road and HLA-B51: historical and geographical perspectives. Tissue Antigens. 1999;54:213–20.
3. Maldini C, Lavalley MP, Cheminant M, de Menthon M, Mahr A. Relationships of HLA-B51 or B5 genotype with Behçet's disease clinical characteristics: systematic review and meta-analyses of observational studies. Rheumatology (Oxford). 2012;51:887–900.
4. Zierhut M, Abu El-Asrar AM, Bodaghi B, Tugal-Tutkun I. Therapy of ocular Behçet disease. Ocul Immunol Inflamm. 2014;22:64–76.
5. Al-Araji A, Kidd DP. Neuro-Behçet's disease: epidemiology, clinical characteristics and management. Lancet Neurol. 2009;8:192–204.
6. Tascilar K, Melikoglu M, Ugurlu S, Sut N, Caglar E, Yazici H. Vascular involvement in Behçet's syndrome: a retrospective analysis of associations and the time course. Rheumatology (Oxford). 2014;53:2018–22.
7. Aguiar de Sousa D, Mestre T, Ferro JM. Cerebral venous thrombosis in Behçet's disease: a systematic review. J Neurol. 2011;258:719–27.

Part III
The Apex to the Saddle

Case 21

History

This 18 year old lady presented to the ophthalmic department with a slowly progressive horizontal diplopia on looking to the right side. There was a 4 week history of a mild but latterly increasing right periorbital headache. There were no other symptoms and she was otherwise well. She had recently started a university course.

Examination

The central acuities were 6/5 N5, with normal color vision on both sides. Trigeminal sensation was normal. Abduction was limited on the right side on right horizontal gaze. There were no other abnormal neurological signs. The systemic examination was also normal.

D.P. Kidd, *Neuro-Ophthalmology*, DOI 10.1007/978-1-4471-2410-8_21

Clinical Evaluation

This is a healthy young lady with a worrying story; a progressive disorder latterly with pain. There are no other abnormal signs to allow a more clear anatomical localization but the presence of pain would make an anteriorly placed disorder – within the orbit, at the apex or at the cavernous sinus – more likely. A skull base lesion would be associated with a Vth and a VIIth, and a lesion further behind – within the cerebellopontine angle or the brainstem – would be associated with a VIIth and hearing loss and/or ataxia. The differential diagnosis is as noted in Appendix 3. Neoplastic causes and inflammatory lesions would be most likely; imaging is warranted as the first and main investigation.

Investigations

ESR, blood count and biochemical screening were unremarkable.

An MRI scan of the orbits (Fig. 21.1) revealed a lesion adjacent to the cavernous sinus on the right side which enhanced avidly following injection of gadolinium.

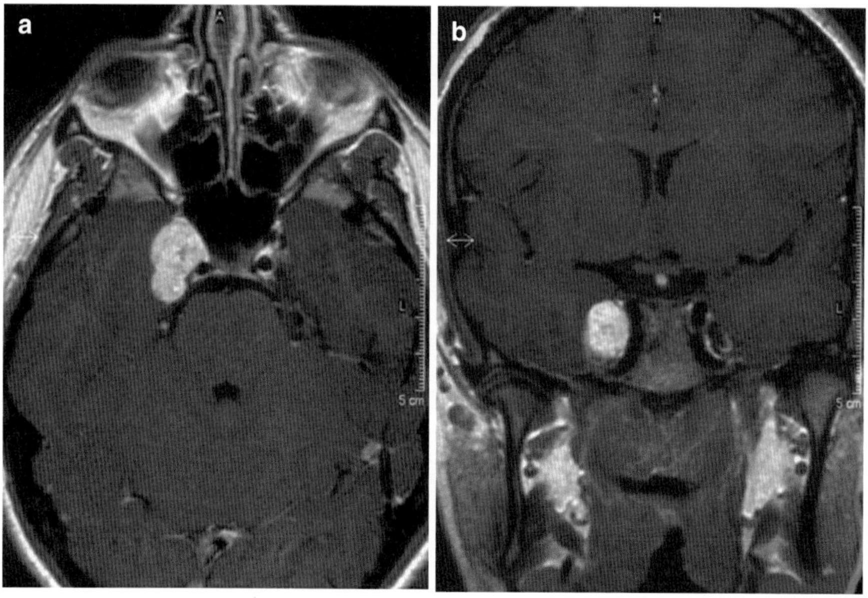

Fig. 21.1 T1 weighted enhanced MRI (**a**) axial and (**b**) coronal images showing a large lesion adjacent to the cavernous sinus on the right side, which is expansile but not associated with meningeal enhancement or "tail"

The radiological differential diagnosis is of neoplastic and inflammatory disorders:

Schwannoma	Sarcoidosis
Meningioma	Idiopathic orbital inflammatory syndrome
Plasmacytoma	Rosai–Dorfman syndrome
Lymphoma	Erdheim–Chester disease
	Mucocoele
	TB

A long discussion was made as to the pros and cons of surgical removal; it was considered easy by the Neurosurgeons, although with a risk of surgical adverse events, whereas radiotherapy on its own was considered inadvisable owing to the wide differential diagnosis and the risks of late effects of radiotherapy, particularly pituitary failure in someone so young. A biopsy was undertaken.

This showed a moderately cellular tumor comprised of interlacing fascicles of spindle shaped cells (Fig. 21.2).

She proceeded to conformal fractionated radiotherapy and received 50Gy in 28 fractions. Her tumor has not grown since although her pituitary function has diminished requiring cortisol support, but her periods are normal.

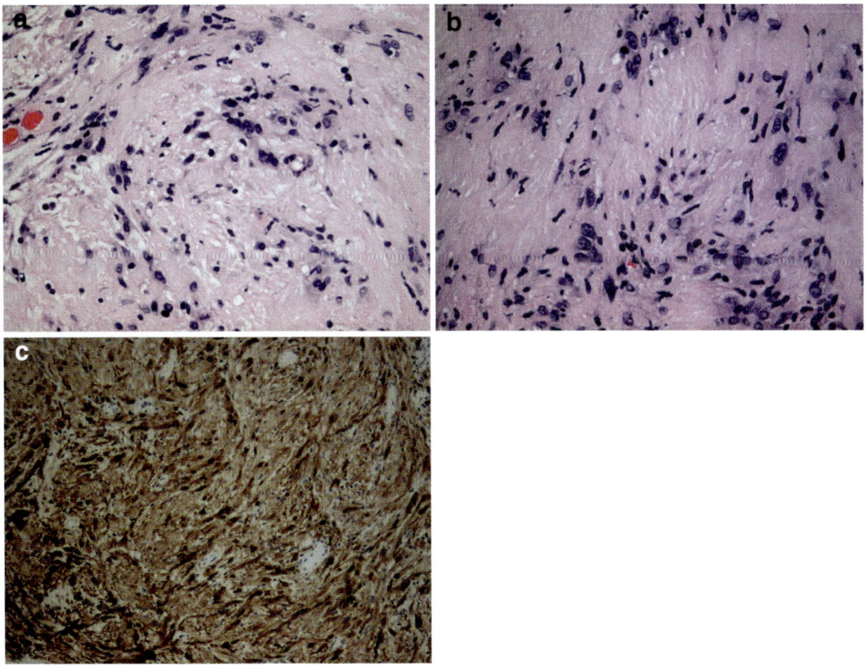

Fig. 21.2 Histology. Moderately cellular tumor composed of interlacing fascicles of spindle shaped cells. Mitotic figures are absent. The appearances are of a benign schwannoma of Antoni B architecture (Pathology images courtesy of Dr Malcolm Galloway, Consultant Neuropathologist, Institute of Neurology and the Royal Free Hospital, London, UK)

Discussion

Schwannomas of the Cranial Nerves

Schwannomas are benign, slow growing tumors which comprise less than 10 % of all intracranial tumors. They arise from the glial-schwann cell myelin border. There is a close association between vestibular schwannoma and neurofibromatosis type 2 (in which the tumor is characteristically bilateral), but other cranial nerves have also been involved.

Non-vestibular schwannomas are rare. Those arising from the Vth and VIIIth nerves are by far and away the most common; schwannomas arise from sensory nerves much more often than motor nerves. Those arising from cranial nerves IX to XII tend to develop at the skull base or foramen magnum, or extracranially [1]. They present with dysfunction of the nerve from which they arise (although some trigeminal schwannomas have presented with lateral rectus paresis), and when anteriorly placed, for example adjacent to the cavernous sinus, headache is a feature. The radiological differential diagnosis is wide since many lesions appear spherical with a uniform pattern of enhancement, including meningioma and aneurysm.

Those arising from the IIIrd, IVth and VIth nerves are exceedingly rare; only 20 cases of abducens schwannoma have been reported to date. They are seen in the cerebellopontine angle and adjacent to the cavernous sinus or orbital apex [2]. Occasionally they arise within the cavernous sinus, and they have also been seen within the orbit.

Early Neurosurgical reports and series suggested a low risk of recurrence and low surgical morbidity, but radiotherapy has superseded surgery as the treatment of choice with "tumor control" achieved in 97 % of one series in vestibular schwannoma [3], and a reduction in size of trigeminal schwannomas in 93 % of another [4]. In one small series of abducens schwannomas arising from the cavernous sinus [5] three were stable without signs of recurrence and one developed an optic neuropathy and worse diplopia as the tumor underwent cystic degeneration.

References

1. Sarma S, Sekhar LN, Schessel DA. Nonvestibular schwannomas of the brain: a seven year experience. Neurosurgery. 2002;50:437–48.
2. Nakamura M, Carvahlo GA, Samii M. Abducens nerve schwannoma: a case report and review of the literature. Surg Neurol. 2002;57:183–8.
3. Boari N, Bailo M, Gagliardi F, Franzin A, Gemma M, del Vecchio A, Bolognesis A, Picozzi P, Mortini P. Gamma knife radiosurgery for vestibular schwannoma: clinical results at long-term follow-up in a series of 379 patients. J Neurosurg. 2014;121(Suppl):123–42.
4. Pan L, Wang EM, Zhang N, Zhou LF, Wang BJ, Dong YF, Dai JZ, Cai PW. Long-term results of Leksell gamma knife surgery for trigeminal schwannomas. J Neurosurg. 2005;102(Suppl):220–4.
5. Hayashi M, Chernov M, Tamura N, Yomo S, Ochia T, Naquai M, Tamura M, Izawa M, Muraqaki Y, Iseki H, Okada Y, Takakura K. Gamma knife surgery for abducens nerve schwannoma: report of four cases. J Neurosurg. 2010;113:136–43.

Case 22

History and Examination

A 68 year old lady with no significant past medical history presented after the abrupt onset of a central visual defect in the right eye. There had been a 3 month history of right periorbital pain which had increased of late. There were no other symptoms and she was otherwise well. She took no regular medications. She was seen in her local ophthalmic emergency department.

Initial examination: the examination findings were of central acuities 6/5 N5 with normal color vision on the left and counting fingers, no color vision and a relative afferent pupillary defect on the right. There was swelling of her right optic disc. The ocular media were clear and the retinae normal. There were no cotton wool spots or intraretinal hemorrhages. There was a centrocecal scotoma on the right side (Fig. 22.1).

Initial management: Imaging was considered to be normal and a diagnosis of giant cell arteritis was made; she was commenced on high dose oral corticosteroids. Neither the orbital pain nor the vision improved over the course of 3 days and she was therefore referred for a neuro-ophthalmology opinion to the Royal Free Hospital.

The examination findings were unchanged and the pain remained severe. There was no limitation of eye movements and no other abnormal neurological signs.

D.P. Kidd, *Neuro-Ophthalmology*, DOI 10.1007/978-1-4471-2410-8_22

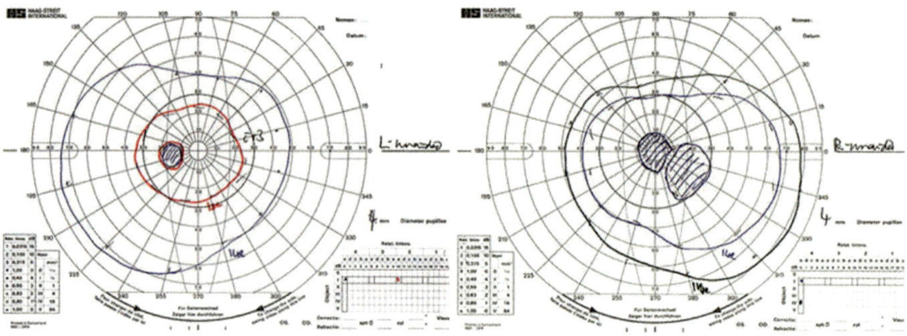

Fig. 22.1 Goldman visual field showing a centrocecal scotoma on the right side

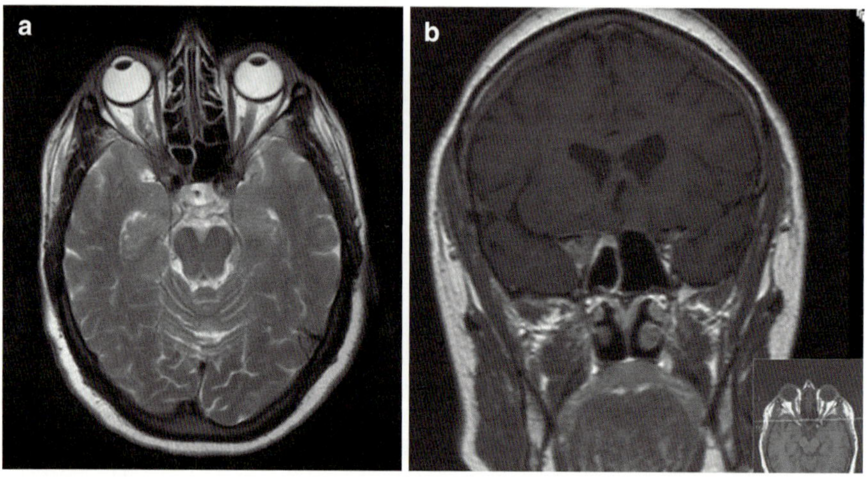

Fig. 22.2 T2 weighted axial (**a**) and T1 weighted enhanced coronal (**b**) MR images of orbits showing a right orbital apex mass which surrounds the optic nerve (Reproduced with permission from O'Toole et al. [1])

Further Investigations

Her ESR was 40, CRP 5. Biochemical screening was normal and serum ACE was not raised. She did not have ANCA, ENA or other auto antibodies.

Imaging was repeated (Fig. 22.2) and revealed an orbital mass surrounding the optic nerve at the apex.

A CSF examination was unremarkable, with four lymphocytes and normal protein and glucose content. There were no malignant cells on cytological examination.

A Chest X-ray was normal and a CT scan of the chest abdomen and pelvis also within normal limits.

A right temporal artery biopsy showed no evidence for vasculitis.

Further Management

Infiltration by metastatic carcinoma, lymphoma or granulomatous disease were considered to be the most likely causes of the clinical syndrome; it was considered essential to obtain a histological diagnosis, and a right orbital decompression was performed through the lateral orbital wall. No solid tumor or inflammatory mass was seen, but pus was aspirated, with fungal hyphi seen on cytopathology (Fig. 22.3), which grew *Aspergillus Fumigatus* at culture.

Her postoperative course was stormy with the development of a fungal meningitis and cerebral infarction, presumably due to arteritis. She was treated with intravenous amphotericin and improved but with no return of vision and a left hemiparesis.

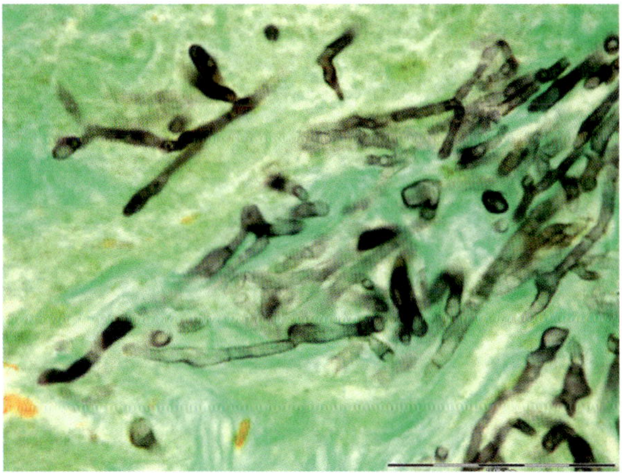

Fig. 22.3 Photomicrograph showing numerous branching septate hyphae (Grocott's methamine silver stain, objective 60) (Reproduced with permission from O'Toole et al. [1])

Discussion

This elderly lady presents with a painful optic neuropathy, and correctly giant cell arteritis was first considered. Imaging although considered normal did in fact show a lesion of the orbital apex which would not be associated with the first diagnosis and further investigations were unhelpful in determining an underlying systemic infective or neoplastic cause. The causes of painful and non-painful orbital apex syndromes are noted in table 1 of Appendix 3. A neoplastic cause (a metastasis from an unknown primary or less likely lymphoma) was considered to be most likely, then an infective disorder, of which bacterial infections including TB would be much more likely than a fungal infection. It was thought that a pathological examination of the tissue was the only way to determine the diagnosis.

Infection of the paranasal air sinuses by fungal pathogens such as Aspergillus is common in immunocompromised patients, in particular those with diabetes, on long-term steroids and those with lymphoreticular disorders and immunodeficiency. Non-invasive aspergillosis remains localized to the sinuses or to the lung, whereas the invasive form is associated with ulceration and tissue destruction, and hematogenous spread. A subacute invasive form may also arise in which angiitis and granulomatous inflammation develops leading to fibrosis.

When the infection spreads from the paranasal air sinuses it leads to an inflammatory orbital apex syndrome with a painful optic neuropathy and ophthalmoparesis [2, 3]. It may also be associated with the development of a chronic hypertrophic pachymeningitis [4].

Open craniotomy is invariably complicated by the development of a fungal meningoencephalitis and cerebral vasculitis [2, 3]. The mortality rate is very high. However, when the orbital lesion is associated with the presence of sinus disease and the tissue sample acquired via an endoscopic approach, the surgical morbidity and mortality is markedly reduced.

In an Indian case series the majority of cases was associated with Aspergillus species [5] whilst in an Australian series around a third were due to Aspergillus, and a third to zygomycetes [6].

Treatment is with intravenous anti-fungal agents, followed by oral itraconazole or variconazole; some cases have responded to oral treatment alone [6].

References

1. O'Toole L, Acheson JA, Kidd D. Orbital apex lesion due to Aspergillosis presenting in immunocompetent patients without apparent sinus disease. J Neurol. 2008;255:1798–801.
2. Hedges TR, Leung LE. Parasellar and orbital apex syndrome caused by aspergillosis. Neurology. 1976;26:117–20.
3. Fernando SSE, Lauer CS. Aspergillus infection of the optic nerve with mycotic arteritis of cerebral vessels. Histopathology. 1982;6:227–34.
4. Ismail AR, Clifford L, Meacock WR. Compressive optic neuropathy in fungal hypertrophic cranial pachymeningitis. Eye. 2007;21:568–9.

5. Pushker N, Meel R, Kashyap S, Bajaj MS, Sen S. Invasive aspergillosis of orbit in immunocompetent patients: treatment and outcome. Ophthalmology. 2011;118:1886–91.
6. Thurtell MJ, Chiu AL, Goold LA, Akdal G, Crompton JL, Ahmed R, Madge SN, Selva D, Francis I, Ghabrial R, Ananda A, Gibson J, Chan R, Thompson EO, Rodriguez M, McCluskey PJ, Halmagyi GM. Neuro-ophthalmology of invasive fungal sinusitis: 14 consecutive patients and a review of the literature. Clin Experiment Ophthalmol. 2013;41:567–76.

Case 23

History

This 74 year old lady presented to the emergency department following an abrupt onset very severe headache with nausea. At the same time she noted horizontal double vision which had worsened over the following 24 hours. The headache was right sided, throbbing and severe. It radiated into the right eye. There was a previous history of common migraine without visual aura, which had affected either side for many years. Generally it had responded well to sumatriptan.

There was a past medical history of hypercholesterolemia, but no symptomatic atheromatous disease and no hypertension. She was a non-smoker.

Examination

The anterior visual pathways and discs were normal. There was a failure of abduction of the right eye. The other eye movements were normal. Levator function was symmetrical. The right pupil was smaller than the left. Trigeminal function was unimpaired. The lower cranial nerves and the remainder of the neurological examination were normal.

D.P. Kidd, *Neuro-Ophthalmology*, DOI 10.1007/978-1-4471-2410-8_23

Evaluation

This lady wakes with a very painful diplopia which does not happen in her regular migraines, and the pain was more severe than average, and sufficient to consider it necessary to present herself to the emergency department. There they considered migraine and a "microvascular" sixth, and, finding no evidence for a stroke, allowed her home with a referral to the neuro-ophthalmology clinic. The examination shows an isolated sixth neuropathy without evidence for trigeminal involvement, although the pain is strongly suggestive of trigeminal involvement. In general the presence of ipsilateral pain suggests an anteriorly placed lesion, although it is hard to define accurately its locality without other abnormal signs. A posteriorly placed lesion, in the brainstem for example, would not be associated with pain and there would be other brain stem or long tract signs.

Anisocoria is common and increasingly common in older patients, in whom 30% have unequal pupils. In this case the right pupil is smaller than the left; it is important to identify which if any is abnormal – is the right abnormally small or the left abnormally large? Examination of the pupils in light and dark (see Appendix 2) may be helpful.

Investigations are warranted; a space occupying lesion, for example a pituitary adenoma with hemorrhage (pituitary "apoplexy"), a meningioma arising from the sphenoid ridge, metastatic disease to the orbit, orbital apex or cavernous sinus, an inflammatory or infective lesion arising from the sinuses and extending into the orbit, a skull base lesion from infection and tumor, infiltration from the posterior nasal space (for example nasopharyngeal carcinoma, lymphoma and secondary tumor) and giant cell arteritis should all be considered in the acute phase.

Investigation

The pupillary assessment was informative; the right pupil was smaller than the left in normal background illumination and the disparity was less in very bright conditions (when an indirect ophthalmoscope was shone on the pupils), and became more distinct in darkness. Although there was no ptosis, the pupillary changes imply involvement of the sympathetic outflow on the right side. She may

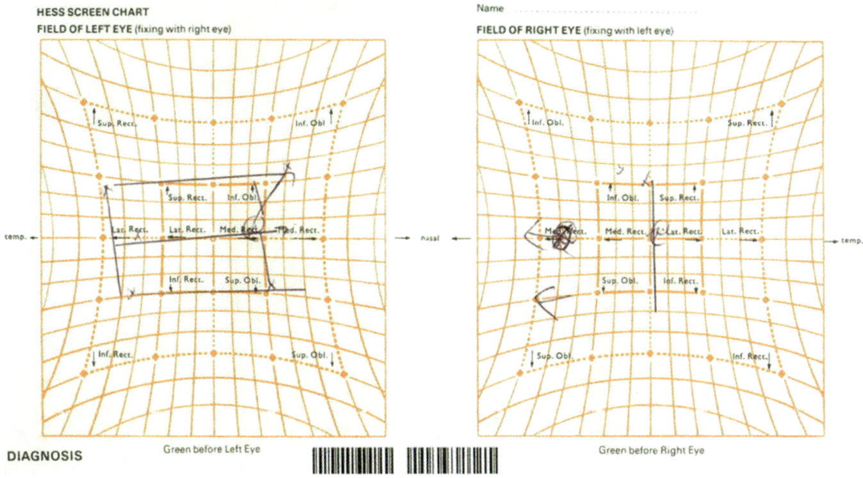

Fig. 23.1 Lees screen test showing failure of abduction of the right eye

therefore have a Horner's syndrome; the coexistence of Horner's syndrome and a sixth neuropathy means that the lesion must lie within the cavernous sinus (see below).

Full blood count and biochemical screening was normal. ESR and CRP were not raised. An orthoptic examination confirmed a right sixth neuropathy (Fig. 23.1). An MRI scan of orbits (Fig. 23.2) showed enlargement of the right cavernous sinus with erosion of the anterior clinoid process on the right. A CT angiogram showed a partially thrombosed aneurysm of the internal carotid artery within the cavernous sinus (Fig. 23.3).

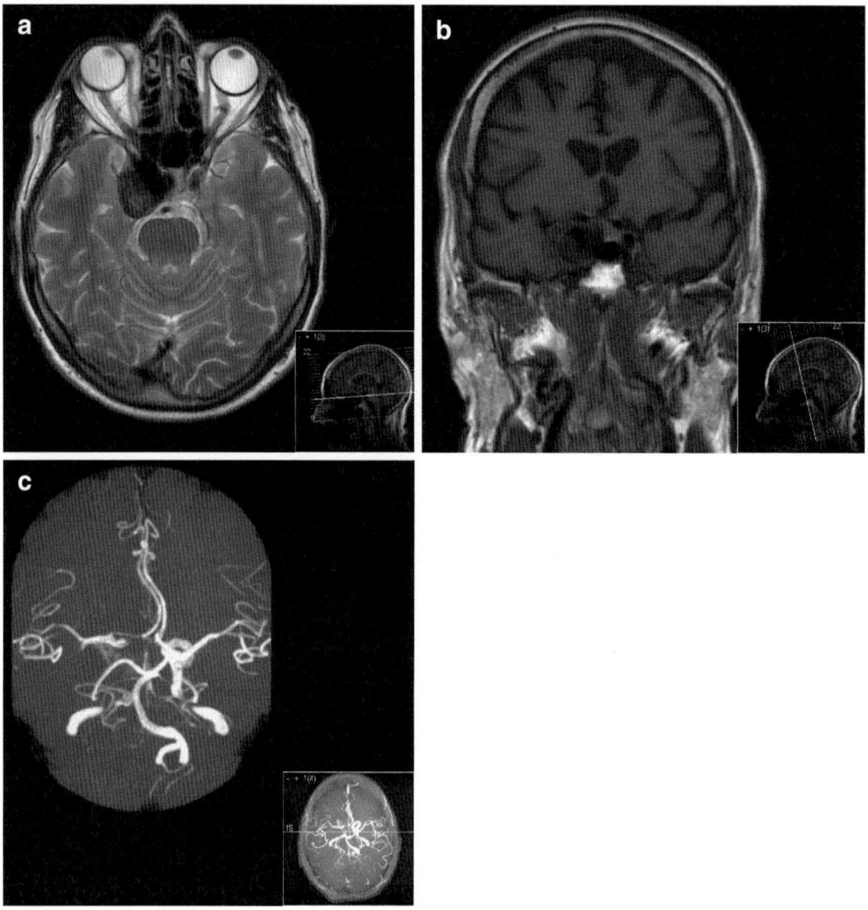

Fig. 23.2 MRI of orbits showing a large mass centered on the right cavernous sinus which obliterates Meckel's cave. The area of abnormality shows reduced signal on the T2 weighted sequences (**a**), with concentric mild T1 shortening in the lateral aspect in keeping with partial thrombosis within a cavernous segment internal carotid artery aneurysm (**b**). The intracranial MRA (**c**) shows some disturbance of signal and likely underscores the true patent lumen of the aneurysm

Management

It was recommended that she be referred to the interventional vascular neuroradiology team in order that a stenting procedure be undertaken. She declined but both imaging and clinical examinations have remained stable.

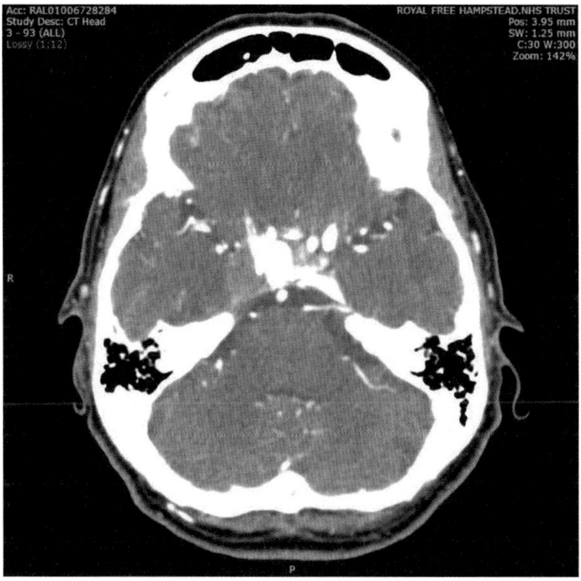

Fig. 23.3 CT of orbits: there is expansion of the right cavernous sinus with moderately hyperdense material, with a degree of the medial extension towards the sella turcica. There is accompanying erosion of the right anterior and posterior clinoid processes, and attenuation of the superior aspect of the petroclival junction. This demonstrates a partially thrombosed large intracavernous aneurysm, measuring 20 mm in maximum dimension in the sagittal plane

Discussion

Intracavernous internal carotid artery aneurysms account for only around 5 % of all intracranial aneurysms and 14 % of those arising from the carotid artery [1]. They are very much more common in women over the age of 50 years than men. They develop within the sinus and grow to occupy its entire space, acquiring a dural extra wall in doing so, with the result that rupture is exceedingly uncommon. They have laminar clot within, which may cause TIAs. The aneurysm may grow so large as to compress the orbital apex, causing optic neuropathy, and erosion into the sphenoid sinus, leading to epistaxis, and even into the pituitary fossa. Intracavernous aneurysms may be bilateral.

The presenting feature is almost always diplopia due to ophthalmoparesis, and a sixth is the most common feature, since the abducens nerve passes through the lateral wall of the sinus (Fig. 23.4) adjacent to the artery. The oculosympathetic pathway passes from the artery to the abducens nerve within the cavernous sinus before moving to the ophthalmic division of the trigeminal nerve and passing into the orbit. The overlying oculomotor and trochlear nerve become compressed at a later stage. Trigeminal involvement occurs early with the presence of pain, which is often episodic and lancinating like trigeminal neuralgia, but objective diminishment of ophthalmic and maxillary division sensation is uncommon and often late.

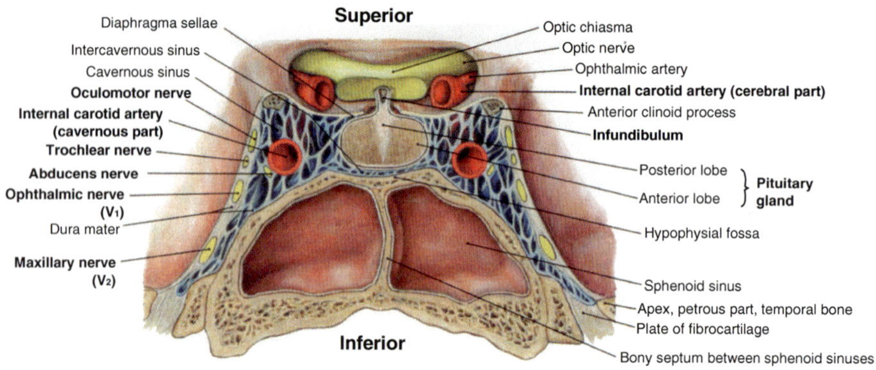

Fig. 23.4 Cross sectional diagram of the cavernous sinus showing its relationship to the IIIrd, IVth, VIth and Vth nerves, and the internal carotid artery (Reproduced with permission from Paulsen and Waschke [4])

Complications

For the reason noted above, the risk of rupture of such aneurysms is small, but if the aneurysm expands outside the limits of the sinus into the subarachnoid space then subarachnoid hemorrhage may arise. Intralobar hemorrhage has also occurred. TIAs may arise though a stenosed artery, and stroke has been reported. When the aneurysm ruptures within the sinus a carotico-cavernous fistula (CCF) develops, venous pressure within the orbit increases, leading to venous engorgement causing conjunctival chemosis, proptosis (which is often pulsating), worsening diplopia and visual loss [2]. The speed of onset depends on the flow; high flow CCFs have an explosive onset, often associated with pulsatile exophthalmos and an audible orbital bruit, and alarming chemosis with "arterialized" conjunctival and episcleral vessels, and low flow fistulas develop sometimes over months.

Treatment

If the clinical features are not progressive and there is no pain it may be safe to observe with interval imaging. Modern endovascular treatments are however increasingly used to treat and on occasion to allow improvement in the clinical features [3] with selective coiling and stent insertions, which are associated with low morbidity [3]. A more old fashioned carotid occlusion may also be performed, after balloon occlusion during angiography allows an assessment of the collateral circulation before it is performed.

References

1. Newman SA. Aneurysms. In: Miller NR, Newman NJ, editors. Walsh and Hoyt's clinical neuro-ophthalmology. 6th ed. Philadelphia: Lippincot Williams and Wilkins; 2005. p. 2188–92.
2. Miller NR. Carotid-cavernous sinus fistulas. In: Miller NR, Newman NJ, editors. Walsh and Hoyt's clinical neuro-ophthalmology. 6th ed. Philadelphia: Lippincot Williams and Wilkins; 2005. p. 2263–83.
3. Penchet G, Mourier K. Collaborative retrospective multicentre series of giant intracavernous carotid aneurysms. Neurochirurgie. 2015;61:366–70; epub Mar 21.
4. Paulsen F, Waschke J. Sobotta Atlas of Human Anatomy, 15th ed. Munich: ©Elsevier GmbH, Urban & Fischer; 2011.

Case 24

History

This 68 year old lady developed double vision on looking up. It worsened very slightly over a 3 month period and she consulted an Ophthalmologist who found no abnormalities, but who referred her to an Orthoptist who did. She was referred in turn to the Neuro-ophthalmology clinic. There had been some discomfort around the left eye for a couple of years which she felt was not painful, just noticeable. There was no numbness and her vision was the same in both eyes.

She took medication for hypertension and was not known to be diabetic. She was otherwise well and continued to work as a receptionist.

Examination

The central acuities and color vision were normal. The pupillary responses were symmetrical. The visual fields were full and the discs normal. Examination of the eyes revealed a right over left hyperphoria in the primary position which increased on upgaze. Downgaze was normal and on the Hess chart (Fig. 24.1) there was a limitation of adduction not seen on cover testing. Examination of facial sensation was normal and the other cranial nerves also unimpaired.

D.P. Kidd, *Neuro-Ophthalmology*, DOI 10.1007/978-1-4471-2410-8_24

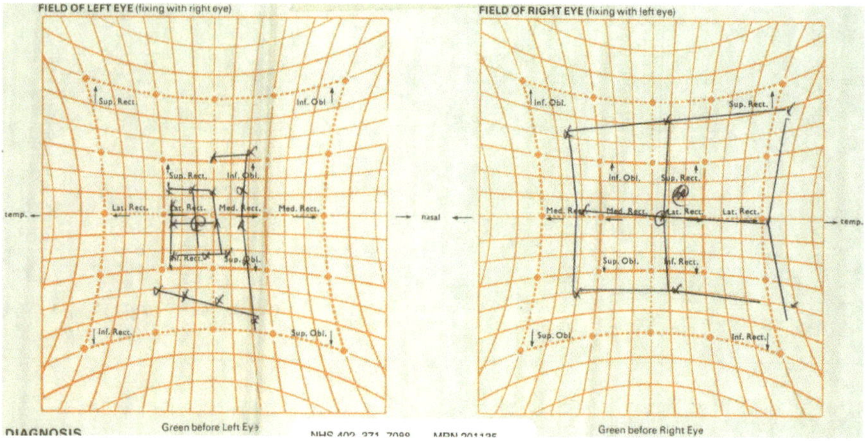

Fig. 24.1 Lees screen test chart showing underaction of elevation and medial rectus on the left side

Evaluation

This lady present with a left sided predominately superior division third neuropathy which is pupil-sparing. The third nerve divides at the orbital apex into superior and inferior divisions, the latter passing into the orbit to innervate the medial and inferior recti and the inferior oblique muscles, the former to the levator palpebrae superioris and superior rectus muscles. Since the clinical features in this lady involves the superior division and the nerve to medial rectus, the lesion must lie anteriorly, near to or at the superior orbital fissure but not within the orbit itself. It must be superiorly placed since there is no evidence for an optic neuropathy.

The differential diagnosis is noted in Appendix 3, and there are no other signs which would help to localize the disorder more closely. Imaging was performed.

Investigations

The MRI scan showed a reasonably large mass centered on the left cavernous sinus which extends medially over the suprasellar cistern just below the optic chiasm and forwards to the orbital apex (Fig. 24.2). Following gadolinium the mass shows uniform enhancement. The intracavernous carotid artery looks attenuated, but is patent.

Management

This is a cavernous sinus meningioma; inflammatory disorders such a sarcoidosis and orbital inflammatory disease, and infections such as tuberculosis and a sphenoid sinus mucocoele would be unlikely at her age and in the context of her being otherwise so well. Indeed, screening blood investigations were normal.

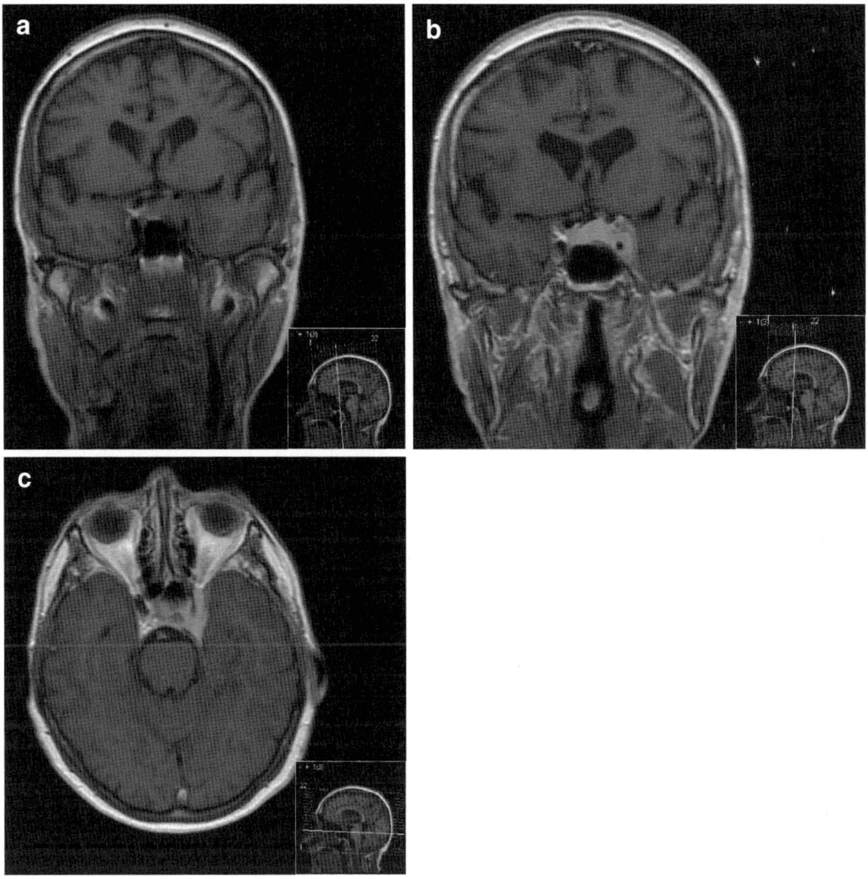

Fig. 24.2 T1 weighted coronal MRI (**a**) before and (**b**) after administration of contrast showing a homogeneous well-circumscribed mass arising from the left cavernous sinus, extending to the suprasellar cistern superiorly and the orbital apex anteriorly. The lesion enhances vividly (**b**, **c**) and is typical of a meningioma

It was recommended that the lesion be observed untreated, that surgery not be performed for fear of damaging the adjacent neurological structures, the carotid artery and the pituitary, and that radiotherapy be undertaken were the lesion to be seen to enlarge.

Over a 4 year follow up period she has remained the same and the meningioma has not enlarged on MRI.

Discussion

Skull Base Meningiomas

Meningiomas account for 20 % of all brain tumors. They arise from cap cells in the arachnoid which line the outer surface of the arachnoid layer of the dura. In one series of 262 cases 46 % arose from the convexity, falx or tentorium and the remainder from the skull base [1]. Meningiomas are twice as common in women as men, and their prevalence increases with advancing age. Most grow between 0.02 and 0.24 cm per year. Because they are so slowly growing they tend not to present until late middle age. Most grow circumferentially; they are firm and indeed often calcified. Some are highly vascular and may bleed spontaneously. Meningioma *en plaque* are much less common than meningioma *en masse*, accounting for less than 10 % of meningiomas, but are common at the sphenoid ridge; here they infiltrate the dura in thin sheets, then pass into the underlying bone. In time they induce a prominent hyperostosis, more prominent than their *en masse* counterparts, leading to a progressive proptosis without other abnormal neurological signs. They cannot be removed, and recurrence rates are high and early [2].

Skull base meningiomas arise from the olfactory groove, the sphenoid ridge, the clivus, the cerebellopontine angle and the foramen magnum (Fig. 24.3). Sphenoid ridge meningiomas may be lateral or middle, and medially placed meningiomas involve the cavernous sinus. All parts of the parasellar region may be involved.

Meningiomas are radiosensitive and there are now numerous series published which demonstrate a response rate of 40 % for tumor shrinkage, but more importantly 75–90 % progression-free survival rates at 10 years when stereotactic radiosurgery is employed [3–5]. Irradiation doses of 12–16 Gy appear to be effective, with a lower incidence of radiation-associated complications (25 % *vs* 60 % for microsurgical excision [6]).

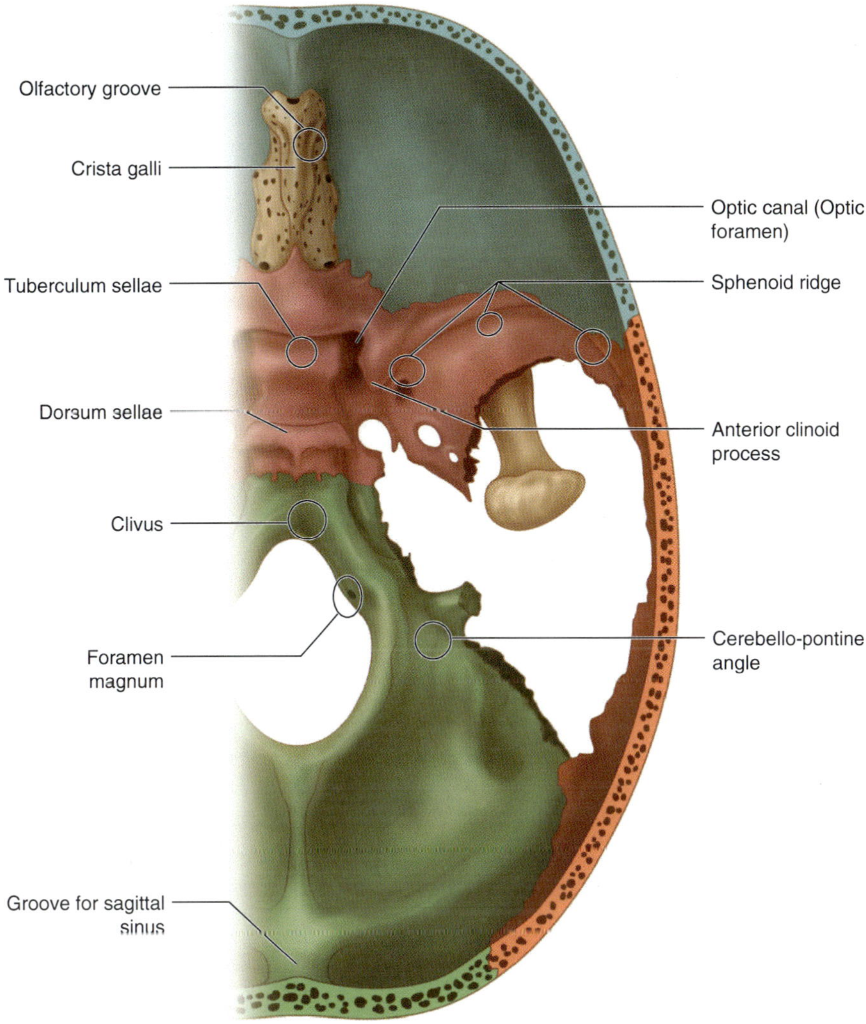

Fig. 24.3 Drawing of the skull base showing the common sites from which meningiomas of the skull base develop (see Table 24.1) (Adapted from Anderson [8]: figure 7–38)

Cavernous Sinus Meningioma

Cavernous sinus meningiomas are uncommon, accounting for only 1 % of intracranial tumors, but are important to Neuro-ophthalmologists as the clinical signs involve exclusively cranial nerves II to VI. They are impossible to remove, and any attempt at a surgical debulking or aggressive resection inevitably causes an increase in neurological impairment. The rate of recurrence is high, albeit 20 years after surgery [3–5].

Meningiomas express somatostatin receptors, and PET tracer studies such as Ga-68-DOTA-TATE show binding and tracer uptake within meningiomas which would not be seen in other tumors, such as metastasis for example [7]. These scans can be used to increase diagnostic certainty through imaging, plan treatment and avoid the risk of acquiring a tissue diagnosis prior to treatment.

Table 24.1 Skull base meningiomas and their neuro-ophthalmic consequences

The olfactory groove	8 %		Anosmia (unilateral then complete)
			Seizures, incontinence, abulia
			Foster Kennedy syndrome: ipsilateral optic atrophy with contralateral papilloedema
			Unilateral optic neuropathy
			Bilateral optic neuropathy with binasal field loss
The sphenoid ridge	16 %	Outer third	Seizures, mass effect, UMN VII
			Proptosis due to hyperostosis
			Temporal hyperostosis
			Diplopia on lateral gaze
			Insidious optic atrophy
		Middle third	Proptosis
			Outer third syndrome
			Inner third syndrome
		Inner third	Superior orbital fissure syndrome
			Cavernous sinus syndrome
			Proptosis (hyperostosis)
			Proptosis (venous congestion)
The parasellar region	12 %		Chiasmal syndrome
			Optic tractopathy
The clivus	Rare		V, VI, VII, VIII
			Hydrocephalus
			Cerebellopontine angle syndrome
The cerebellopontine angle	13 %		Unilateral VII, VI, V ataxia
			Spasticity
			Hydrocephalus
The foramen magnum	3 %		Cough headache
			Tingling on head movement
			Downbeat nystagmus
			Upper cord lesion

Aberrant Regeneration of the Oculomotor Nerve

When the integrity of a nerve is disrupted axons passing through it must regenerate. When they do not follow their previous path axons destined for one muscle may pass instead to another, leading to a disturbance of function. This is known as synkinesis, and is common in facial neuropathy. When the oculomotor nerve is affected for example by an aneurysm or by trauma (including neurosurgery) synkinesis may develop, and when this occurs without a history of an initiating event, care must be taken to look for a cause, since the cause is often an unrecognized cavernous sinus meningioma or aneurysm.

Commonly the lid elevates when the eye moves down or adducts, or a depression of the lid occurs in abduction. Pupillary meiosis may occur when the eye is depressed or adducted.

References

1. Condra KS, Buatti JM, Mendenhall WM, Friedman WA, Marcos Jr RB, Rhoton AL. Benign meningiomas: primary treatment selection affects survival. Int J Radiat Oncol Biol Phys. 1997;39:427–36.
2. Mirone G, Chibbaro S, Schiabello L, Tola S, George B. En plaque sphenoid wing meningiomas: recurrence factors and surgical strategy in a series of 71 patients. Neurosurgery. 2009;65:100–8.
3. Klinger DR, Flores BC, Lewis JJ, Barnett SL. The treatment of cavernous sinus meningiomas: evolution of a modern approach. Neurosurg Focus. 2013;35:E8.
4. Mendenhall WM, Friedman WA, Amdur RJ, Foote KD. Management of benign skull base meningiomas: a review. Skull Base. 2004;14:53–60.
5. Vera E, Iouiescu JB, Raper DMS, Madhavan K, Lally BE, Morcos J, Elhammady S, Sherman J, Komotar RJ. A review of stereotactic radiosurgery practice in the management of skull base meningiomas. Skull Base. 2014;75:152–8.
6. Sughrue ME, Rutkowski MJ, Aranda D, Barani IJ, McDermott MW, Parsa AT. Factors affecting outcome following treatment of patients with cavernous sinus meningiomas: clinical article. J Neurosurg. 2010;113:1087–92.
7. Klingenstein A, Haug AR, Miller C, Hintschich C. Ga-68-DOTA-TATE PET/CT for discrimination of tumors of the optic pathway. Orbit. 2015;34:16–22.
8. Anderson JE. Grant's atlas of anatomy. 7th ed. Baltimore: Williams and Wilkins; 1978.

Case 25

History

This 27 year old lady was 8 weeks postpartum when she developed a painful tooth. She sought the advice of her dentist who recommended that a premolar tooth be removed and this occurred under local anesthetic reportedly uneventfully.

Shortly afterwards she noticed mild respiratory symptoms with cough and some sputum, then fever. A day later she noticed headache, increasing photophobia, then vomiting. She was admitted to her local hospital.

Previously well, she took no regular treatment. The pregnancy and birth had gone well and she was breast feeding normally. The baby had not had any infective illness.

Examination

She was drowsy and photophobic, tachypoeic and distressed. She was febrile: 39.5 °C. There was obvious neck stiffness and Kernig's sign was positive. There were no other neurological signs in the emergency department.

D.P. Kidd, *Neuro-Ophthalmology*, DOI 10.1007/978-1-4471-2410-8_25

Initial Investigations

Her pO_2 was 7.5, CRP 308, WCC raised with a neutrophilia. A chest X Ray showed patchy shadowing.

A CT scan of the brain was considered to be normal and they proceeded to a spinal fluid examination. The pressure was not measured. Investigations: CSF protein was raised at 2.0 g/dl, the CSF white cell count was 140; 90 % monocytes, 10 % neutrophils and the glucose differential 2.0/5.7 mmol/l. CSF gram stain was negative.

She was treated with Ceftriaxone 2 g bd intravenously, and blood and CSF cultures awaited.

Clinical Course

She deteriorated; there was more drowsiness and the signs of meningism increased. She developed double vision. She transferred to the Royal Free Hospital.

Examination at the Royal Free: she was drowsy, febrile and tachypnoeic. She orientated in time and place, but distressed and in pain. There was a right sided proptosis and there was an esotropia due to a lateral rectus weakness on the right side. The central acuities were normal on bedside testing and there was no afferent pupillary defect.

There were no other abnormal neurological signs.

Clinical Evaluation

This young lady presents post-partum with an infective illness characterized first by an upper respiratory tract infection and sore throat then alarmingly with the development of headache, drowsiness and meningism. Clearly this is a bacterial infection and evidently she has developed meningitis. Her initial emergency treatment was prompt and correct. The CSF shows increased white cell count and protein, and a reduced glucose differential; however the white cells are predominately monocytes, and the glucose although reduced is still 2.0 mmol/l, unlike that seen in a bacterial meningitis.

What, then of the development of double vision and proptosis? It is very common to develop cranial neuropathy during acute bacterial meningitis; VIIIth, VIth, IIIrd and IInd are most common, but proptosis suggests an orbital disorder. Abscess should be considered, but the presence of proptosis and an ipsilateral VIth strongly suggests a disorder of the cavernous sinus, and, in the context of an acute infection, cavernous sinus thrombosis. Further and urgent investigations are warranted.

Further Investigations

The CRP remained raised and she required 35% oxygen to maintain reasonable saturations. A CT scan of the chest revealed patchy infiltrations but no mediastinal lymphadenopathy or neoplastic lesion. Serum ACE was normal, and ANA and ANCA were negative.

An MRI scan of the orbits confirmed thrombosis of the right cavernous sinus (Fig. 25.1).

A Gallium-67 scan (Fig. 25.2) showed no evidence for an underlying systemic inflammatory disorder or neoplasia but uptake within the skull base on the right side. The radiologists gave a differential diagnosis of infection, neoplasia including lymphoma, and sarcoidosis.

Blood cultures grew Fusobacterium necrophorum.

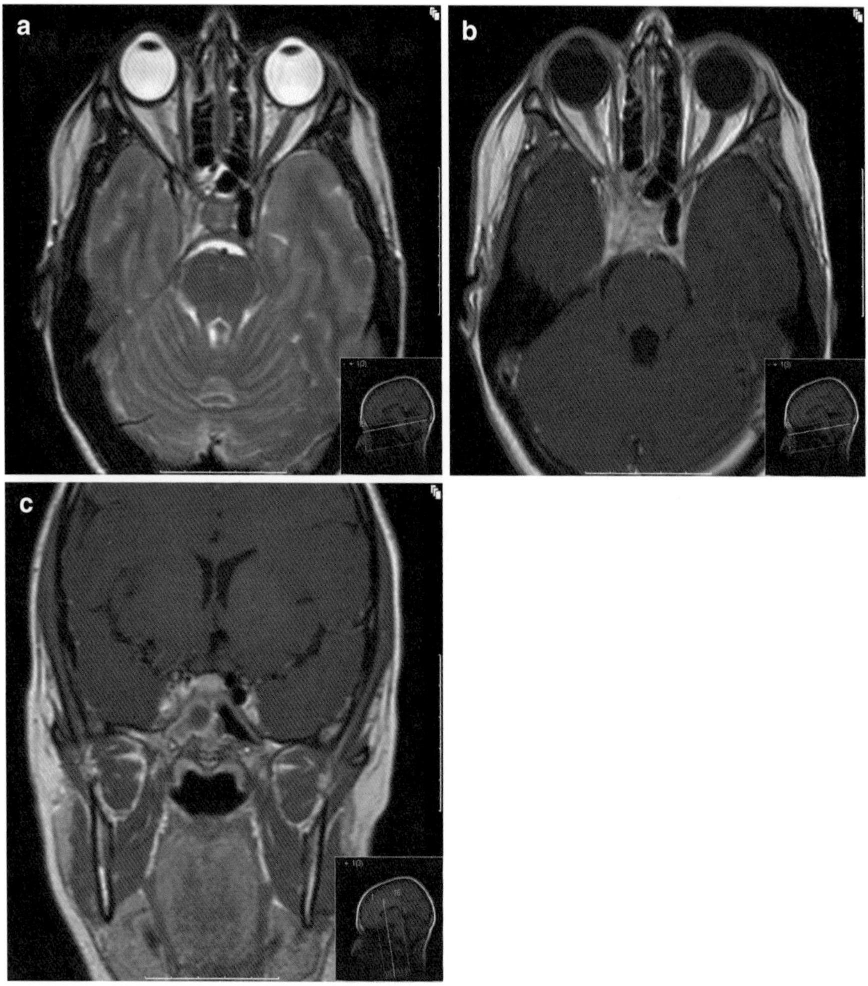

Fig. 25.1 (**a**) Axial T2 weighted MRI scan of orbits showing widening of the cavernous sinus on the right with reduced caliber of the intracavernous right internal carotid artery with high signal in the lumen due to slow "trickle" flow; (**b**) axial and (**c**) coronal T1 weighted MRI following injection of contrast showing the same features, and (**c**) a small signal void corresponding to the superior limb of the vessel, possibly representing retrograde arterial flow in the supraclinoid segment (With thanks to Dr Lloyd Savy, Consultant Neuroradiologist, Royal Free Hospital)

Management

The bacterial infection showed sensitivity to Amoxicillin and doxycycline and she was treated with 1 g tds intravenously of the former and 200 mg od orally of the latter. She received low molecular weight heparin and then oral warfarin. She improved; the headache resolved and the proptosis disappeared although the VIth was slow to recover. Her blood indices normalized.

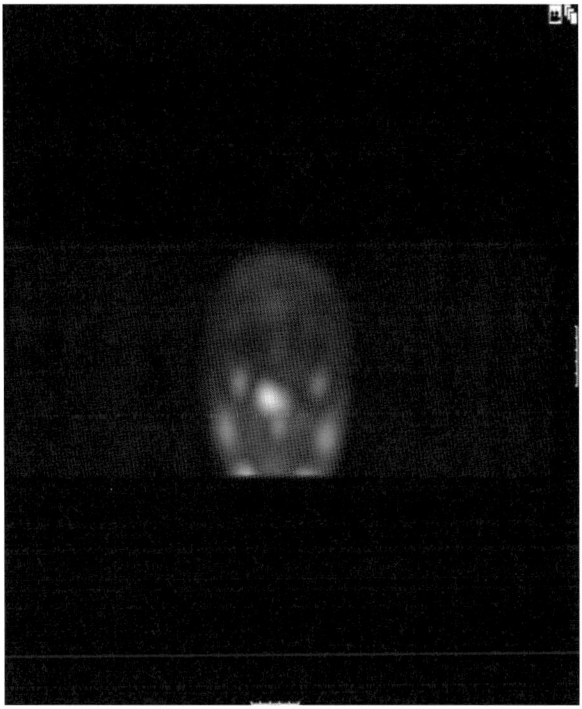

Fig. 25.2 Uptake of Gallium-67 within the lesion on the right side, in keeping with infection

Discussion

Cavernous Sinus Thrombosis

The cavernous sinus drains the orbit of blood, so when it is thrombosed venous pressure rises leading to proptosis, conjunctival chemosis and dilatation of the retinal veins. Pain is very common and ophthalmoparesis progressively worsens; the lateral rectus first and then all the muscles. Optic neuropathy through thrombosis of the posterior ciliary arteries, central retinal artery or ophthalmic artery is also common. Pain occurs in 90 % of cases. Most are caused by infection; aseptic cases are most rare and are seen after trauma including surgery [1].

Typically the septic cases are associated with an infection in the head and neck; sinusitis, dental infection, otitis media, pharyngeal and tonsillar infections, and even skin infections such as furunculosis and erysipelas. Most cases are caused by streptococcus and staphylococcus *sp*. It is clear that the route of infection is a direct one, through the facial vein to the pterygoid plexus and thence to the cavernous sinus.

Imaging shows an expansion of the cavernous sinus, in particular a convexity replacing the normal concavity, and evidence for venous hypertension, in particular a dilatation of the superior ophthalmic vein, and proptosis. In septic cases there is often direct evidence for the infection, including meningeal enhancement [2].

Treatment is with antibacterial therapy, and although mortality has reduced from 80 to 20 %, it remains a grave disease, and many fail to respond to treatment even when the diagnosis and appropriate treatment is stared promptly. Spread to the other eye may occur, and there is a high morbidity in survivors, with diplopia and optic neuropathy.

Lemierre's Syndrome

Lemierre's syndrome is a disorder related to oropharyngeal sepsis in which thrombosis of the internal jugular vein occurs. In the pre-antibiotic era the disorder was common and uniformly fatal [3]. Nowadays the incidence is three per million, but much more common in young adults (the median age is 20 years). Men are affected more often than women. Eighty percent of cases are caused by Fusobacterium necrophorum, an anaerobic Gram-negative bacillus which accounts for less than 1 % of bacteraémias [3].

The disorder begins 1–2 weeks after a sore throat with increasing fever, rigors and constitutional symptoms; anaerobic septicemia occurs, leading to hematogenous septic spread, particularly in the lungs, leading to pulmonary abscess, or empyema. Pulmonary embolism is also common. Septic arthritis and liver abscess has also been seen. One recent case was associated with a frontal lobe abscess [4].

The organism causing the pharyngotonsillitis spreads into the retropharyngeal space, a thrombophlebitis and thrombosis of the peritonsillar veins occurs, which then propagates to the internal jugular vein. The thrombus then continues to propagate, through the petrosal sinuses to the cavernous sinus itself.

In Kuppalli's review 22 cases with neurological involvement were identified; of these 10 were associated with cavernous sinus thrombosis, 5 with venous sinus thrombosis, 6 with cerebral infarction and 8 with cerebral abscess, bacterial encephalitis or subdural empyema [4]. They also note that those not associated with Lemierre's syndrome are also associated with cerebral complications, including abscess and venous sinus thrombosis, and also a carotid arteritis leading to cerebral infarction. These were associated with suppurative middle ear disease rather than pharyngotonsillitis.

Metronidazole and Ceftriaxone are the treatments of choice, and anti-microbial resistance is said to be rare. Anticoagulation is not recommended [4].

References

1. Desa V, Green R. Cavernous sinus thrombosis: current therapy. J Oral Maxillofac Surg. 2012;70:2085–91.
2. Olson KR, Freitag SK, Johnson JM, Branda JA. Case records of the Massachusetts General Hospital: case 36–2014. An 18 year old woman with fever, pharyngitis and double vision. N Engl J Med. 2014;371:2018–27.
3. Riordan T. Human infection with Fusobacterium necrophorum (necrobacillosis), with a focus on Lemierre's syndrome. Clin Microbiol Rev. 2007;20:622–59.
4. Kuppalli K, Livorsi D, Talati NJ, Osborn M. Lemierre's syndrome due to Fusobacterium necrophorum. Lancet Infect Dis. 2012;12:808–15.

Case 26

History

This lady was 40 when she presented with a mild visual blurring. There had been headaches for some time, which were sharp and stabbing, in the temporal regions on both sides, with a more mild background throbbing which followed. These occurred most weeks and lasted for a day or two before resolving. There had been no previous history of headaches, for example in adolescence.

Previously well, there were no other symptoms. She was assessed in her local ophthalmic department, imaging arranged and then referred to the Royal Free Hospital.

Examination

The central visual acuities were 6/9, N6 in both eyes. The color vision was normal. The pupillary responses were symmetrical. The visual fields (Fig. 26.1) showed a bilateral upper quadrantinopia which was symmetrical. The ocular media were clear and the discs were symmetrically pale in the temporal regions. There were no other abnormal neurological signs.

D.P. Kidd, *Neuro-Ophthalmology*, DOI 10.1007/978-1-4471-2410-8_26

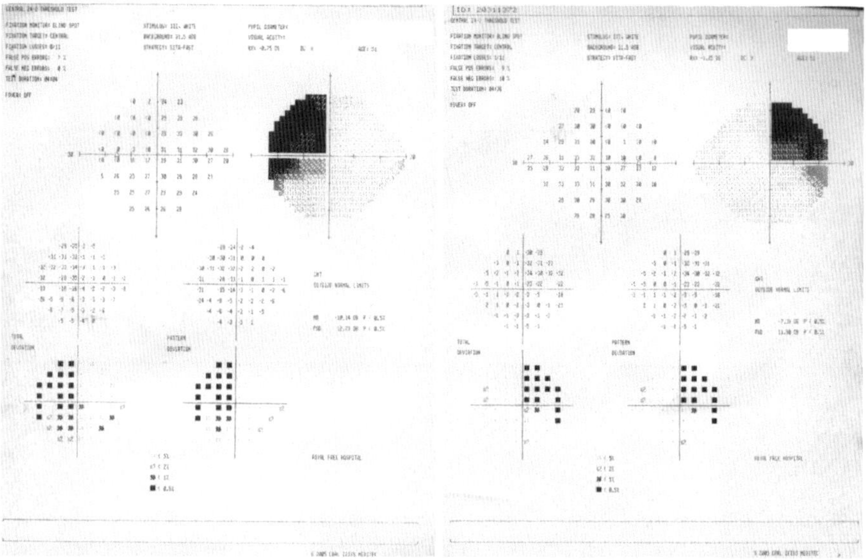

Fig. 26.1 Humphrey visual fields at presentation

Evaluation

There is no clear evidence for an optic neuropathy in that the color vision and pupillary responses are symmetrical. However there is evidence for a disorder of the optic chiasm in that there is a bilateral field defect which is bitemporal in distribution. A disorder of the pituitary fossa is likely, ascending from below and in doing so causing the upper fields to be lost before the lower (see Appendix 1). An MRI scan would be the first correct investigation.

Investigation

The MRI scan (Fig. 26.2) showed a cyst arising from the pituitary fossa ascending to and compressing the optic chiasm in the midline. There is no abnormal enhancement and no mass within or adjacent to the lesion, but there is enhancement of the cyst wall.

Screening blood investigations were normal. Pituitary tests showed a normal prolactin and cortisol, and normal FSH, LH, IGF-1 and thyroid function.

Management

The MRI appearances are typical of a Rathke's cleft cyst. Since she was symptomatic and in particular since there was a visual field defect she underwent a trans-sphenoidal aspiration of the cyst and her vision improved incompletely. The cyst was monitored carefully and recurred 3 years later, requiring a second procedure. Her fields deteriorated slightly (Fig. 26.3) and have not substantially improved.

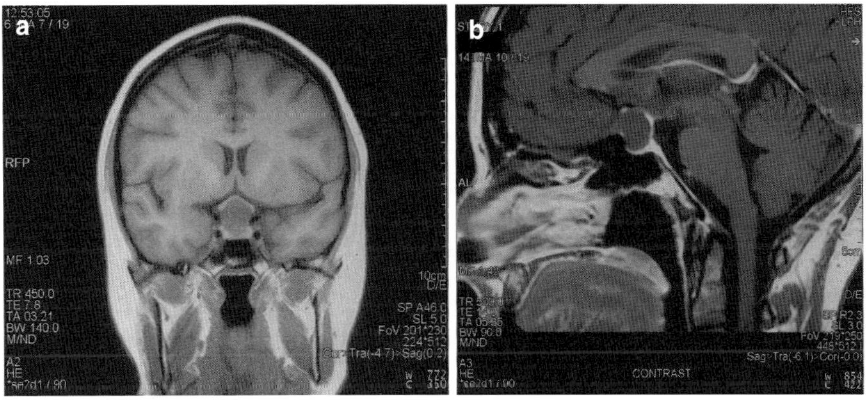

Fig. 26.2 (**a**) T1 weighted coronal MRI scan showing a cyst arising from the pituitary fossa and extending upwards to elevate the chiasm in the midline; (**b**) T1 weighted sagittal MRI following administration of contrast showing uptake of contrast agent within the wall of the cyst but not within

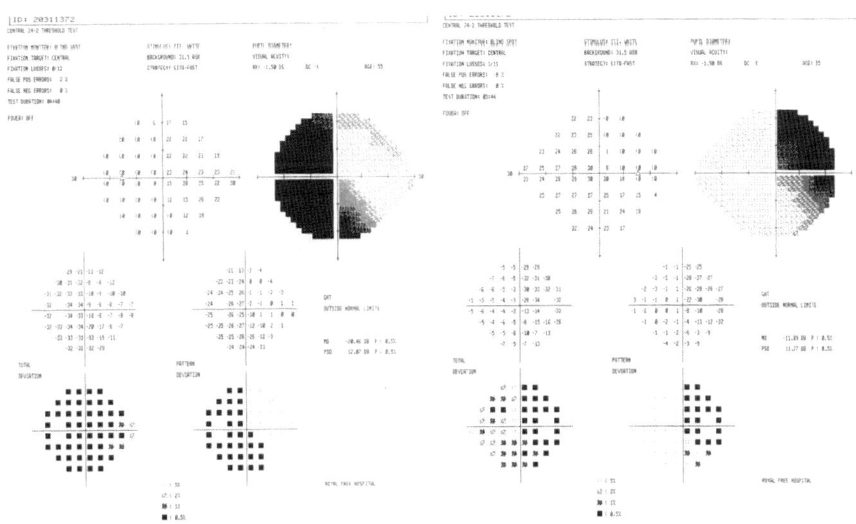

Fig. 26.3 Humphrey visual fields after the second surgery

Discussion

The Embryological Development of the Pituitary Gland

Cells within the oral ectoderm proliferate and form a pouch, the hypophyseal placode, which invaginates then separates from the oral ectoderm and migrates upwards as Rathke's pouch through the craniopharyngeal canal until it comes into contact with the ventral diencephalon (Fig. 26.4 [1] and [2]). Cells within the anterior wall of Rathke's pouch differentiate to form the adenohypophysis whilst those within the posterior wall form the pars intermedia (Fig. 26.4 [3]). The neurohypophysis arises from the ventral diencephalon which also forms the hypothalamus, the third ventricle and the optic chiasm. The cleft which separates the adenohypophysis from the neurohypophysis is Rathke's cleft.

It is assumed that the various cystic structures which may develop in this area all share the same basic pathogenesis; cells originating in Rathke's pouch persist and retain the ability to develop epithelial structures. So Rathke's cleft cysts, dermoid

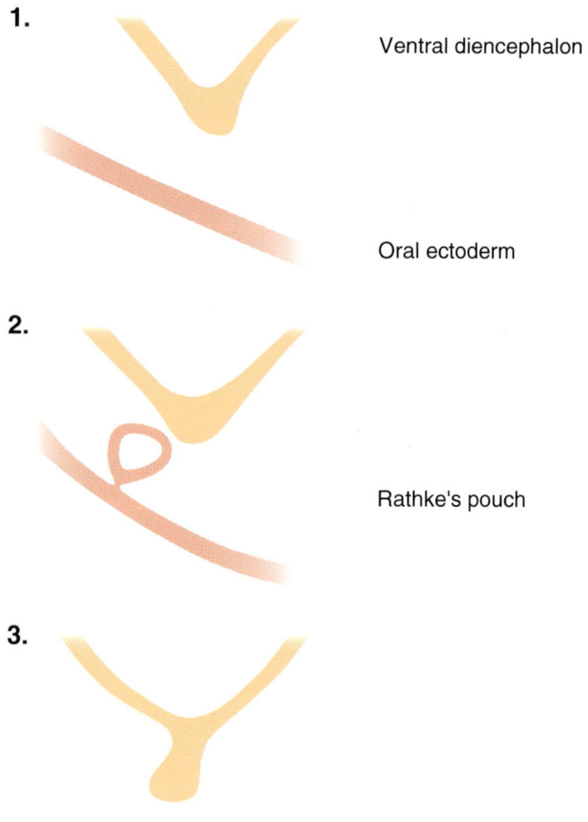

Fig. 26.4 Embryology of the pituitary gland and hypothalamus

and epidermoid cysts, and papillary and adamantinomatous craniopharyngiomas all have the same origin. Lesions which share histological appearances of more than one of these lesions are often seen.

Rathke's Cleft Cysts

Rathke's cleft cysts are more common in women and the mean age at presentation is 30–50 years. They present uncommonly in childhood, and therefore develop slowly over decades. The cyst has a thin wall and is filled with thick, gelatinous material. The wall is composed of cuboidal or columnar epithelium, cilia and mucous secreting cells, and squamous metaplasia is common. The cystic fluid contains cholesterol and protein.

Headache is the most common presenting symptom, in 40 % of cases; it does not correlate with cyst size or location [2], although is more common when there is MRI evidence for more dense fluid (hyperintensity on T1 weighted imaging).

Visual field defects obviously do correlate with the size and location of the cyst [3]. Endocrine dysfunction may occur and is said to result most often from hyperprolactinemia [1]. Diabetes insipidus is uncommon.

Occasionally cysts rupture and induce a chemical meningitis rather like pituitary apoplexy.

When small they are seen as intrasellar cystic lesions which displace the pituitary. As they enlarge they fill the pituitary fossa and assume a dumbbell shape, as in this case. When identified as a pituitary "incidentaloma" they should be observed if asymptomatic; one study showed that only 30 % of 61 enlarged [4]. The treatment for those which are causing field defects is surgical; there is a high rate (25 %) of post-operative CSF leak, but recurrence is uncommon (18 % in [4]). Intrasellar lesions may be approached trans-sphenoidally whereas suprasellar lesions must be operated on through a frontal craniotomy.

Craniopharyngioma

As noted above these lesions too are derived from embryological remnants of Rathke's pouch. Unlike RCC they possess mitotic activity and are more likely to provoke neurological impairments. There is a bimodal prevalence; the childhood form presents at a median age of 8, and the adult form over the age of 50 years.

The childhood form is an adamantinoma with cyst formation and is associated with a mutation in the beta-catenin gene, which is not present in the adult form, whose histological appearances are those of a papillary squamous tumor.

Children present with hypothalamic disturbances, including growth delay and obesity. Both patient groups present with headache and visual field defects. Most are suprasellar in site; an intrasellar cyst is less common. Treatment is surgical and because recurrence rate is high, post-operative radiotherapy is given at diagnosis. A high dose (54 Gy) is required to control disease. Gamma knife and proton beam therapy is also increasingly used. Radiotherapy-associated pituitary failure, vascular disease and neurological deficits are important considerations, particularly in children receiving treatment.

References

1. Larkin S, Karavitaki N, Ansorge O. Rathke's cleft cyst. Handb Clin Neurol. 2014;124:255–69.
2. Nihsioka H, Haraoka J, Izawa H, Ikeda Y. Headaches associated with Rathke's cleft cyst. Headache. 2006;46:1580–6.
3. Nishioka H, Haraoka J, Izawa H, Ikeda Y. Magnetic resonance imaging, clinical manifestations and management of Rathke's cleft cyst. Clin Endocrinol (Oxf). 2006;64:184–8.
4. Aho CJ, Liu C, Zelamn V, Couldwell WT, Weiss MH. Surgical outcomes in 118 patients with Rathke's cleft cysts. J Neurosurg. 2005;102:189–93.
5. Muller HL. Craniopharyngioma. Handb Clin Neurol. 2014;124:135–253.

Case 27

History and Examination

This 44 year old lady was referred to her local ophthalmic department having noticed that her vision in the right eye appeared to be more dull than that in the left. The examination showed normal central acuities and a constricted right field (Fig. 27.1). There was thought to be a relative afferent pupillary defect. The right optic disc was seen to be uniformly pale.

Imaging was performed promptly (Fig. 27.2) and she was referred directly to the Neurosurgeons at the Royal Free Hospital. The nature of the lesion was uncertain, but it was thought likely to be a craniopharyngioma. Screening blood investigations including pituitary hormone levels were normal.

She underwent an extended endoscopic trans-sphenoidal debulking of the lesion. At surgery the lesion was found to be adherent to the right optic nerve and chiasm and was dissected away as much as possible (Fig. 27.3).

There were post-operative problems with hydrocephalus and a parietal hemorrhage following insertion of an external ventricular drain. She was left with no vision in the right eye and a left hemianopia.

D.P. Kidd, *Neuro-Ophthalmology*, DOI 10.1007/978-1-4471-2410-8_27

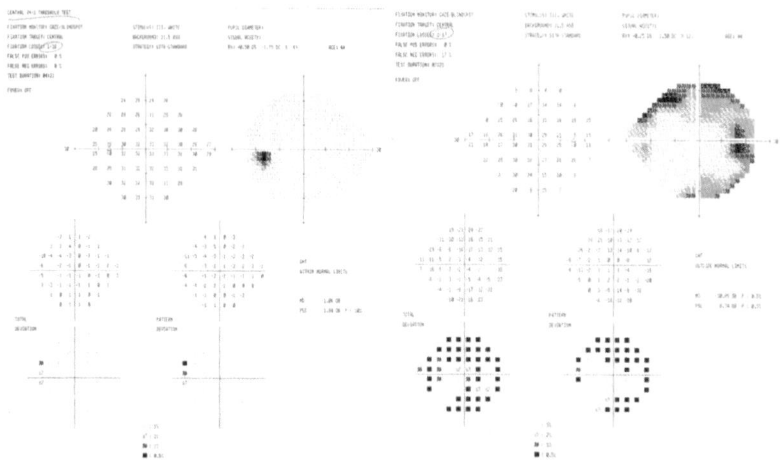

Fig. 27.1 Humphrey visual field showing a right sided constriction

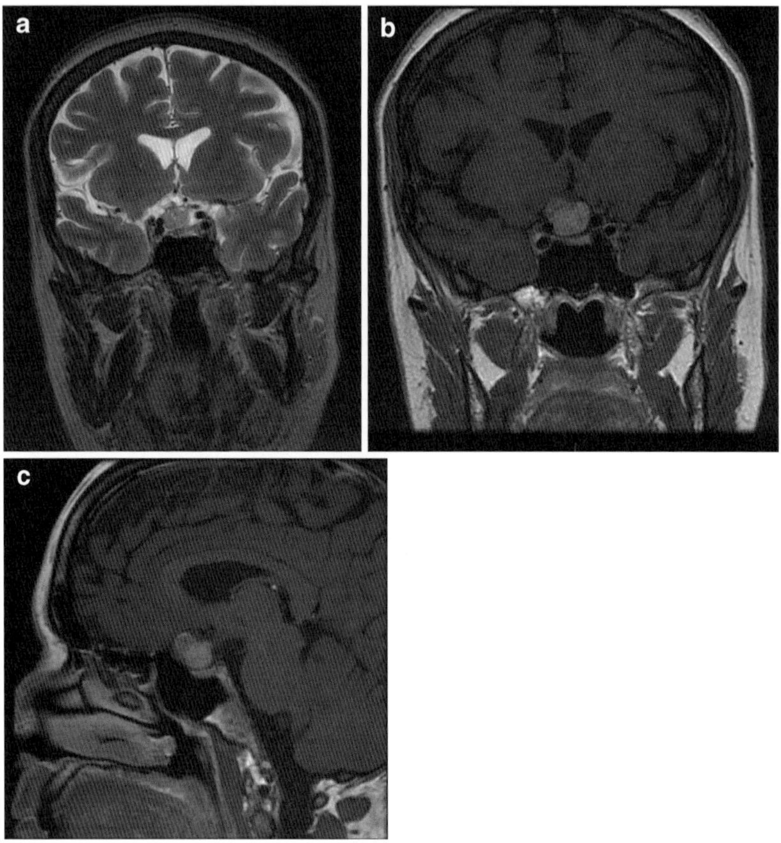

Fig. 27.2 MRI: (**a**) T2 weighted and (**b**) T1 weighted contrast enhanced coronal scans showing a large lesion which is separate from the anterior pituitary and displaces the stalk to the left. The pituitary fossa is not enlarged (**c**). It appears to be arising from the right optic nerve. The lesion exhibits uniform enhancement with Gadolinium

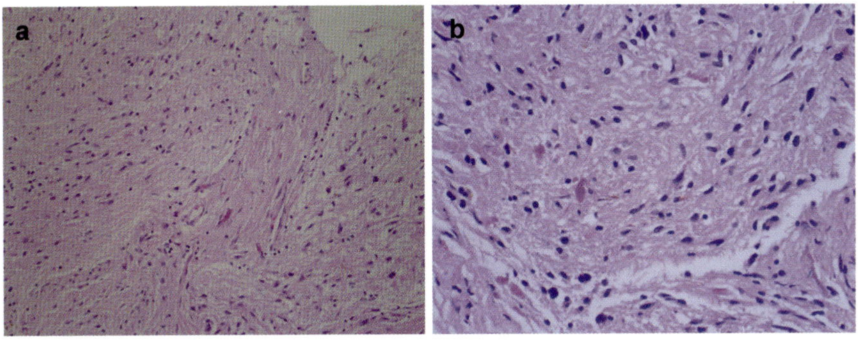

Fig. 27.3 (**a**) Hematoxylin and eosin stained section showing an astrocytic tumor containing Rosenthal fibers. The bipolar morphology of many of the tumor cells is seen, with thin hair like process emanating from opposite ends of the cells. (**b**): In this higher power image the presence of Rosenthal fibers is highlighted. In this area of the tumor the cells are set more haphazardly within a fibrillary stroma. These are the features of a pilocytic astrocytoma, WHO grade I (Pathology images courtesy of Dr Malcolm Galloway, Consultant Neuropathologist, Institute of Neurology and the Royal Free Hospital, London, UK)

Discussion

Pilocytic Astrocytoma

Pilocytic astrocytomas are more common in children. They may arise in all parts of the brain; in one series of 100 patients 76 were younger than 18 and none of the adults was older than 45 [1]; 26 were found in the brain stem, 23 in the cerebellum, 22 in the chiasm and 22 in the hemisphere of whom 12 were situated within the thalamus. Most show a cyst on MRI with an enhancing mural nodule. This enhancement confers concern that the lesion is more aggressive i.e., malignant than it actually is. However the same series showed that in no case in which the enhancement pattern or the presence of central necrosis implied an aggressive histological feature was there evidence for anaplasia on histological analysis of the biopsy carried out [1].

This is particularly important in the case of astrocytomas of the chiasm which present in adulthood; with increasing age the likelihood of the lesion being a highly aggressive glioblastoma multiforme also increases. Such cases are exceedingly rare; the author has seen only one. These patients present with a rapidly progressive unilateral or bilateral visual loss without proptosis, and often with pain. The histological features are of an anaplastic glioblastoma, very different to the benign pathology of the pilocytic astrocytoma seen in childhood gliomas associated with or independent from neurofibromatosis-1 (see Case 16) [2, 3]. Patients with malignant glioma of the optic nerve or chiasm do not respond to radiotherapy or chemotherapy and invariably die within 2 years of symptom onset [4, 5].

The treatment of less aggressive astrocytomas of the anterior visual pathway should not involve surgery; inevitably there is loss of vision in the affected eye, and surgical morbidity may be even greater, as unfortunately in this case. The diagnosis should be made reliably without recourse to biopsy. Chemotherapy using vincristine and carboplatin is associated with a progression-free response of some 75 % [5]. Temozolamide is also used. Radiotherapy is used for chemotherapy-unresponsive or recurrent disease [5].

In malignant glioma radiotherapy and chemotherapy have shown a palliative effect in prolonging but not influencing survival [4].

References

1. Kumar AJ, Leeds NE, Kumar VA, Fuller GN, Lang FF, Milas Z, Weinberg JS, Ater JL, Sawaya R. Magnetic resonance imaging features of pilocytic astrocytoma of the brain mimicking high-grade gliomas. J Comput Assist Tomogr. 2010;34:601–11.
2. Pecen PE, Bhatti MT. Clinical reasoning: a 61 year old woman with a swollen optic nerve and progressive visual loss. Neurology. 2014;82:e205–9.
3. Nagaishi M, Sugiura Y, Takano I, Tanaka Y, Suzuki K, Yokoo H, Hyodo A. Clinicopathological and molecular features of malignant optic pathway glioma in an adult. J Clin Neurosci. 2015;22:207–9.
4. Wabbels B, Demmler A, Seitz J, Woenckhaus M, Bloss HG, Lorenz B. Unilateral adult malignant optic nerve glioma. Graefes Arch Clin Ophthalmol. 2004;242:741–8.
5. Shapey J, Danesh-Meyer HV, Kaye AH. Diagnosis and management of optic nerve glioma. J Clin Neurosci. 2011;18:1585–91.

Case 28

History

This 45 year old lady presented with a 9 month history of increasing thirst and polyuria. She attended her GP who arranged blood investigations. These showed a normal sugar but a high sodium. Further investigations including the finding of a high serum osmolality and a low urine osmolality led to the diagnosis of diabetes insipidus.

There were occasional headaches but no visual symptoms.

An MRI was performed and she was referred to the pituitary clinic.

Examination

There were no abnormal neuro-ophthalmic signs; the fields were full and the anterior visual pathways normal. The endocrine examination was normal.

D.P. Kidd, *Neuro-Ophthalmology*, DOI 10.1007/978-1-4471-2410-8_28

Investigations

On desmopressin 10 μg her urea and electrolytes and urine and serum osmolalities were normal. Thyroid function, LH, FSH and cortisol were normal. The prolactin was raised at 968 mIU/l. IGF-1 was normal at 19 nmol/l. Serum ACE, αFP and βHCG were all normal.

The MRI showed an enhancing lesion of the pituitary and its stalk (Fig. 28.1).

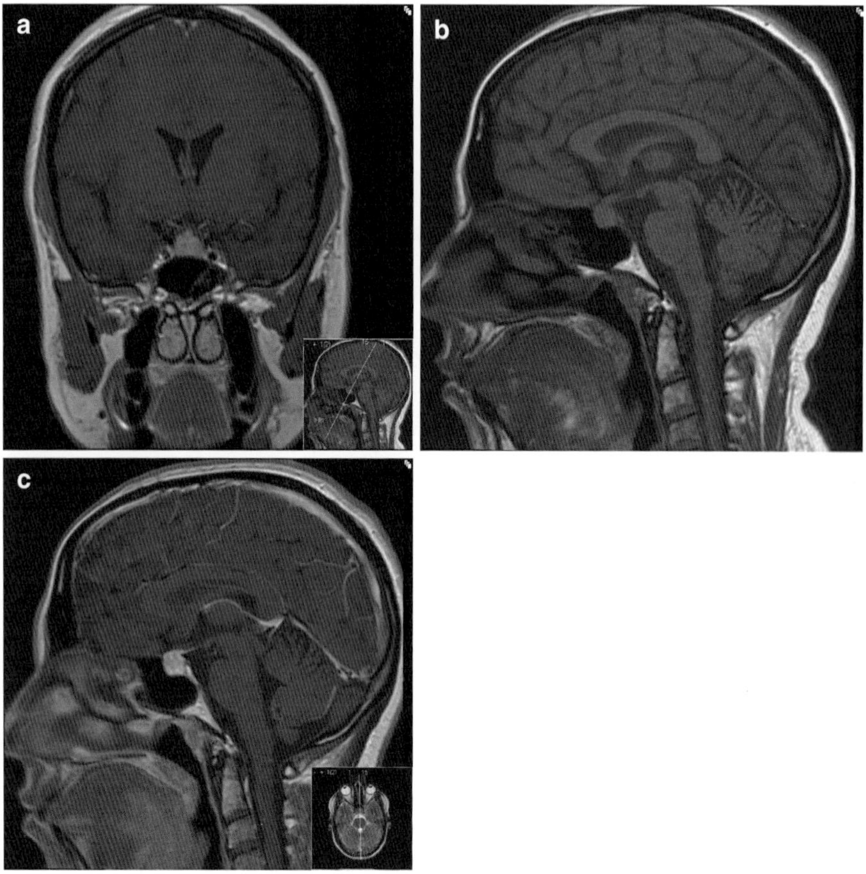

Fig. 28.1 T1 weighted coronal and sagittal MRI (**a**, **b**) showing a mass arising from the pituitary fossa which uniformly enhances following administration of contrast (**c**) and which rises to but does not compress the chiasm. Notice that the normal brightness of the posterior pituitary is absent. The anterior aspect of the pituitary stalk is enlarged and also enhances

Evaluation

This lady presents with symptoms of insufficiency of the posterior pituitary and endocrine investigations led to the diagnosis of diabetes insipidus. There were headaches but no other neurological symptoms; nonetheless imaging of the pituitary was warranted and led to the discovery of the causative mass within the pituitary fossa. Endocrine investigations show that the prolactin is modestly raised but not as high were the lesion to be a prolactin secreting microadenoma. In any case such lesions would not present in this way (since 90 % of vasopressin is synthesized in the hypothalamus). Rathke's cleft cyst, chordoma and meningioma would also be unlikely for the same reason. Choristomas such as dermoid and epidermoid cysts would show differing imaging characteristics and germ cell tumors are unlikely with normal αFP and βHCG. Craniopharyngioma, a benign tumor arising from Rathke's pouch remnants, and more common in children and the elderly with a bimodal peak of prevalence, may be associated with diabetes insipidus at onset (in 33 % of one large series [1]), but almost all also have signs of anterior pituitary dysfunction at the same time. Inflammatory processes and infection may present thus, however.

She underwent a trans-sphenoidal pituitary biopsy.

The histological appearances were of a lymphocytic infiltration within the pituitary tissue (Fig. 28.2).

Table 28.1 Causes of diabetes insipidus [2]

Neoplastic	Craniopharyngioma Germinoma Pituitary adenoma/surgical removal of Pinealoma Infiltration by leukemia and lymphoma
Head injury	
Infection	Toxoplasma CMV Tuberculosis Listeria
Inflammations	Erdheim Chester disease Granulomatous hypophysitis Lymphocytic hypophysitis IgG4 disease
Idiopathic	
Inherited	
Nephrogenic	

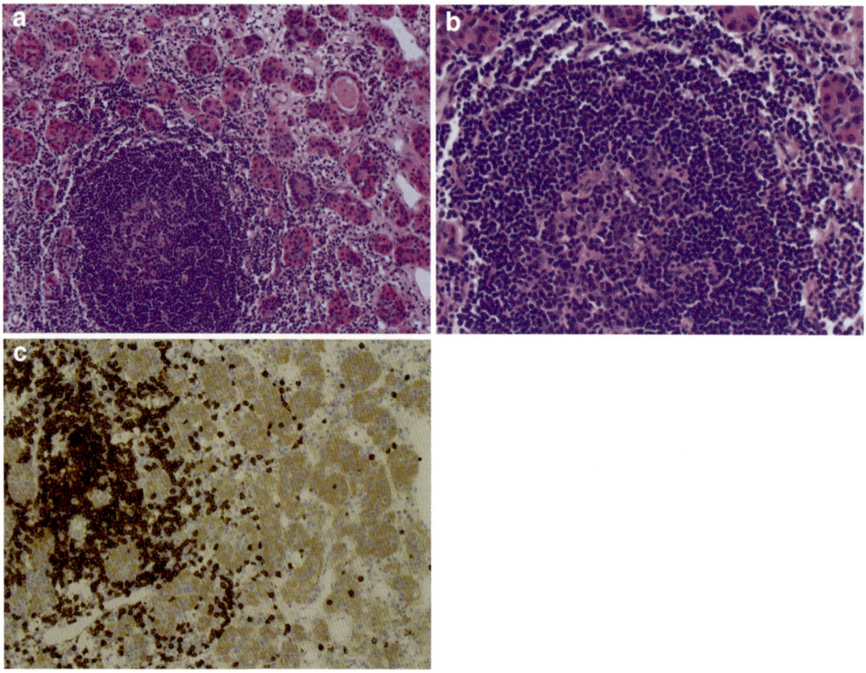

Fig. 28.2 Hematoxylin and eosin stained sections (**a** ×20, **b** ×40) showing a prominent aggregate of lymphocytes within the adenohypophysis. Lymphocytes are also present between the surviving nests of endocrine cells. The stroma is fibrotic. CD3 immunostain shows that there is a T lymphocytic infiltration (**c**). The features are those of lymphocytic hypophysitis (Pathology images courtesy of Dr Malcolm Galloway, Consultant Neuropathologist, Institute of Neurology and the Royal Free Hospital, London, UK)

Discussion

Lymphocytic hypophysitis is a most uncommon condition, thought to have an incidence of 1 per 9×10^6 per year [3]. It is more common in women and indeed shows a striking relationship to the third trimester of pregnancy and the post-partum period. It may affect the anterior pituitary alone, the posterior pituitary or both (lymphocytic panhypophysitis (LPH)). The condition accounts for less than 1 % of all pituitary surgeries [3].

Fifty percent of patients have another auto-immune disease, particularly Hashimoto's thyroiditis (Graves' disease is less commonly associated). It is thought that the early immune activation is against specific cell types, particularly ACTH and TSH, before the inflammatory response spreads to involve the whole pituitary.

The presenting features may be acute or subacute, as in this case, or chronic, when a progressive selective (particularly ACTH deficiency) or panhypopituitarism develops with fibrosis and an empty sella. In the acute form spread of inflammatory tissue to the adjacent cavernous sinus or floor of the middle cranial fossa may simulate a progressive pachymeningitis.

There is no way aside from a pituitary biopsy to diagnose the disorder with certainty; various anti-pituitary antibodies have been identified but none appears to be pathogenic and the sensitivity and specificity of the assays are low (normal patients may also possess these antibodies) [4].

The condition, particularly that involving the neurohypophysis alone, is often self-limiting, with a restoration of normal pituitary function or with isolated or more widespread hormone deficiency [4], whilst in chronic cases the disease is progressive leading to fibrosis, empty sella and panhypopituitarism. There are no helpful data on which to recommend treatment; it is acknowledged that surgery should be limited to biopsy alone since the prevalence of post-operative hormone deficiency and diabetes insipidus is high, and it is not clear from other papers that steroids and immune suppression alter the course of progressive disease. One did show an improvement in hormone levels and a reduction in pituitary size in around half of a cohort of seven treated with 120 mg oral methylprednisolone for 2 weeks followed by a taper over a further four [5].

Other Causes of Auto-immune Hypophysitis

Lymphocytic hypophysitis related to the recently characterized IgG4 disease, in which there is an intense infiltration of IgG4 positive plasma cells and a raised serum IgG4, seems to occur in elderly men and is sensitive to glucocorticoids [6]. The condition may be associated with IgG4 related disease elsewhere (for example liver, pancreas and the orbit) but may be isolated.

Cases of hypophysitis associated with Pit-1 antibodies seemingly separate to other pituitary antibodies have also been reported [7], and also cases related to the use of the anti-CTLA-4 monoclonal antibody Ipilimumab used in the treatment of metastatic melanoma.

Granulomatous hypophysitis may be associated with systemic disease such as sarcoidosis, granulomatosis with polyangiitis and with tuberculosis and syphilis infection. A recent review of the 82 cases reported in the world literature [8] showed that the disorder is also more common in young women but is less often associated with other auto-immune diseases. The presenting features are of pituitary dysfunction and the visual effects of the pituitary mass. It appears that pituitary failure is less common than in the lymphocytic variety. Those untreated by steroids appeared to fare as well those who were, but in either group the requirement for hormone replacement therapy was 90 %. Recurrence rate after excision or biopsy was low.

The term xanthomatous hypophysitis was coined in 1998 when pituitary tissue was seen to contain foamy histiocytes with S68 and S100 immunohistochemical properties [9] in three female patients with pituitary masses but only minor endocrine dysfunction; indeed normal pituitary tissue was observed within the inflammatory infiltration. This appears to be a separate and most uncommon disease entity, although other cases show a combination of granulomatous inflammation and this histiocytic disorder.

The histiocytic disorders Erdheim-Chester disease and Langerhan's cell histiocytosis commonly present with parasellar lesions and indeed diabetes insipidus, but are uniformly systemic diseases with a wide involvement of other tissues at presentation [10]. Rosai-Dorfman disease [11] may also involve the parasellar region.

References

1. Kendall-Taylor P, Jonsson PJ, Abs R, Erfurth EM, Koltowska-Haggstrom M, Price DA, Verhelst J. The clinical, metabolic and endocrine features and the quality of life in adults with childhood-onset craniopharyngioma. Eur J Endocrinol. 2005;152:557–67.
2. Oiso Y, Robertson GL, Norgaard JP, Juul KV. Clinical review: treatment of neurohypophyseal diabetes insipidus. J Clin Endocrinol Metab. 2012;98:3958–67.
3. Falomi A, Minarelli V, Bartoloni E, Alunno A, Gerli R. Diagnosis and classification of autoimmune hypophysitis. Autoimmun Rev. 2014;13:412–6.
4. De Bellis A, Ruocco G, Battaglia M, Conte M, Coronella C, Tirelli G, Bellastella A, Pane E, Sinisi AA, Bellastella G. Immunological and clinical aspects of lymphocytic hypophysitis. Clin Sci. 2008;114:413–21.
5. Kristof RA, van Roost D, Klingmuller D, Springer W, Schramm J. Lymphocytic hypophysitis: non-invasive diagnosis and treatment by high dose methylprednisolone pulse therapy? J Neurol Neurosurg Psychiatry. 1999;67:398–402.
6. Shimatsu A, Oki Y, Fujisawa I, Sano T. Pituitary and stalk lesions (infundibulo-hypophysitis) associated with immunoglobulin G4-related systemic disease: an emerging clinical entity. Endocr J. 2009;56:1033–41.
7. Takahashi Y. Autoimmune hypophysitis: new developments. Handb Clin Neurol. 2014;124:417–22.
8. Hunn BHM, Martin WG, Simpson S, McLean CA. Idiopathic granulomatous hypophysitis: a systematic review of 82 cases in the literature. Pituitary. 2014;17:357–65.
9. Fokerth RD, Price DL, Schwartz M, Black PM, De Girolami U. Xanthomatous hypophysitis. Am J Surg Pathol. 1998;22:736–41.
10. Mazor RD, Maneich-Mazor M, Shoenfeld Y. Erdheim-Chester disease: a comprehensive review of the literature. Orphanet J Rare Dis. 2013;8:1750–72.
11. Kidd D, Miller NR, Revesz T. Neurological complications of Rosai-Dorfman syndrome. Neurology. 2007;67:1551–5.

Case 29

History

This 45 year old man was healthy and kept himself fit and had no relevant past medical history. He developed a seemingly mild upper respiratory tract infection and after a prolonged coughing fit noted eye pain. This became more severe and was lancinating and felt as if it were arising from within the center of the eye.

On the following day his wife noted that his left eyelid looked different, and he went to two different emergency departments and was reassured. When the pain became more severe he attended the Royal Free Hospital and, pleasingly, was not turned away.

Neurological Examination

This was normal save for a pupillary inequality and a 2 mm left ptosis (Fig. 29.1). The disparity in pupil size increased in darkness.

D.P. Kidd, *Neuro-Ophthalmology*, DOI 10.1007/978-1-4471-2410-8_29

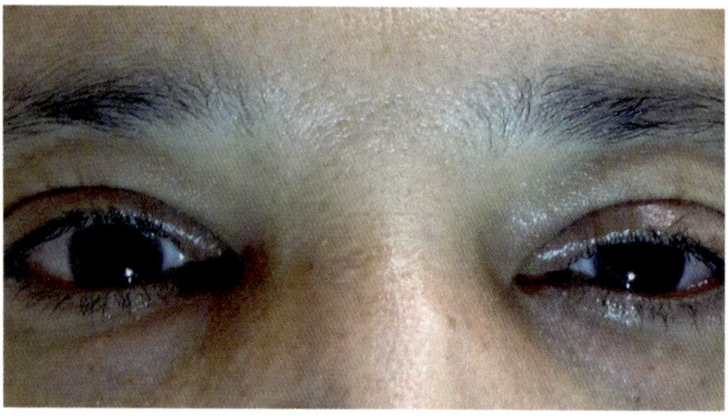

Fig. 29.1 The patient's pupils (Reproduced with his permission)

Clinical Evaluation

The patient has a left Horner's syndrome.

Eight percent of the normal population has unequal pupils. It is thought to be due to an asymmetry of autonomic flow on either side of the body. The prevalence doubles in elderly populations. The techniques of examining the pupils are noted in Appendix 2; in simple or physiological anisocoria the pupillary inequality remains proportionately the same in light and dark illumination. However in Horner's syndrome there is an unopposed parasympathetic drive to the pupil, leading to it being held in a miosed state in both light and dark, so when the normal pupil dilates in darkness the abnormal one remains smaller. There is however a dilatation after a time; when the lights are turned out the normal pupil will immediately dilate, and on the other side the pupil will begin to dilate incompletely several seconds afterwards. This can be measured using infrared pupillography or more simply by taking two photographs of the eyes, 5 and 15 seconds after turning off the lights and measuring the pupil diameter in each case. This "dilatation lag" is pathognomonic of an oculosympathetic disorder.

In Horner's syndrome sympathetic underactivity leads to paralysis of the smooth muscles of the eyelid innervated by the sympathetic nerves. In the upper eyelid this is Muller's muscle. There is also smooth muscle in the lower lid, so that the upper lid falls partially and the lower lid lifts slightly. This causes the *apparent* enophthamos noted by Horner.

The vasomotor effects vary according to the site of the lesion and when it occurs. In the acute stage there may be an increases in skin temperature with flushing of the face on the affected side; with time (because of denervation hypersensitivity) the affected side become paler and colder owing to vasoconstriction.

The pharmacological testing to confirm and localize the site of the sympathetic disorder is noted in Appendix 2.

The Sympathetic Pathway

The first order neuron arises in the posterolateral hypothalamus and pass down through the brain stem laterally to the ciliospinal center of Budge in the intermediolateral column of the spinal cord at C8 – T1. The second order neuron arises from the ciliospinal center and passes out of the spinal canal passes over the apex of the lung to the stellate ganglion, thence to the carotid artery sheath to the superior cervical ganglion.

The third order neuron arises in the superior cervical ganglion and passes in the wall of the internal carotid artery to the cavernous sinus where it joins the abducens nerve then passes to the ophthalmic division of the trigeminal nerve as the nasociliary nerve, then on their own as the two long ciliary nerves to the anterior segment and the iris.

Within the brain the lesions are commonly tumors and hemorrhage. Within the brain stem infarction, demyelination and vascular malformations are common causes, and in the cord vascular lesions and demyelination.

Pre-ganglionic (Second Order) Neuron

Tumors of the lung ("pancoast") and mediastinum
Rowland Payne syndrome: an ipsilateral Horner's syndrome with phrenic, vagus and recurrent laryngeal nerve palsy, due to primary and secondary tumors and infections of the lung and lymph nodes including tuberculosis
Schwannoma, paraganglioma, neurofibroma involving the cervical sympathetic chain
Lesions due to anesthetic and surgical procedures including catheterization, chest drain insertion, pacemaker implantation and carotid endarterectomy.

Post-ganglionic (Third Order) Neuron

Cervical carotid artery dissection
Lesions of the cavernous sinus (especially aneurysm of the carotid artery)
Cluster headache (5–25 % of cases are associated with Horner's syndrome and may be transient or permanent)
"Raeder's paratrigeminal syndrome" (Table 29.1)

Table 29.1 Clinical features associated with Horner's syndrome

Central lesions (first order neuron)	
Hypothalamus	Contralateral hemiparesis
Thalamus	Contralateral hemisensory loss
Midbrain	Contralateral IV
Medulla	The lateral medullary syndrome of Wallenberg
Cervical cord	Other features of a cord lesion

Investigations

He underwent an MRI scan of the brain, and subsequently vascular imaging of the neck (Figs. 29.2 and 29.3).

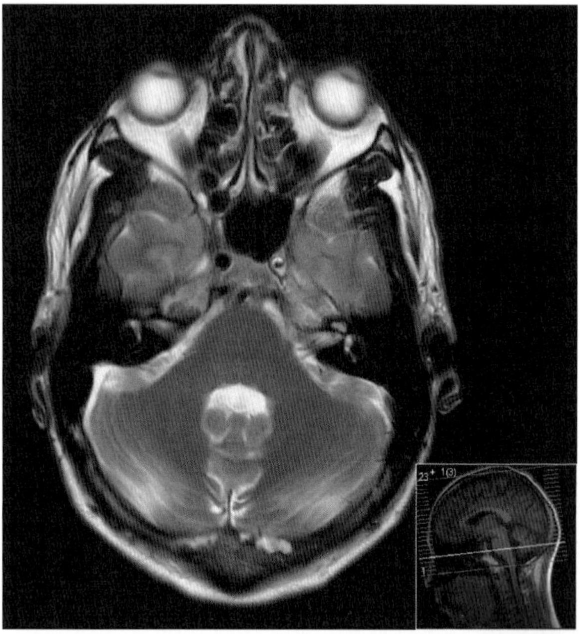

Fig. 29.2 MRI: there is abnormal signal within the left internal carotid artery with a crescentic appearance and a reduction in the lumen of the artery

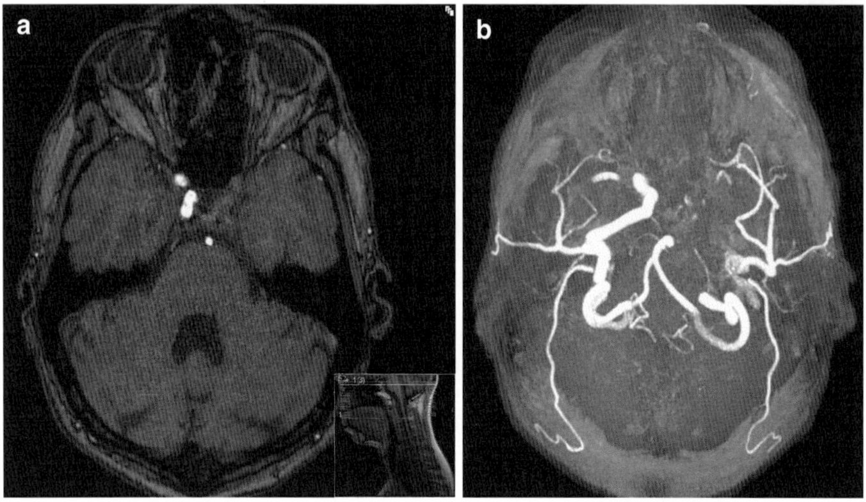

Fig. 29.3 MRA of the carotid artery and circle of Willis showing dissection of the left internal carotid artery from C2 to the cavernous segment, with very little flow through the string-like lesion. There is evidence for good collateral and retrograde flow from the posterior communicating arteries and the supraclinoid segment of the carotid artery

Management

It was recommended that he be discharged on oral aspirin rather than be admitted for intravenous then oral anticoagulation. At that time the literature showed points against and in favor of anticoagulation and indeed a multi-center trial has very recently shown no advantage in anticoagulation over provision of antiplatelet agents [1]. However, he awoke on the following day with a right sided weakness and an expressive dysphasia. Thankfully he returned quickly and within the stipulated time window to allow him to receive intravenous thrombolysis. His MRI scan showed restricted diffusion within the territory of the left middle cerebral artery (Fig. 29.4) prior to thrombolysis. After treatment the scan returned to normal and 4 days later had no abnormal neurological signs save for the left Horner's syndrome.

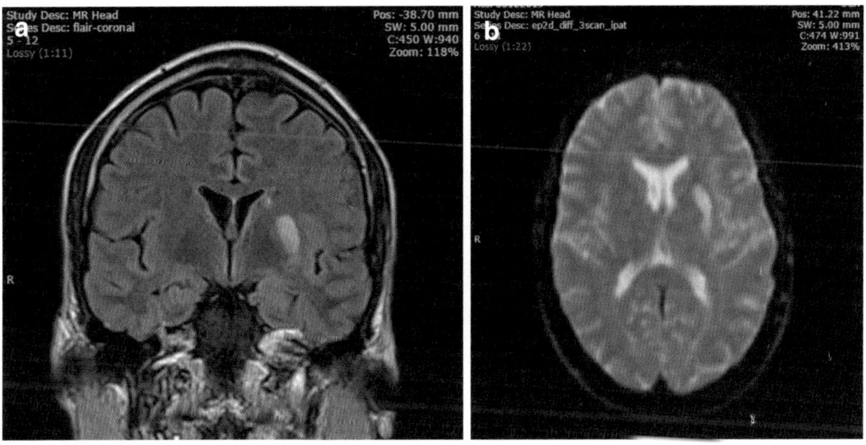

Fig. 29.4 MRI scan of the brain: (**a**) coronal FLAIR sequence showing increased signal within the left corona radiata, and (**b**) diffusion weighted imaging showing restricted diffusion throughout the territory of the left middle cerebral artery

Discussion

Most carotid artery dissections arise just above the carotid bifurcation. The incidence is 3 per 10^5 population per year, more than that of vertebral artery dissection (1 per 10^5 per year) [2]. It is thought that most have an underlying connective tissue disorder which renders the artery at risk of dissection when a traumatic stretching occurs, for example blunt trauma, whiplash and even sneezing or coughing as in this case. The prevalence of an inherited connective tissue disorder such as Ehlers-Danlos syndrome is however very low.

Patients affected present with pain and Horner's syndrome as in this case, transient ischemic attacks of the anterior circulation including amaurosis fugax, and with stroke and central retinal artery occlusion. Rarely a XIIth neuropathy may arise (presumably as a result of ischemia) on the same side.

Stroke occurs as a result of embolism from the site. It accounts for 10–20 % of strokes in a young age group, including children, although only 2–3 % of all strokes [2]. In the CADISS trial 4 % had stroke after diagnosis and no significant difference between the two treatments was identified [1]. Another study showed that 38 % of patients with cervical carotid artery dissection had Horner's syndrome and that subgroup of patients in general had a better outcome [3]. Factors associated with delayed stroke (*ie* after diagnosis, as in this case) include occlusion of the dissected artery and multiple dissections [4]. Patients with Horner's syndrome were less likely to have delayed stroke. In that study of 945 patients 339 had no stroke, 382 had stroke at diagnosis and 224 had delayed stroke.

Thrombolysis, when acute cerebral infarction occurs, is safe, although was only used in 11 % of the patients studied [5].

Cervical carotid and vertebral artery dissections may spread intracranially; spontaneous intracranial artery dissection is rare, and said to be more common in children and in Asian populations, and may present with ischemic complications or subarachnoid hemorrhage. Aneurysm formation may occur, and morbidity and mortality is much higher than in patients with cervical dissections [6].

References

1. CADISS trial investigators, Markus HS, Hayter E, Levi C, Feldman A, Venables G, Norris J. Antiplatelet treatment compared with anticoagulation treatment for cervical artery dissection (CADISS): a randomised trial. Lancet Neurol. 2015;14:361–7.
2. Debette S, Leys D. Cervical artery dissections: predisposing factors, diagnosis and outcome. Lancet Neurol. 2009;8:668–78.
3. Lyrer PA, Brandt T, Metso TM, Metso AJ, Kloss M, Debette S, Leys D, Caso V, Pezzini A, Bonati LH, Thijs V, Bersano A, Touzé E, Gensicke H, Martin JJ, Lichy C, Tatlisumak T, Engelter ST, Grond-Ginsbach C. Cervical Artery Dissection and Ischemic Stroke Patients (CADISP) Study Group. Clinical import of Horner syndrome in internal carotid and vertebral artery dissection. Neurology. 2014;82:1653–9.

4. Lichy C, Metso A, Pezzini A, Leys D, Metso T, Lyrer P, Debette S, Thijs V, Abboud S, Kloss M, Samson Y, Caso V, Sessa M, Beretta S, Lamy C, Medeiros E, Bersano A, Touze E, Tatlisumak T, Grau A, Brandt T, Engelter S, Grond-Ginsbach C, Cervical Artery Dissection and Ischemic Stroke Patients-Study Group. Predictors of delayed stroke in patients with cervical artery dissection. Int J Stroke. 2015;10:360–3.
5. Engelter ST, Dallongeville J, Kloss M, Metso TM, Leys D, Brandt T, Samson Y, Caso V, Pezzini A, Sessa M, Beretta S, Debette S, Grond-Ginsbach C, Metso AJ, Thijs V, Lamy C, Medeiros E, Martin JJ, Bersano A, Tatlisumak T, Touzé E, Lyrer PA, Cervical Artery Dissection and Ischaemic Stroke Patients-Study Group. Thrombolysis in cervical artery dissection – data from the Cervical Artery Dissection and Ischaemic Stroke Patients (CADISP) database. Eur J Neurol. 2012;19:1199–206.
6. Debette S, Compter A, Labeyrie MA, Uyttenboogaart M, Metso TM, Majersik JJ, Goeggel-Simonetti B, Engelter ST, Pezzini A, Bijlenga P, Southerland AM, Naggara O, Béjot Y, Cole JW, Ducros A, Giacalone G, Schilling S, Reiner P, Sarikaya H, Welleweerd JC, Kappelle L, de Borst GJ, Bonati LH, Jung S, Thijs V, Martin JJ, Brandt T, Grond-Ginsbach C, Kloss M, Mizutani T, Minematsu K, Meschia JF, Pereira VM, Bersano A, Touzé E, Lyrer PA, Leys D, Chabriat H, Markus HS, Worrall BB, Chabrier S, Baumgartner R, Stapf C, Tatlisumak T, Arnold M, Bousser MG. Epidemiology, pathophysiology, diagnosis, and management of intracranial artery dissection. Lancet Neurol. 2015;14:640–54.

Case 30

History

This 30 year old lady had been troubled by headaches for 6 months when she noticed a visual impairment on one side. She sought the advice of her optometrist who was alarmed that her acuities had decreased over the previous year. She was referred to the local ophthalmology department.

There were no other symptoms save for amenorrhea for the previous 8 months. Her past medical history was otherwise unremarkable.

Examination

Her central acuities were 6/60 right and 6/12 left. There was no color vision and there was a right relative afferent pupillary defect. There was a complete bitemporal hemianopia (Fig. 30.1). The ocular media were clear but the discs were pale.

There were no other abnormal neurological signs.

D.P. Kidd, *Neuro-Ophthalmology*, DOI 10.1007/978-1-4471-2410-8_30

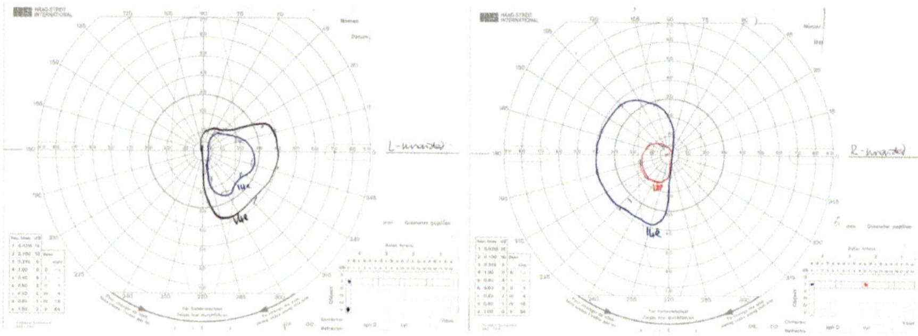

Fig. 30.1 Goldman visual fields showing a complete bitemporal hemianopia

Clinical Evaluation

A straightforward clinical syndrome of headache and visual loss with the identification of a bitemporal hemianopia which very strongly suggests a chiasmal disorder. The amenorrhea must surely be connected; a pituitary disorder would be the most likely cause. The initial examination would be an urgent MRI of the pituitary fossa and a series of endocrine blood investigations.

Investigation

An MRI scan of the sellar region showed a cystic suprasellar mass which extended down into the pituitary stalk (Fig. 30.2).

Screening blood investigations were normal. Pituitary hormones revealed a slightly raised prolactin but no other abnormalities.

It was felt to be a craniopharyngioma or Rathke's cleft cyst, and a debulking procedure undertaken urgently.

The histological diagnosis was a suprasellar germinoma (Fig. 30.3).

Her vision had not improved post-operatively, and she was referred for radiotherapy. She received 50 Gy in 15 fractions. Her vision has not deteriorated and imaging has shown stable appearances over the ensuing 6 years.

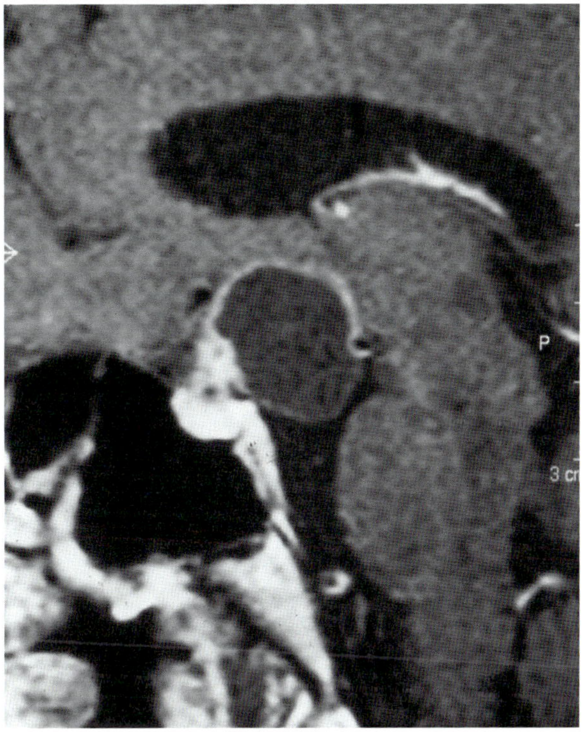

Fig. 30.2 T1 weighted sagittal MRI showing a large cystic lesion behind the pituitary extending up to and compressing the chiasm and third ventricle

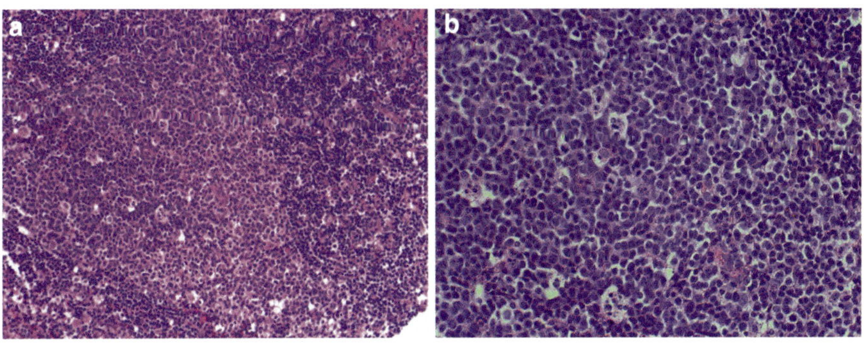

Fig. 30.3 Hematoxylin and eosin stained section showing mitotically active tumor cells. The neoplastic cells are larger than the reactive lymphocytes to the right hand side of the image. The presence of a prominent reactive lymphocytic infiltrate within the tumor is a common feature of germinomas. Reticulin staining showed extensive fibrosis. Immunohistochemistry revealed no hormone expression. They were negative for LCA, ACHL-1 and L26 and were positive for PLAP and C-kit, and CAM 5.2. They were negative for alpha fetoprotein and beta HCG (Pathology images courtesy of Dr Malcolm Galloway, Consultant Neuropathologist, Institute of Neurology and the Royal Free Hospital, London, UK)

Discussion

Suprasellar Germinomas

Primary intracranial germ cell tumors account for only 1 % of all brain tumors seen in adulthood. 65 % are germinomas; teratoma, embryonal carcinoma, yolk sac tumors, choriocarcinomas and tumors of mixed cell type account for the remainder. Most present in the second and third decades of life; the pineal and the suprasellar regions are most often affected [1]. The tumor markers β–HCG, α-fetoprotein, CEA and SP-1 are often present in germ cell tumors, although not in germinoma.

In children the tumors present with visual loss and hydrocephalus, and endocrine disorders including precious puberty, hypopituitarism and diabetes insipidus. In young adulthood they present more often with pituitary failure or hydrocephalus.

Occasionally germinomas may be incorrectly diagnosed as an inflammatory hypophysitis since they may be associated with prominent fibrous tissue and even granulomatous inflammation [2].

Germinomas respond well to radiotherapy with a low risk of recurrence [1, 3].

References

1. Kyritsis AP. Management of primary intracranial germ cell tumors. J Neurooncol. 2010;96:143–9.
2. Utsuki S, Oka H, Tanizaki Y, Kondo K, Kawano N, Fujii K. Pathological features of intracranial germinomas with reference to fibrous tissue and granulomatous change. Brain Tumor Pathol. 2005;22:9–13.
3. Oka H, Kawano N, Tanaka T, Utsuki S, Kobayashi I, Maezawa H, Fujii K. Long-term functional outcome of suprasellar germinomas: usefulness and limitations of radiotherapy. J Neurooncol. 1998;40:185–90.

Case 31

History

This 40 year old man was born in Africa and had moved to the UK a year before the onset of his disorder. He presented with a 2 month history of headache which was right sided and periorbital. His GP prescribed antibiotics for a putative sinus infection without benefit. Over 6 weeks his headache worsened and felt generally unwell. There were night sweats and chest pains. He developed numbness over the top half of the right side of his face.

When he developed horizontal double vision he attended the emergency department of his local hospital and was admitted, then transferred to the Royal Free Hospital for further investigations.

His past medical history was unremarkable and he took no regular medications. There had been no weight loss.

Examination

The anterior visual pathways were normal. There was no proptosis. There was a right sixth neuropathy (Fig. 31.1), and upper and middle division trigeminal sensory loss. The lower cranial nerves were normal.

The systemic examination including chest and abdomen was normal. There were palpable cervical and inguinal lymph nodes. The ocular media and retinae were normal.

D.P. Kidd, *Neuro-Ophthalmology*, DOI 10.1007/978-1-4471-2410-8_31

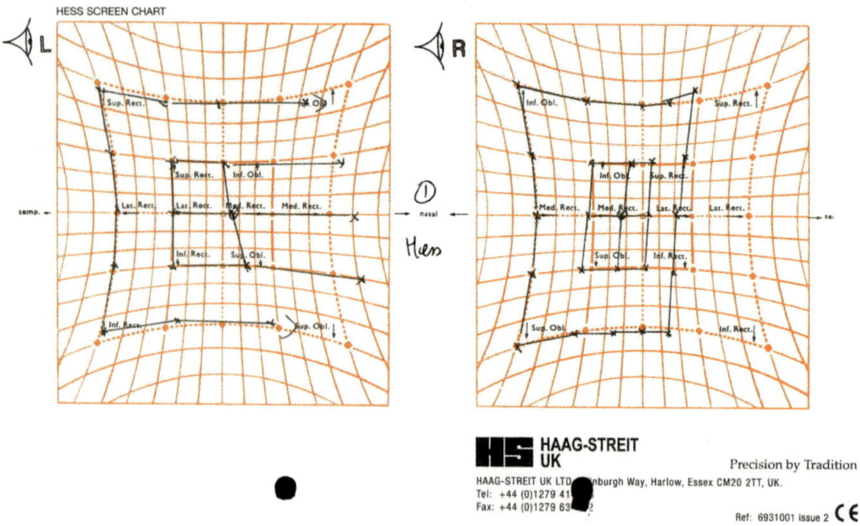

Fig. 31.1 Lees screen test chart showing acute right sided lateral rectus weakness

Clinical Evaluation

This man presented with a subacute worsening neurological disorder with prominent systemic features, particularly night sweats. There was lymphadenopathy.

The neuro-ophthalmic signs of normal visual function, ophthalmoparesis and both upper and middle division trigeminal involvement point to a lesion of the cavernous sinus rather than the orbital apex (see Appendix 3). There is clear evidence for a systemic disorder bearing in mind the lymphadenopathy and the constitutional symptoms.

The differential diagnosis would be wide, encompassing infective diseases, most particularly tuberculosis and HIV, inflammatory disorders such as sarcoidosis and vasculitis, and neoplastic disease for example lymphoma. A wide ranging series of investigations is required initially.

Investigations

Bloods: full blood count was normal, including white cell count and lymphocyte count; ESR 34; biochemical screening revealed normal renal and liver functions; serum calcium was normal and ACE 38.

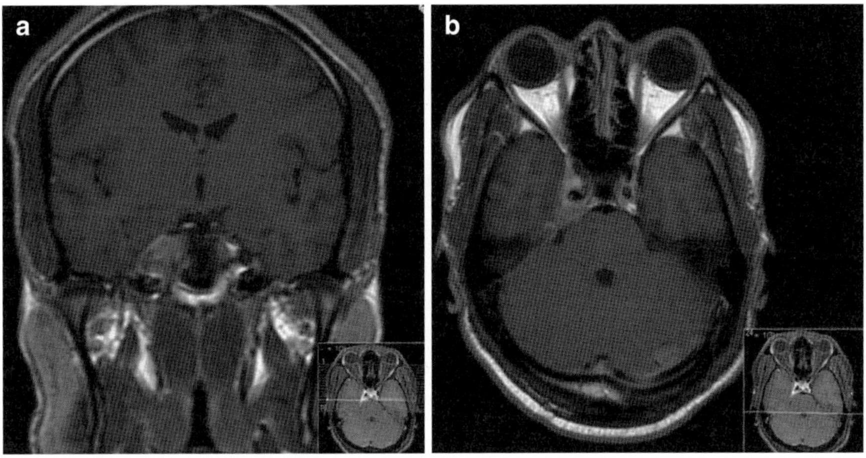

Fig. 31.2 MRI: (**a**) T1 weighted axial scan showing an expansile lesion contiguous with the meninges arising from the right cavernous sinus and extending into Meckel's cave, along the petrous ridge and as far as the pre-pontine cistern, which enhances (**b**). On the left there is additional meningeal enhancement adjacent to the temporal and occipital lobes

Serological tests: HIV, HSV, HHV6 and EBV were negative. ANA, ENA and ANCA were negative. Borrelia and syphilis titers were not raised.

A chest x-ray was normal.

MRI scan showed an enhancing mass involving the right cavernous sinus (Fig. 31.2).

CT PET scan showed uptake of tracer in the petrous region on the right side and within several lymph nodes (Fig. 31.3).

The CSF was under raised pressure at 28 cm. The protein was 0.55 g/dl. There were ten white cells, and cytological analysis revealed these to be lymphocytes. No malignant cell was seen. The sugar differential was normal at 3.5/5.5. Oligoclonal bands were absent.

A cervical node was biopsied and was seen to contain non-caseating granulomas, with histiocytes, giant cells and plasma cells. No acid fast bacilli or fungal hyphi were seen on staining, and no tuberculous or fungal growth was identified subsequently.

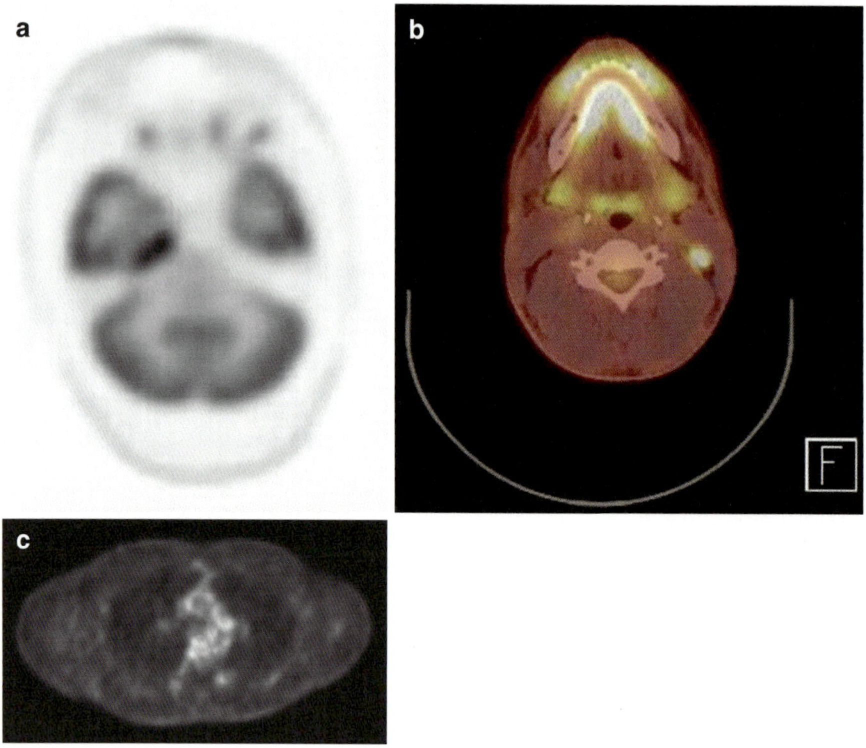

Fig. 31.3 CT PET: There is uptake of FDG tracer in the regions of enhancement seen on the MRI in the right petrous ridge (**a**). There was uptake in the neck on both sides (**b**), within lymph nodes and the left submandibular gland. In the thorax there was only minor uptake in the right hilar glands. The abdomen and pelvis were normal

Management

The histological appearances, the PET scan and chest imaging appearances and the normal blood investigation results suggested that the lesion was not an infective one but systemic sarcoidosis. He was treated with intravenous then oral steroids and his night sweats resolved, the headache abated and the double vision reduced then resolved. Oral methotrexate was prescribed after 2 months and continues. The steroids were withdrawn over 9 months and he returned to normal. So too did the MRI (Fig. 31.4). He remains on oral methotrexate 10 mg once per week and is well.

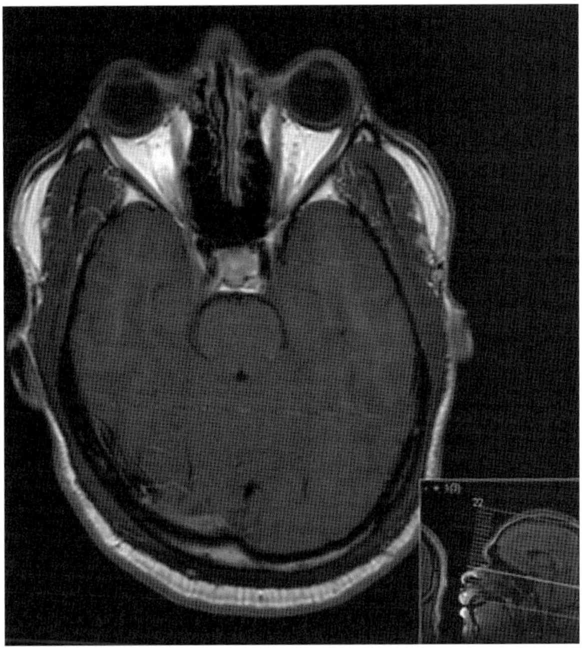

Fig. 31.4 T1 weighted MRI scan after treatment showing resolution of the inflammatory mass

Discussion*

Sarcoidosis forms a spectrum of auto-inflammatory disorders of unknown etiology characterized by the development of immune activation leading to an immunological cascade which results in an inflammatory infiltration with granuloma formation and later fibrosis. Any tissue may be affected, the lungs, skin, liver and joints being the most frequently so [1].

The disorder is more common in women than men, and predominately a disease of young adulthood but affects all age groups [2, 3]. There is a higher prevalence in African Americans, and the disease may be more severe in this ethnic group [2, 4].

Ophthalmic complications of the disease arise in some 10–50 % [5–7], with 12 % in the ACCESS study [2]; not all patients show the characteristics of a granulomatous uveitis [8]. Anterior uveitis is the most common, with mutton fat keratic precipitates and Koeppe iris nodules, a vitritis leading to the string of pearls, periphlebitis, candle wax drippings and choroidal involvement all well known [5–11]. The development of keratoconjunctivitis sicca appears to be almost inevitable. The prognosis for visual recovery in those with intraocular inflammation is in general good [9–11] with correct treatment.

Involvement of the nervous system accounts for 5–10 % of published retrospective series [12]. It may arise at any point during the disease, and all regions of the

*Part of this discussion appears in Kidd DP et al. Optic neuropathy in systemic sarcoidosis. *Neurology, Neuroimmunology and Neuroinflammation.* 2016;3:e270.

nervous system may be affected. However, involvement of the parasellar region is uncommon; of the four recently published series of neuro-ophthalmic complications of sarcoidosis [13–16], 3/13 [14], 1/20 [15] and 1/15 [16] showed a lesion involving or adjacent to the cavernous sinus.

Treatment is with corticosteroids in the first instance, but neurological involvement aside from that due to a mononeuropathy with meningoencephalitis, always requires additional oral or intravenous immunosuppression. Those with relapsing or resistant disease respond well to TNFα blockade.

References

1. Iannuzzi MC, Rubicki BA, Teirstein AS. Sarcoidosis. N Engl J Med. 2007;357:2152–65.
2. Baughman RP, Teirstein AS, Judson MA, Rossman MD, Yeager H, Bresnitz EA, et al. Clinical characteristics of patients in a case control study of sarcoidosis. Am J Respir Crit Care Med. 2001;164:1885–9.
3. Pietinalho A, Hiraga Y, Hosoda Y, Lofroos AB, Yamaguchi M, Selroos O. The frequency of Sarcoidosis in Finland and Hokkaido, Japan: a comparative epidemiological study. Sarcoidosis. 1995;12:61–7.
4. Rybicki BA, Major M, Popovich Jr J, Mailiarik MJ, Iannuzzi MC. Racial differences in sarcoidosis incidence: a 5 year study in a health maintenance organization. Am J Epidemiol. 1997;145:234–41.
5. Jabs DA, Johns CJ. Ocular involvement in sarcoidosis. Am J Ophthalmol. 1986;102:297–301.
6. Karma A, Huhti E, Poukkula A. Course and outcome of ocular sarcoidosis. Am J Ophthalmol. 1988;106:467–72.
7. Rothova A. Ocular involvement in sarcoidosis. Br J Ophthalmol. 2000;84:110–6.
8. Herbort CP, Rao NA, Mochizuki M, members of Scientific Committee of First International Workshop on Ocular Sarcoidosis. International criteria for the diagnosis of ocular sarcoidosis: results of the first international workshop on ocular sarcoidosis. Ocul Immunol Inflamm. 2009;17:160–9.
9. Dana MR, Merayo-Lloves J, Schaumberg DA, Foster CS. Prognosticators for visual outcome in sarcoid uveitis. Ophthalmology. 1996;103:1846–53.
10. Edelstein C, Pearson A, Joynes E, Stanford MR, Graham EM. The ocular and systemic prognosis of patients presenting with sarcoid uveitis. Eye (Lond). 1999;13:748–53.
11. Lobo A, Barton K, Minassian D, du Bois RM, Lightman S. Visual loss in sarcoid-related uveitis. Clin Experiment Ophthalmol. 2003;31:310–6.
12. Kidd D, Beynon HLC. Neurological complications of systemic sarcoidosis (review). Sarcoidosis Vasc Diffuse Lung Dis. 2003;20:85–94.
13. Frohman LP, Guirgis M, Turbin RE, Bielory L. Sarcoidosis of the anterior visual pathway: 24 new cases. J Neuroophthalmol. 2003;23:190–7.
14. Heuser K, Kerty E. Neuro-ophthalmological findings in sarcoidosis. Acta Ophthalmol Scand. 2004;82:723–9.
15. Lamirel C, Badelon I, Gout O, Berthet K, Héran F, Laloum L, Cochereau I, Gaudric A, Bousser MG, Vignal-Clermont C. Manifestations neuro-ophtalmologiques révélatrices d'une neurosarcoidose. J Fr Ophthalmol. 2006;29:241–9.
16. Koczman JJ, Rouleau J, Gaunt M, Kardon RH, Wall M, Lee AG. Neuro-ophthalmic sarcoidosis: the University of Iowa experience. Semin Ophthalmol. 2008;23:157–68.

Case 32

History and Examination

This lady was 19 and at University when she presented with a progressive visual loss in the left eye. Her local ophthalmology service found bitemporal field defects (Fig. 32.1) and an MRI was performed (Fig. 32.2a–c), with the result she was referred to our Neurosurgery department.

There were no other symptoms and she was otherwise healthy and well.

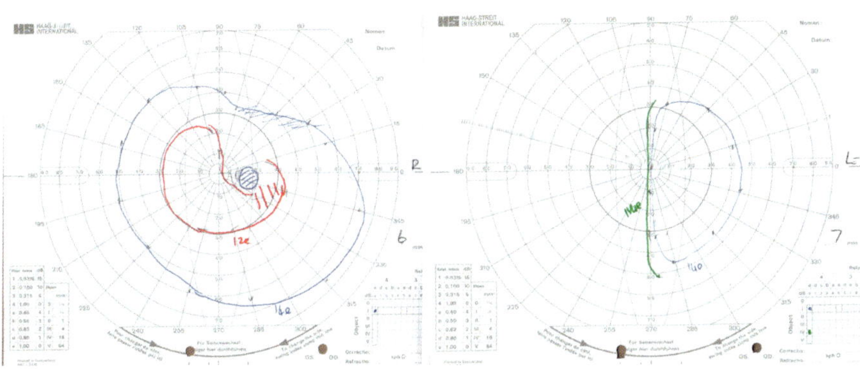

Fig. 32.1 Goldman fields showing a bitemporal pattern field loss, hemianopic on the left and an upper quadrantinopia on the right

D.P. Kidd, *Neuro-Ophthalmology*, DOI 10.1007/978-1-4471-2410-8_32

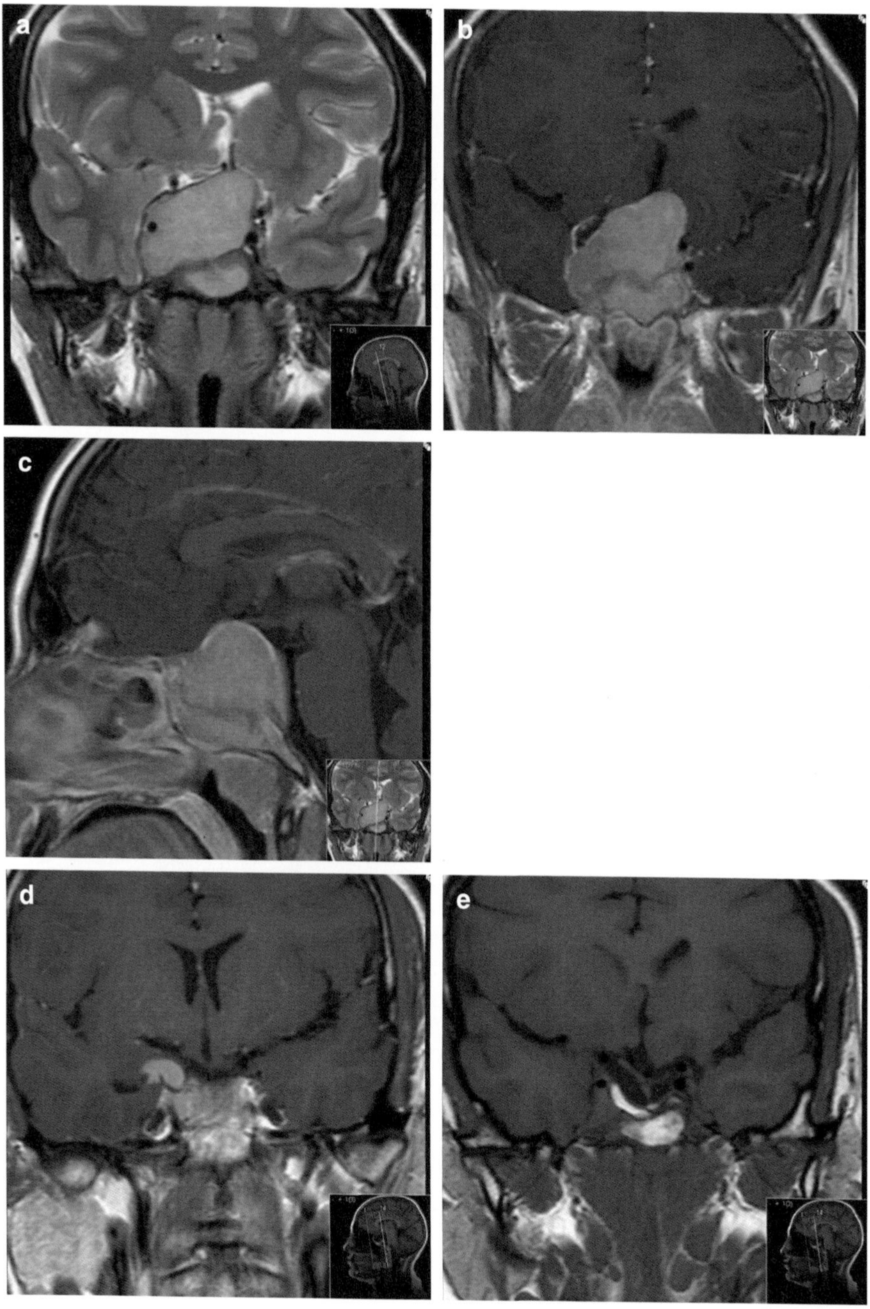

Fig. 32.2 (**a**) Coronal T2 weighted MRI at diagnosis, showing an enormous lesion arising from the pituitary fossa and extending up to cause the chiasm to splay and to compress the third ventricle. The lesion shows uniform enhancement (**b**, **c**) with gadolinium. MRI more recently, showing (**d**) invasion of the right mesial temporal lobe, and (**e**) "tenting" of the chiasm

Clinical Evaluation

A visual disorder in which the visual field on both sides is affected particularly in the temporal fields must be related to a disorder of the chiasm. A pituitary adenoma is the most common cause but there are many other pathological processes to consider (Table 32.1).

She underwent a series of endocrine investigations (Table 32.2) and when the prolactin was not found to be raised the lesion was removed through a trans-sphenoidal approach (Fig. 32.3). There was a brief disorder of urine concentration treated with ddAVP and she noted her vision to improve. She was discharged on hydrocortisone replacement and followed up.

Post operatively her vision improved to 6/6 and 6/18 over 6 weeks, but then she noticed it deteriorating again. Her TSH and T4 remained elevated; further imaging showed a cystic recurrence of the lesion, which was again decompressed through a trans-sphenoidal approach. She was referred for radiotherapy and received 20 Gy over 4 weeks.

Thereafter her vision and her fields were stable, but imaging revealed a recurrence 2 years later and she underwent a third hypophysectomy. Thereafter her TSH has remained normal.

Four years later she developed brief absences preceded by a sense of déjà vu which increased in frequency and resolved using Lamotrigine which she continues. Her scans shows invasion of the adjacent mesial temporal lobe (Fig. 32.2d).

Table 32.1 Differential diagnosis of a mass lesion arising from the pituitary fossa [1]

Neoplastic	Inflammatory	Infective	Vascular
Pituitary adenoma	Sarcoidosis	Pyogenic abscess	Aneurysm
Pituitary carcinoma	Erdheim Chester	Tuberculosis	Cavernoma
	Lymphocytic hypophysitis		
Granular cell tumor	ANCA positive vasculitis		
Astrocytoma of the stalk	Sphenoid sinus mucocoele		
Hypothalamic glioma			
Hemangioblastoma			
Germ cell tumors			
Esthesioneuroblastoma			
Meningioma			
Chordoma			
Hemangiopericytoma			
Chondrosarcoma			
Paraganglioma			
Craniopharyngioma			
Lymphoma			
Metastasis: carcinoma, leukemia, lymphoma			
Rathke's cleft cyst			
Choristoma eg epidermoid cyst			

Her vision deteriorated again more recently without evidence for tumor recurrence but note that the chiasm has become stretched downwards through tethering (Fig. 32.2e). Further surgery was not recommended, being considered a greater risk for her remaining vision than leaving it alone, and her field has stabilized.

Table 32.2 Initial endocrine investigation results

Urea 3.7	TSH 4.32
Na 141	T4 39.2
K 4.1	Prolactin 401
SC 49	Cortisol 109
FBC normal	Serum osmolality 287
ESR 3	Urine osmolality 649

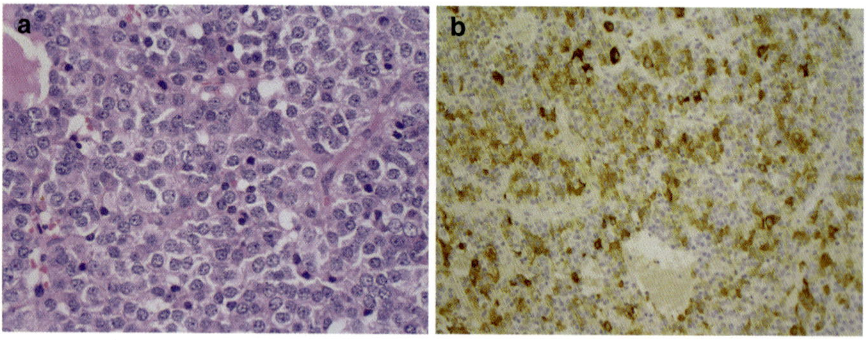

Fig. 32.3 (**a**) Hematoxylin and eosin stained section showing a pituitary tumor composed of expanded nests of neuroendocrine tumor cells with round monomorphous nuclei and variable amounts of cytoplasm. Mitotic activity is inconspicuous, and there is no necrosis. (**b**) On immunocytochemistry many of the cells are positive for TSH. A few were positive for growth factor but there is no staining for FSH, LH, ACTH or prolactin. Although the cytological features are not overtly atypical, it should be noted that even without histological atypia, some pituitary adenomas may pursue an aggressive clinical course (Pathology images Courtesy of Dr Malcolm Galloway, Consultant Neuropathologist, Institute of Neurology and the Royal Free Hospital, London, UK)

Discussion

Field Defects in Pituitary Disorders

In a series of 91 consecutive patients with pituitary tumor [2] 37 had normal visual fields. Forty-one percent of those with abnormal fields had bitemporal field defects of whom 50 % had normal central acuity. Thirty-three percent had unilateral defects of which the majority were temporal hemi- or quadrantic defects, but altitudinal defects were also seen. Bilateral homonymous defects were seen in 13 %.

What field defect develops depends on the site of the compression of the chiasm; anteriorly placed lesions will cause a unilateral optic neuropathy, often with a junctional temporal scotoma, lesions of the body of the chiasm will cause bitemporal defects, and lesions of the posterior angle will show bitemporal hemianopic scotomas or tract lesion defects (Fig. 32.4). The reasons for this are noted in detail in reference [3].

Following surgery the majority of patients show a significant improvement in acuity and field [4].

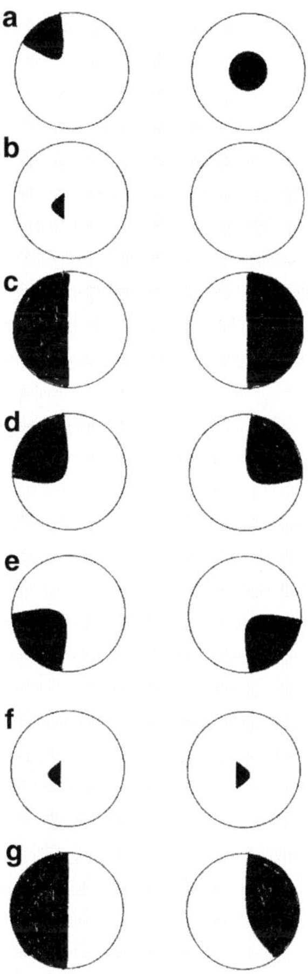

Fig. 32.4 Visual field defects seen in chiasmal disorders: (**a**) ipsilateral central field defect and contralateral junctional scotoma in a lesion involving the anterior angle of the chiasm
(**b**) also at the anterior angle, when only the crossing macular fibers are affected
(**c**) bitemporal hemianopia when the body of the chiasm is affected
(**d**) and (**e**) bitemporal upper and lower quadrantinopia when the lesion compresses the chiasm from below and above respectively
(**f**) bitemporal hemianopic scotomas when a lesion involves the posterior angle of the chiasm
(**g**) a non-congruous hemianopia occurs when the tract is affected (Reproduced with permission from Kidd [3])

Pituitary Adenoma

Pituitary tumors account for 10 % of all intracranial tumors. Ninety percent secrete hormones, and the majority are microadenomas (measuring 10 mm or less). They present with the endocrinological consequences most commonly. Non-secreting adenomas account for only 10 % of all pituitary adenomas and so are large at the time of diagnosis and tend to present with visual loss [5, 6].

Prolactin	Prolactinoma
Corticotrophin	Cushing's disease
Somatotrophin	Acromegaly
TSH	TSH-oma

Prolactinomas account for 40 % of all pituitary tumors and usually present with galactorrhea and amenorrhea. Only 10 % are macroadenomas, which can enlarge appreciably in pregnancy. They respond well to treatment with dopamine agonists, and even large tumors tend not to require surgery [7].

Corticotrophin and somatotrophin secreting tumors cause Cushing's disease and acromegaly/gigantism respectively. Corticotrophin releasing tumors are small and intrasellar; only 5 % are macroadenomas, but most nonetheless are removed [8]. Somatotrophin releasing tumors may be small or large, and are also removed at surgery, and treated with radiotherapy with recurrence. Somatostatin analogs and cabergoline reduce IGF-1 levels. Tumors frequently produce prolactin as well as somatotrophin [9].

Most can be removed through a trans-sphenoidal approach [6]; the remainder are removed or debulked through a frontal craniotomy. In general recurrence relates to the size of the tumor at presentation and to the degree of removal at first surgery. Clearly it is less easy to remove large invasive adenomas than small ones which are confined to the sella turcica. Non-secreting adenomas and prolactinomas have been found to recur most often, and tend to do so between 1 and 5 years after first surgery. Hormone secreting adenomas can however be monitored endocrinologically post-operatively.

Twenty to eighty percent of non-functioning adenomas recur [10] but 90 % stop growing after radiotherapy. The problem is that there is a high risk of pituitary failure after radiotherapy, even at low dose (14–20 Gy) and there are neurological complications to optic nerve, tract and chiasmal function as well.

Prolactinomas are not often resistant to dopamine agonists and so surgery is required less often, but in these and in corticotrophin and somatotrophin secreting tumors a higher dose of radiotherapy is required (around 24 Gy) although the response rates are also high at 90 % [11, 12]. The modern techniques of gamma knife radiosurgery and cyberknife appear to be better tolerated with a lower rate of pituitary and neurological long term complications. The response rate seems to be higher with cyberknife [12].

In this case the TSH and free T4 were raised and so it was no surprise that the tumor expressed immunocytochemical reactivity to TSH. TSH-secreting tumors are rare, accounting for only 2 % of pituitary tumors; 75 % present with thyrotoxicosis and 25 % with visual loss [13]. Eighty percent are macroadenomas. Thyrotoxicosis is associated with thyroid gland hypertrophy, simulating Graves's disease, but treatment of putative thyrotoxicosis fails to induce a lowering of TSH levels. The pituitary lesions are large at presentation, and often invade the cavernous sinus, which makes surgical removal difficult [14]. Some series have reported a low rate of recurrence when the tumor is removed in entirety [15], but all series report that recurrence is common when debulking rather than removal is carried out [13–15].

These tumors sometimes have more than one secreting cell type, and prolactin or growth hormone may also be released. Such tumors may therefore respond to treatment with dopamine agonists, and many centers have used somatostatin analogs with some reports of success [16]. One series showed normalization of TSH prior to surgery in 73 % of cases and tumor shrinkage in 60 % [17].

Prevalence of Headache in Pituitary Disorders

Headache is common in pituitary adenoma, to the extent that an appreciable number of pituitary "incidentalomas" are found when imaging is carried out for the assessment of headache. In one study 71 were identified in a 5 year period [18], of whom 48 were pituitary adenomas and 9 Rathke's cleft cysts. Twenty-nine percent subsequently underwent surgery. In a study of 84 patients headache was not related to tumor size or to invasion of trigeminal structures [19]; most headaches showed features of migraine or cluster headache. Patients with hormone secreting microadenomas often showed features of short lasting unilateral neuralgiform headache with conjunctival injection and tearing (SUNCT). Only half improved with treatment, and disability related to headache was appreciable.

Prevalence of Epilepsy in Pituitary Disorders

There is no published study which has assessed the prevalence of epilepsy in pituitary tumors which invade adjacent temporal cortex, but one study found that of 29 patients with MRI evidence for temporal invasion five had suffered seizures of mesial temporal type [20]. Furthermore those whose macroprolactinomas has diminished in size with dopamine agonist therapy noted a reduction in seizure frequency.

References

1. Powell M. Disorders of the sella and parasellar region. In: Kidd DP, Newman NJ, Biousse V, editors. Neuro-ophthalmology. Philadelphia: Butterworth – Heinemann; 2008. p. 242.
2. Ogra S, Nichols AD, Stylli S, Kaye AH, Savino PJ, Danesh-Meyer HV. Visual acuity and pattern of visual field loss at presentation in pituitary adenoma. J Clin Neurosci. 2014;21:735–40.

3. Kidd DP. The optic chiasm. In: Kennard C, Leigh JR, editors. Neuro-ophthalmology. Handbook of clinical neurology, vol. 102. Amsterdam: Elsevier; 2011. p. 186.
4. Powell M. Recovery of vision following transsphenoidal surgery for pituitary adenomas. Br J Neurosurg. 1995;9:367–73.
5. Wilson CB. Endocrine-inactive pituitary adenomas. Clin Neurosurg. 1992;38:10–31.
6. Powell M. Disorders of the sella and parasellar region. In: Kidd DP, Newman NJ, Biousse V, editors. Neuro-ophthalmology. Philadelphia: Butterworth – Heinemann; 2008. p. 243–5.
7. Schleckte JA. Prolactinoma. N Engl J Med. 2003;349:2035–41.
8. Tritos NA, Biller BM. Cushing's disease. Handb Clin Neurol. 2014;124:221–34.
9. Chanson P, Salenave S, Kamenicky P. Acromegaly. Handb Clin Neurol. 2014;124:197–219.
10. Roelfsema F, Biermsz NR, Pereira A. Clinical factors involved in the recurrence of pituitary adenomas after surgical remission: a structured review and meta-analysis. Pituitary. 2012;15:71–83.
11. Gopalan R, Schlesinger D, Vance ML, Kaws E, Sheehan J. Long-term outcomes after gamma knife radiosurgery for patients with non-functioning pituitary adenoma. Neurosurgery. 2011;69:284–93.
12. Kim W, Clelland C, Yang I, Pouratian N. Comprehensive review of stereotactic radiosurgery for medical and surgically refractory pituitary adenomas. Surg Neurol. 2012;3 Suppl 2:S79–89.
13. Brucker-Davis F, Oldfield EH, Skarulis MC, Doppman JL, Weintraub BD. Thyrotropin-secreting pituitary tumors: diagnostic criteria, thyroid hormone sensitivity, and treatment outcome in 25 patients followed at the National Institutes of Health. J Clin Endocrinol Metab. 1999;84:476–86.
14. Clarke MJ, Erickson D, Castro MR, Atkinson JL. Thyroid-stimulating hormone pituitary adenomas. J Neurosurg. 2008;109:17–22.
15. Malchiodi E, Profka E, Ferrante E, Sala E, Verrua E, Campi I, Lania AG, Arosio M, Locatelli M, Mortini P, Losa M, Motti E, Beck-Peccoz P, Spada A, Mantovani G. Thyrotropin-secreting pituitary adenomas: outcome of pituitary surgery and irradiation. J Clin Endocrinol Metab. 2014;99:2069–76.
16. Neggers SJCMM, van der Lely AJ. Medical approach to pituitary tumors. Handb Clin Neurol. 2014;124:303–16.
17. Fukuhara N, Horiguchi K, Nishioka H, Suzuki H, Takeshita A, Takeuchi Y, Inoshita N, Yamada S. Short-term preoperative octreotide treatment for TSH-secreting pituitary adenoma. Endocr J. 2015;62:21–7.
18. Esteves C, Neves C, Augusto L, Menzes J, Pereira J, Bernardes I, Fonseca J, Carvahlo D. Pituitary incidentalomas: analysis of a neuroradiological cohort. Pituitary. 2014;18(6):777–81.
19. Levy MJ, Matharu MS, Meeran K, Powell M, Goadsby PJ. The clinical characteristics of headache in patients with pituitary tumours. Brain. 2005;128:1921–30.
20. Deepak D, Daousi C, Javadpour M, MacFarlane IA. Macroprolactinomas and epilepsy. Clin Endocrinol (Oxf). 2007;66:503–7.

Case 33

History

This 44 year old lady awoke with blurred vision in the central field on the right. There was no ocular pain, nor pain on eye movements. She was seen in the emergency department of her local hospital and was reassured. Over the following week her vision improved and she was well for about 2 months when she developed a recurrence of the disorder, but associated with pain on eye movements, and a mild orbital ache. There was some flickering of light in the abnormal visual field. She was referred to the Royal Free Hospital.

Examination

On examination she saw 6/24 with absent color vision on the right and a diffuse central field defect (Fig. 33.1a), 6/5 with normal color vision and field on the left. There was a right sided relative afferent pupillary defect. The ocular examination was normal, but there was temporal pallor of the right disc. The left side was normal. There were no other abnormal neurological signs.

D.P. Kidd, *Neuro-Ophthalmology*, DOI 10.1007/978-1-4471-2410-8_33

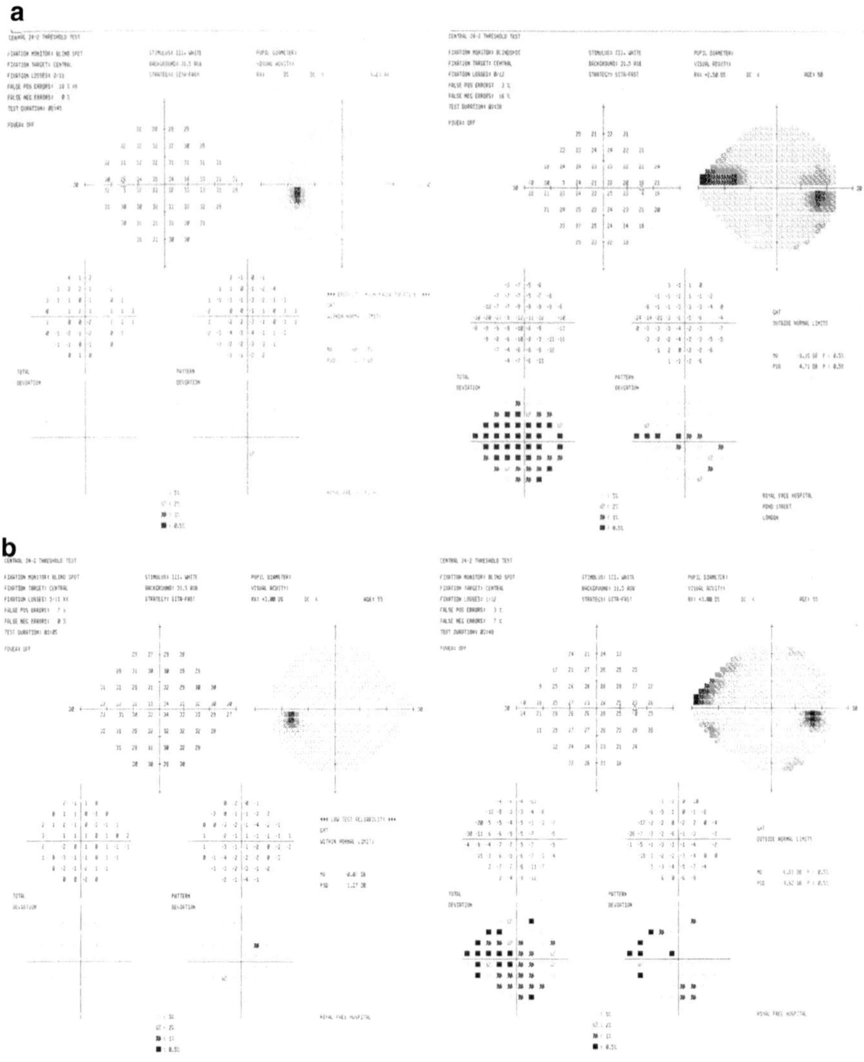

Fig. 33.1 Humphrey visual field (**a**) before and (**b**) after surgery showing a right sided defect

Evaluation

She has a painful optic neuropathy which may have relapsed. Imaging is warranted in this case because of the previous brief and self-limiting disorder, because of the presence of pain, and because there had been no prior neurological symptoms at her age. In addition, on further enquiry there had been a long history of asthma and

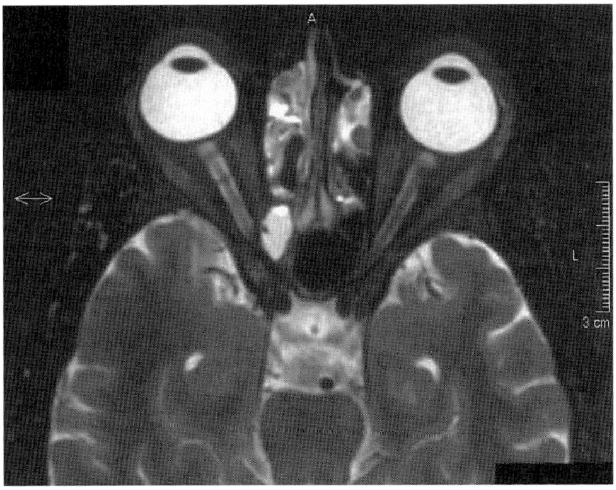

Fig. 33.2 T2 weighted axial MRI showing a high signal mass arising from the posterior ethmoid air cells on the right and extending into the orbital apex causing compression of the right optic nerve

respiratory problems, and she had been treated at the Royal Brompton Hospital with oral and inhaled steroids for many years. We wondered whether or not there may have been an infective disorder arising from the sinuses.

Investigations

Screening blood investigations were normal, although she was noted to have a mild eosinophilia. Serological tests for Aspergillus and mucormycosis were however negative and the ESR and CRP not raised.

Imaging showed a lesion arising from the posterior ethmoid air sinus compressing the medal aspect of the right optic nerve at the orbital apex (Fig. 33.2).

Management

During this time her vision had deteriorated further, to perception of hand movements, and she was referred urgently to the Royal National Nose Throat and Ear hospital for decompressive surgery. This occurred through an endoscopic transnasal approach. Her vision improved to 6/12 with abnormal color vision and a pale disc, and an improved visual field (Fig. 33.1b).

Discussion

Mucocoele of the Paranasal Air Sinuses

Mucocoeles are slowly growing expansile lesions of the paranasal air sinuses which arise when the sinus ostium is blocked by secretions. They are lined by respiratory epithelium and are filled by mucus secretions [1]. The frontal sinuses are the most commonly affected (65 %) followed by the ethmoids (20–30 %). The maxillary sinuses are affected in 10 % of cases and the sphenoid in only 3 %. Over time mucocoeles may erode adjacent bone and protrude and grow into surrounding neurological structures [2].

There is a clear association with chronic rhinosinusitis and many patients have already undergone one or more ENT surgical procedures. It also complicates skull fractures and occurs in fibrous dysplasia for example in the McCune-Albright syndrome.

Frontal mucocoele: if the mucocoele extends backwards over and into the orbit the eye becomes displaced and double vision develops. An optic neuropathy may also arise.

Those arising from the ethmoid sinuses may also displace the orbit, but are also associated with an orbital apex syndrome and cavernous sinus syndrome. Isolated third and sixth neuropathies have been reported as well as unilateral and bilateral optic neuropathies, particularly when the mucocoele arises from the posterior cells. 10 % of people have an additional posterior ethmoid air cell (the Onodi cell) which projects laterally and superiorly and lies behind the sphenoid sinus, immediately beneath the optic nerve before it enters the optic canal. Mucocoeles of this sinus are rare, but commonly associated with optic neuropathy, which may be sudden and simulate an acute optic neuritis [3].

Sphenoid sinus mucocoeles are uncommon, but can grow to a large size. The clinical features depend on the direction in which the mucocoele expands; it may do so superiorly causing bilateral optic neuropathy and destroying the pituitary gland, or to one side associated with cavernous sinus syndrome or isolated third, fourth and sixth neuropathies, or anteriorly to the orbital apex and even into the orbit.

Mucocoeles are treated by experienced sinus surgeons; an endoscopic approach carries a much lower surgical morbidity although external neurosurgical approaches are also on occasion needed [4].

References

1. Lee JT, Brunworth J, Garg R, Shibuya T, Keschner DB, Vanefsky M, Lin T, Choi S, Stea R, Thompson LDR. Intracranial mucocele formation in the context of longstanding chronic rhinosinusitis: a clinicopathologic series and literature review. Allergy Rhinol (Providence). 2013;4:e166–75.
2. Delfini R, Missori P, Ianetti G, Ciapetta P, Cantore G. Mucoceles of the paranasal sinuses with intracranial and intraorbital extension: report of 28 cases. Neurosurgery. 1993;32:901–6.
3. Klink T, Pahnke J, Hoppe F, Lieb W. Acute visual loss by an Onodi cell. Br J Ophthalmol. 2000;84:799.
4. Lund VJ. Endoscopic management of paranasal sinus mucocoeles. J Laryngol Otol. 1998; 112:36–40.

Part IV
The Brain Stem

Case 34

History

This 18 year old university student at UCL, presented via the emergency department. There had been a 3 week history of escalating headache which was worse in the morning and increased with coughing, laughing or straining. There was no prior history of headache, and he was normally in good health. He had suffered glandular fever a year previously but had recovered well.

He presented to the emergency department owing to the development of visual blurring and this became considerably worse when he stood up from lying or sitting; his vision would darken for 2 or 3 seconds then brighten again. There were no other symptoms.

Examination

His central visual acuities were 6/6 N5 in both eyes with normal color vision. The visual fields (Fig. 34.1) showed no peripheral constriction but enlargement of the blind spots on both sides symmetrically. There was no relative afferent pupillary defect.

Examination of the discs revealed a chronic moderately severe papilloedema with a splinter hemorrhage adjacent to the right disc and a cotton wool spot superior to the left (Fig. 34.2). The eye movements were normal, although the pursuit upwards was jerky and there was a reduction in the amplitude of OKN on vertical gaze upwards. There were no other abnormal neurological signs.

D.P. Kidd, *Neuro-Ophthalmology*, DOI 10.1007/978-1-4471-2410-8_34

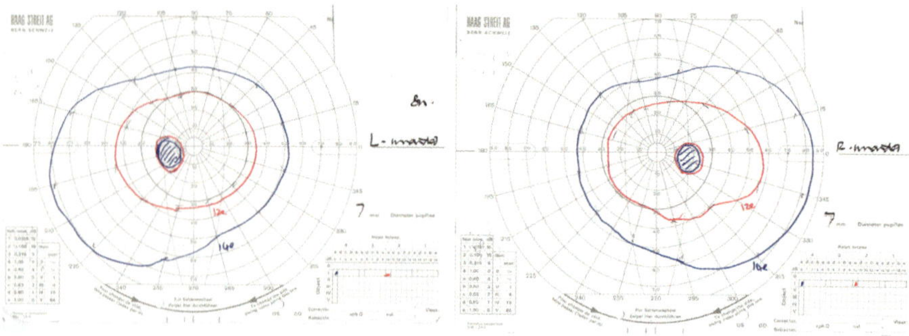

Fig. 34.1 Goldman fields showing enlargement of the blind spots on both sides right more than left, with a slight restriction in peripheral fields

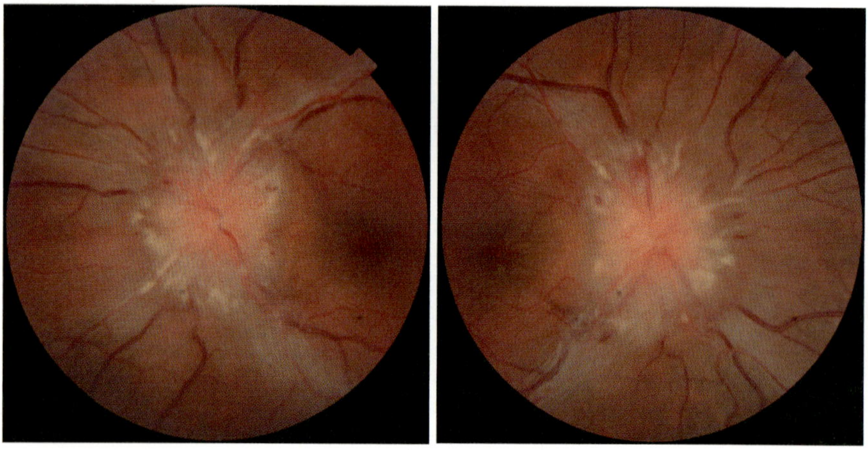

Fig. 34.2 Fundus photographs showing bilateral papilloedema

Clinical Evaluation

Clearly this is an emergency; this young man present with escalating headache and visual symptoms and is seen to have papilloedema. The visual blurring is related to the enlargement of the blind spots; patients can often see their blind spots even when they are of normal size, and it is common that the nasal side, when it increases, becomes visible in papilloedema. There is no evidence for an optic neuropathy, and there is no evidence for a foveal problem, due for example to macular fluid. The visual disorder upon standing is characteristic of transient visual obscuration, a temporary reduction in visual acuity related to high pressure within the optic nerve sheath interfering with axoplasmic flow. It occurs in all types of intracranial hypertension, including idiopathic intracranial hypertension, hydrocephalus, sagittal sinus thrombosis, and also in raised intracranial pressure due to intracerebral mass lesions.

In this case the patient was young, male and thin, and so it was important quickly to proceed to imaging of the brain and venous sinuses. If a mass lesion were not seen, nor hydrocephalus, a venous sinus stenosis or thrombosis should be considered, then a meningitis.

Investigations

Screening blood investigations were uninformative.

An MRI scan of the brain (Fig. 34.3) showed a non-communicating hydrocephalus caused by a lesion of the tectal plate compressing the aqueduct. The lesion did not enhance.

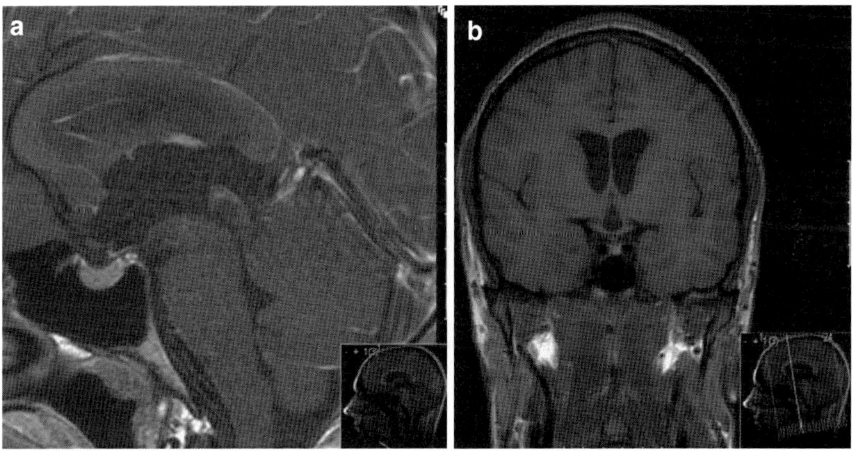

Fig. 34.3 (**a**) T1 weighted sagittal MRI scan showing enlargement of the third and lateral ventricles and a non-enhancing lesion of the tectal plate. Coronal scans (**b**) show the base of the third ventricle prolapsing into the suprasellar cistern

Management

He underwent an endoscopic third ventriculostomy. His hydrocephalus resolved and has not recurred. Cytological examination of the CSF showed no cells, and over a 5 year follow up the brainstem lesion has not enlarged, and he has remained well.

Discussion

This young man was seen in the emergency department on a Wednesday, the neuro-ophthalmology clinic on the next day, had his MRI on the same day, and had neurosurgery on the Friday. This case emphasizes the importance of understanding that the symptoms were evolving and that the signs were developing; there is a very significant risk of permanent visual loss if the source of the raised intracranial pressure is not identified and treated emergently.

Papilloedema arises when raised intracranial pressure prevents or diminishes axoplasmic flow in optic nerve axons. Axoplasm collects at the lamina cribrosa, the axons swell and the disc enlarges. This takes between 1 and 7 days before it is noticeable clinically, although OCT examination of the disc reveals enlargement of the retinal nerve fiber layer at an earlier point [1].

Loss of central visual acuity is usually a very late sign in papilloedema; characteristically there is a peripheral constriction, which allows retention of a normal central acuity, and it may not be identified on a Humphrey visual field, although both Humphrey and Goldman assessments will pick up an enlargement of the blind spot, which occurs when the peripapillary retina becomes filled with fluid. Occasionally this fluid spreads to the macula, causing distortion, and in longstanding cases retinal folds may develop which can also lead to distortion away from foveal vision.

Visual obscuration arises when pressure around the nerve within the optic nerve sheath interferes mechanically with axoplasmic flow; there is normally a pressure gradient between intraocular pressure and retrolaminar pressure (which also allows for venous pulsation in most patients with normal intracranial pressure) and when the patient changes position (commonly standing from lying) there is a net increase in retrolaminar pressure which further impedes axoplasmic flow, resulting in a temporary (lasting a second or 2–20 seconds) loss of optic nerve function [2]. If the cause remains untreated and the pressure is sufficiently high, ischemic change at the disc occurs, leading to nerve fiber bundle defects of the type seen in anterior ischemic optic neuropathy and glaucoma.

In a recent trial of treatment in idiopathic intracranial hypertension 161 of 165 recruited patients were female. The main inclusion criterion was mild (a perimetric mean deviation of −2 to −7 dB) visual loss. In this group 32 % had noted visual loss and 68 % had experienced visual obscurations [3]. Visual acuity was 20/20 (6/6) or better in 71 % and the most common visual field defect was a partial arcuate defect with enlargement of the blind spot. Twelve percent showed enlarged blind spot with a normal surrounding field [4]. High CSF pressure was associated with increasing severity of papilloedema [5].

References

1. Auinger P, Durbin M, Feldon S, Garvin M, Kardon R, Keltner J, Kupersmith M, Sibony P, Plumb K, Wang JK, Werner JS. Baseline OCT measurements in the idiopathic intracranial hypertension treatment trial, part1: quality control, comparisons and variability. Invest Ophthalmol Vis Sci. 2014;55:8180–8.
2. Tso MO, Hayreh SS. Optic disc edema in raised intracranial pressure IV. Axoplasmic transport in experimental papilledema. Arch Ophthalmol. 1977;95:1458–62.
3. Wall M, Kupersmith MJ, Kieburtz KD, Corbett JJ, Feldon SE, Friedman DI, Katz DM, Keltner JL, Schron EB, McDermott MP. The idiopathic intracranial hypertension treatment trial: clinical profile at baseline. JAMA Neurol. 2014;71:693–701.
4. Keltner JL, Johnson CA, Cello KE, Wall M. Baseline visual field findings in the idiopathic intracranial hypertension treatment trial. Invest Ophthalmol Vis Sci. 2014;55:3200–7.
5. Kattah JC, Pula JH, Mejico LJ, McDermott MP, Kupersmith MJ. CSF pressure, papilledema grade, and response to acetozolamide in the Idiopathic Intracranial Hypertension treatment trial. J Neurol. 2015;262:2271–4.

Case 35

History

This 68 year old man presented with a 6 month history of increasing problems with balance and a tendency to fall backwards. There was no weakness or sensory disturbance, no sphincter dysfunction or autonomic instability, and no cognitive symptom. There was a slight tremor of both hands.

He was otherwise well, and neither hypertensive nor diabetic.

Examination

His gait was normal but a little unsteady walking heel to toe. The postural reflexes were unimpaired. There was a mild rather high frequency postural tremor of the hands without rigidity or bradykinesia. There was no ataxia of the limbs. There was no weakness or spasticity and the limb reflexes were normal. Sensation including proprioception was also normal.

His voice was a little hoarse and possibly dysarthric. The jaw reflex was brisker than average.

The eye movements were abnormal with a reduction of vertical gaze on both sides, and the vertical saccades were slow. The horizontal eye movements were full but again the saccadic velocities were reduced. The boundary of the vertical eye movements could be enlarged by moving the head whilst asking him to fixate on a steady target. There was no nystagmus and no square wave jerk.

D.P. Kidd, *Neuro-Ophthalmology*, DOI 10.1007/978-1-4471-2410-8_35

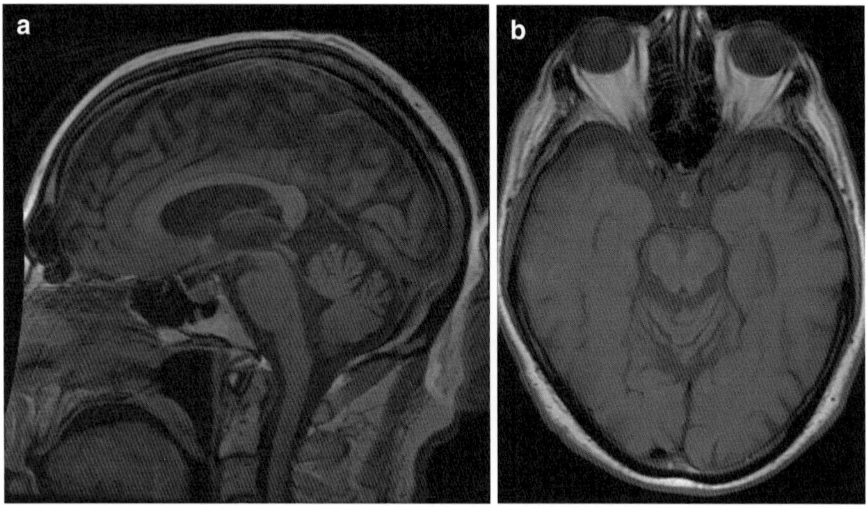

Fig. 35.1 T1 weighted (**a**) sagittal and (**b**) axial MRI scan of brain showing atrophy of the midbrain with normal structure in the pons leading to the "hummingbird" appearance of the brainstem

Clinical Evaluation

A problem with balance with a tendency to fall in an otherwise healthy individual is always significant, even if the examination fails to identity a clear reason for it. In this case there were few abnormal signs when first seen, aside from a disorder of gaze, and this is clearly highly significant. The abnormalities described are in keeping with a supranuclear gaze palsy. The eye movements are conjugate and the saccadic velocities are slow.

Investigations

The screening blood investigations were normal. A serum copper level was normal.

An MRI scan of the brain (Fig. 35.1) was considered to be within normal limits, although the midbrain is seen to be small.

A diagnosis of progressive supranuclear palsy was made, and he was monitored carefully. He did not respond to Amantidine and this was discontinued after a time. He deteriorated, developing a horizontal gaze palsy with square wave jerks, and a more prominent dysarthria. He had to retire from teaching, but continued to write. Dysphagia developed about 3 years after diagnosis.

Discussion

Progressive Supranuclear Palsy

This is a rare disease with an incidence of $1–2 \times 10^5$ per year [1, 2]. The pathological process is deposition of abnormally phosphorylated tau protein which leads to development of neurofibrillary tangles and argyrophyllic inclusions in astrocytes and oligodendrocytes (Fig. 35.2). Neuronal loss ensues, particularly in the brain stem and basal ganglia, and specifically the superior colliculus, oculomotor nuclei, pedunculopontine nuclei, the vestibular nuclei and inferior olives, and the globus pallidus, subthalamic nuclei, substantia nigra and periaqueductal gray matter. The pathological features seen are easily differentiated from other neurodegenerative diseases related to tau deposition, including corticobasal ganglionic degeneration, Pick's disease and others.

Pathological studies of patients with Parkinsonian syndromes has shown that not all those with a typical PSP neuropathology have the typical clinical phenotype; in one series [3] only 54% of 103 cases were thus, with others showing a cross-over between PSP with asymmetric akinetic rigid syndromes. Further subdivisions have led to the definition of a series of subcategories of so-called atypical PSP, including brainstem predominate PSP in which levo-Dopa responsiveness is often, although not always, seen, and with pure akinesia and gait freezing [3], and cortical predominate PSP disorders, whose clinical phenotype precisely correlates with the topographic distribution of the neuropathological features. In the typical PSP cases cortical tau pathology is uncommon; in the cortical predominant atypical subtype cortical tau pathology is greatly more evident, leading to syndromes associated with primary progressive aphasia, corticobasal syndrome, frontal dementia, and primary lateral sclerosis.

The clinical features of the "typical PSP" syndrome involve an early loss of postural reflexes leading to falls (often backwards) and this is related to neuronal loss in the pedunculopontine nuclei. There is an ataxic gait and a symmetrical rigidity which usually affects axial muscles more than those of the limbs.

The neuro-ophthalmic features of typical PSP involve a vertical gaze palsy initially, in which downwards saccadic movements become slow first, then upwards. The saccades are hypometric. Later horizontal movements become slow and hypometric, and square wave jerks, which are horizontal saccadic intrusions which disrupt gaze-holding, are seen. Convergence is reduced but the vestibulo-ocular reflex persists, although in the end all eye movements are lost. Eyelid problems, including apraxia of eyelid opening and blepharospasm, may occur. The neuropathological correlates of these clinical signs are loss of neurons in the superior colliculus and the rostral interstitial nucleus of the medial longitudinal fasciculus in the midbrain and the nucleus raphe interpositus in the pons.

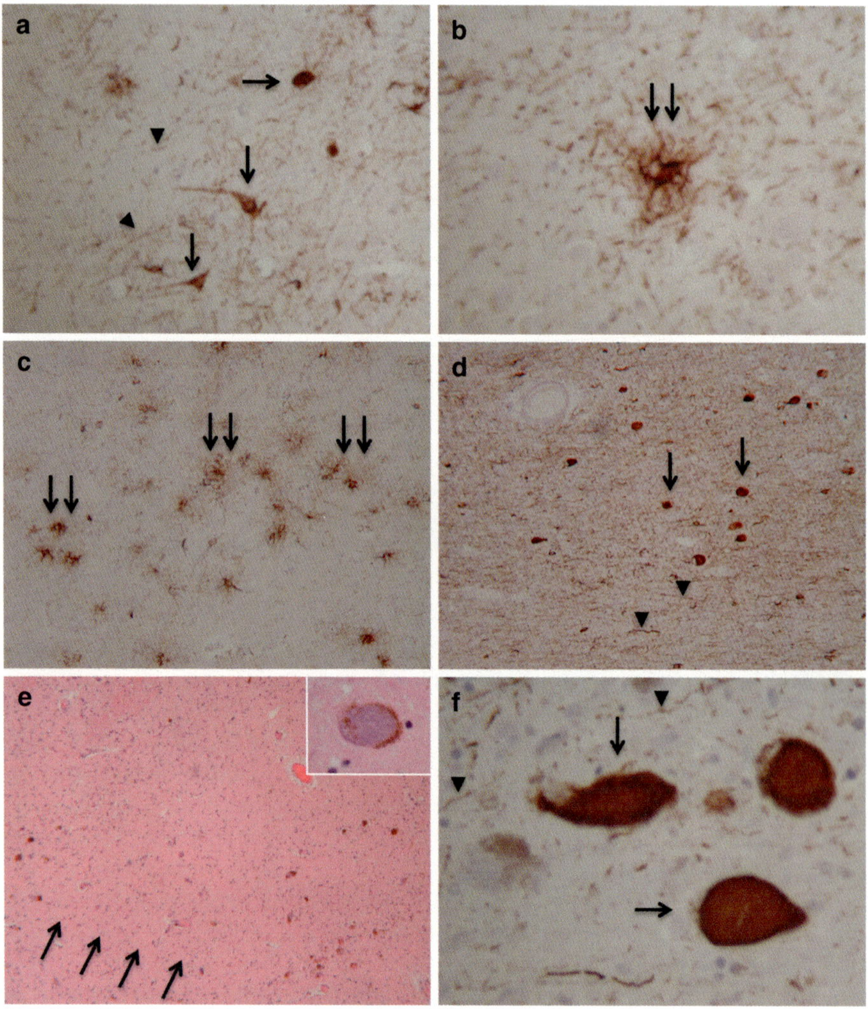

Fig. 35.2 Microscopic findings of progressive supranuclear palsy: Tau immunohistochemistry (**a**–**d**, **f**) highlights the characteristic lesions seen in progressive supranuclear palsy: neurofibrillary tangles (*arrow*), neuropil threads (*arrow head*) (**a**, **d**, **f**) shown in anterior frontal cortex (**a**), subthalamic nucleus (**d**) and substantia nigra (**f**) and the pathognomonic tufted astrocytes (*double arrow*) demonstrated in the anterior frontal cortex (**b**) and caudate nucleus (**c**). Micrograph of the hematoxylin and eosin-stained section of the midbrain (**e**) illustrates severe loss of neurons in the substantia nigra (*arrows*) with the insert showing a 'globose' neurofibrillary tangle in a nigra neuron (Courtesy Prof Tomas Revesz, Dept. Neuropathology, Institute of Neurology)

Dysarthria and dysphagia develop late, alongside a subcortical type slowing of cognitive processing, with apathy and concentrational deficits. The disease course is on average 7–8 years [2].

Imaging shows atrophy of the upper brain stem and periaqueductal gray matter (which can lead to the "hummingbird sign" on sagittal T1 weighted MRI: Fig. 35.1).

References

1. Dickson DW, Ahmed Z, Algom AA, Tsuboi Y, Josephs KA. Neuropathology of variants of progressive supranuclear palsy. Curr Opin Neurol. 2010;23:394–400.
2. Golbe LI. Progressive supranuclear palsy. Semin Neurol. 2014;34:151–9.
3. Williams DR, de Silva R, Paviour DC, Pittman A, Watt HC, Kilford L, Holton JL, Revesz T, Lees AJ. Characteristics of two distinct clinical phenotypes in pathologically proven progressive supranuclear palsy: Richardson's syndrome and PSP-parkinsonism. Brain. 2005;128:1247–58.

Case 36

History

This young man was 18 when he developed his first neurological symptoms; a subacute brain stem disturbance with left sided ataxia, double vision and a sense of rotatory vertigo. He was admitted to hospital and underwent investigations. He received treatment with intravenous corticosteroids and improved.

A year later he developed a subacute ascending numbness to the upper chest with some urinary urgency and a slight impairment of gait. This too resolved.

Over the following years he suffered repeated episodes of similar symptoms, increasingly associated with a gradual accrual of neurological impairment, manifested as an ataxia of gait, spasticity of the lower limbs, urgency of micturition and urge incontinence. After 5 years he was no longer able to walk. He received treatment, but showed no response.

At the age of 22, during a further attack of imbalance, he developed double vision and blurred vision with oscillopsia. This was so severe that he was unable to read or watch television. It affected all directions of gaze. It did not improve.

Examination

His central visual acuity was 6/60 on both sides, without color vision. The pupillary responses were slow but symmetrical. The discs were pale.

The eyes moved constantly and conjugately, at a frequency of about 4 Hz, in all directions of gaze; when he looked right or left they moved horizontally; when up and down the movements were vertical. The velocity of the eye movements was the same in every direction. The saccadic velocities were slow and horizontal movements revealed a bilateral internuclear ophthalmoparesis (in which the adducting eye moved more slowly than the abducting eye on each side) was seen. No torsional movements were observed.

D.P. Kidd, *Neuro-Ophthalmology*, DOI 10.1007/978-1-4471-2410-8_36

There was a slurring cerebellar dysarthria, and a marked bilateral cerebellar tremor on intention. In the limbs there was spasticity and a pyramidal pattern of weakness. The reflexes were abnormally brisk and the plantar responses were extensor.

Clinical Evaluation

The history is typical for a rather aggressive form of the demyelinating disorder multiple sclerosis. His investigations confirmed this; in particular the MRI showed white matter lesions above and below the tentorium, and those above showed a periventricular pattern (Fig. 36.1a). There were numerous lesions within the brainstem (Fig. 36.1b,c). A spinal fluid examination revealed the presence of unmatched oligoclonal bands.

The eye movement disorder is one of nystagmus, and there is neither slow nor fast phase. The nystagmus therefore is a pendular nystagmus, and so this patient has an acquired pendular nystagmus.

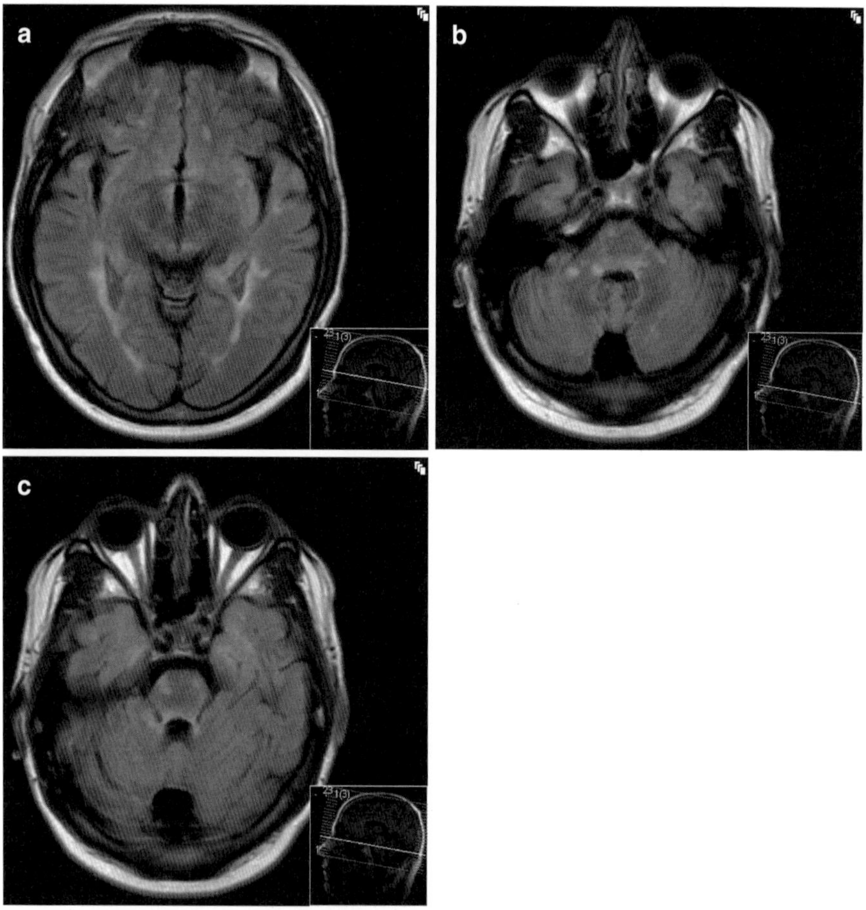

Fig. 36.1 Axial FLAIR MRI scan of brain showing numerous white matter lesions typical of that seen in multiple sclerosis (**a**) in a periventricular pattern and (**b**, **c**) within the brain stem

Acquired Pendular Nystagmus

In pendular nystagmus there is no slow or fast phase and the movements are seen to be pseudo-sinusoidal on an electronystagmogram [1] (Fig. 36.2). There are often horizontal, vertical and tortional components, and this can lead to backwards and forwards movements, convergence and divergence, and, if the vertical and horizontal components are exactly in phase, the movements with be oblique. If out of phase they often appear elliptical, if they are exactly 90° out of phase they will be circular [2] (and see Case 38).

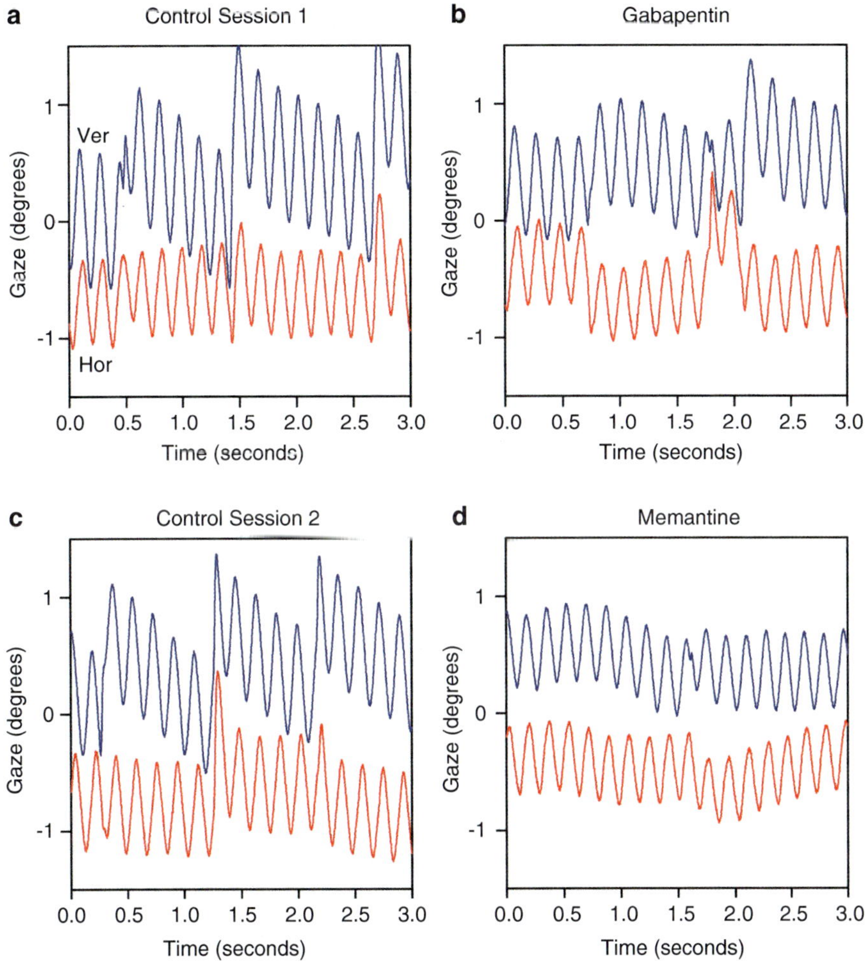

Fig. 36.2 Patients' eye movement velocities were measured using a magnetic search coil technique before and after treatment with Gabapentin and Memantine. The patient shown, who had MS, responded to the latter but not the former (Reproduced with permission from Thurtell et al. [3])

The disorder thus develops when there is a visual deficit and a coexisting brain stem or cerebellar disorder. It is thought to come about through instability of the neural integrator, partly though a lack of visual input and partly through dysfunction of the pathways involved in the pons [2]. One eye is often more affected than the other; usually the one with the more poor vision. In this case the movements were present in all directions of gaze, and symmetrical, presumably because the acuities were equally poor in each eye.

It is seen most often in multiple sclerosis but also in other demyelinating diseases such as Pelizaeus-Merzbacher disease and Cockayne syndrome, in Whipple's disease (when it forms part of the syndrome of oculo-masticatory myorhythmia), and in disorders of the brain stem including stroke and hemorrhage, and in cerebellar degenerations. It may be associated thus with a synchronous palatal tremor, in oculo-palatal tremor [2].

Treatment with gabapentin, baclofen, benzodiazepines and memantine sometimes ameliorates the amplitude of the oscillations, but high doses are required in order to allow an improvement in visual acuity [3]. One study of ten patients found that more than half were shown to have a reduction in amplitude of the oscillations and around half showed an improvement in reading acuity of 0.1 [4]. Some responded to memantine and not gabapentin, and others the opposite.

References

1. Leigh RJ, Zee DS. Diagnosis of central disorders of ocular motility. In: Leigh RJ, Zee DS, editors. The diagnosis of disorders of eye movements. New York: Oxford University Press; 1999. p. 436–8.
2. Thurtell MJ, Leigh RJ. Nystagmus and saccadic intrusions. In: Kennard C, Leigh RJ, editors. Handbook of clinical neurology volume 102: neuro-ophthalmology. Amsterdam: Elsevier; 2011. p. 350–2.
3. Thurtell MJ, Joshi AC, Leone AC, Tomsak RL, Kosmorsky GS, Stahl JS, Leigh RJ. Crossover trial of gabapentin and memantine as treatment for acquired nystagmus. Ann Neurol. 2010;67:676–80.
4. Starck M, Albrecht H, Pollmann W, Dieterich M, Straube A. Acquired pendular nystagmus in multiple sclerosis: an examiner-blind cross-over study of memantine and gabapentin. J Neurol. 2010;257:322–7.

Case 37

History

This lady was 28 when she noticed a slight diminishment of balance when walking, and occasional problems with manual dexterity. These symptoms slowly became more noticeable over a 10 year period.

She was referred with difficulty in focusing and a problem when reading in which as she scanned across the line she would sometimes notice that the words would blur, and occasionally she would lose her place.

She worked as a librarian, so these reading problems were to her more intrusive than the problems with her gait.

There were no other neurological symptoms and at the time she was not aware of any family history of similar problems.

Examination

The central acuities were 6/6 N5 in both eyes. There was normal color vision and the fields were full. The ocular media were clear and the discs normal. The corneae and the retinae in particular were normal.

The eye movements were full and only slightly fragmented. There was no nystagmus and there were no square wave jerks. Examination of saccadic movements revealed a striking slowness to saccadic velocities with a mild hypometria.

Examination of the limbs revealed a bilateral and symmetrical upper and lower limb ataxia with rather brisk reflexes and flexor plantar responses. Strength and sensation were normal. There was a slurring dysarthria and she was unable to walk heel-to-toe.

D.P. Kidd, *Neuro-Ophthalmology*, DOI 10.1007/978-1-4471-2410-8_37

Clinical Evaluation

The history is of a very slowly progressive disorder involving balance and vision. It is too slow for a vascular or inflammatory disorder (even primary progressive MS), although could be caused by a brain stem glioma, which sometimes evolves very slowly indeed. A lesion at the foramen magnum, for example a meningioma or an Arnold Chiari malformation, would cause downbeating nystagmus and would not be associated with slow saccadic velocities. Metabolic disorders such as vitamin deficiency, Wilson's disease, Niemann Pick disease, Gaucher's disease and intoxication with soporific drugs would all be associated with other clinical features.

Investigations

Full blood count and biochemical screening were normal. Copper studies were also normal. Acathocytes were not found on a peripheral blood film. Vitamin levels including vitamin E were normal.

Nerve conduction studies were normal.

An MRI scan of the brain (Fig. 37.1) showed a striking atrophy of the brain stem and cerebellum.

Genetic studies for the spinocerebellar ataxias SCA 1 to 7 revealed an expansion in the SCA 2 locus.

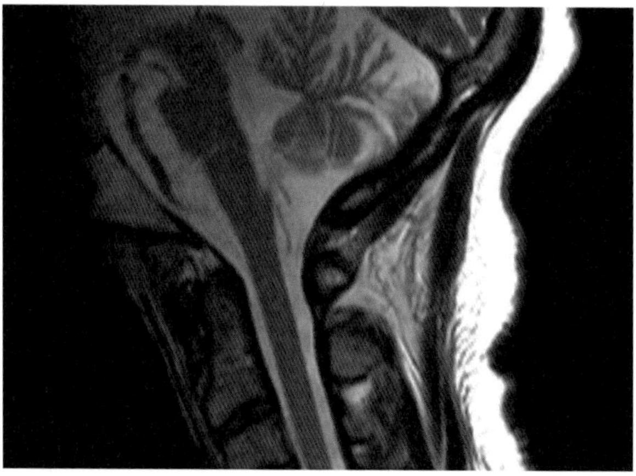

Fig. 37.1 T2 weighted sagittal MRI showing a striking atrophy of the cerebellum and the pons

Disease Progression

Over 10 years since diagnosis the eye movement disorder is unchanged but her gait is poor and she is largely confined to a wheelchair. She had to retire from her job in the library. She developed some spasms and tremors in her jaw for a time but these latterly have resolved. Her cognitive function remains reasonable although formal testing has revealed a subcortical frontal disorganization with poor attention and memory. Her sister was also diagnosed with the condition.

Discussion

She has a spinocerebellar ataxia and the clinical phenotype is typical for the SCA 2 variant. This is an autosomal dominantly inherited disorder. The genetic abnormality is a trinucleotide (CAG) expansion in the Ataxin-2 gene ATXN2. SCA 1, 2, 3, 6, 7 and DRPLA (dentatorubropallidoluysian atrophy) are all caused by a polyglutamine encoding CAG repeat within the respective genes. Each is rare with a prevalence of around 4 per 10^5 in each case. The age of onset for SCA 1, 2 and 3 is in the fourth decade, whilst that of SCA 6, the pure form of cerebellar ataxia, is in the sixth or seventh decade [1, 2]. These four subgroups comprise more than half of all autosomal dominant cerebellar ataxias. The size of the expansion correlates with age of onset [3].

The diagnosis is made genetically; all the cases used to be referred to as ADCA (autosomal dominant cerebellar ataxia) type II. Many share clinical features, but in general those with SCA 1 have pyramidal tract signs whereas peripheral neuropathy and dystonia is more common in SCA 2 and 3. Nystagmus, dysmetric and slow saccadic eye movements and fragmented smooth pursuit occur in all three, but the saccadic velocities are much slower in SCA 2 than in the other groups. Ophthalmoparesis is less common in SCA 2 than in SCA 1 and 3. Those with SCA 6 form a separate group in which there is an older age of onset and a more pure cerebellar ataxia. These patients have less abnormal saccades and a higher prevalence of nystagmus, including downbeating nystagmus [4, 5].

Imaging shows very specific changes, with brain stem and cerebellar atrophy in SCA 1 and 3, and atrophy confined to the cerebellar gray matter in SCA 6 [6]. This is also seen in SCA 2, as shown in the figure.

References

1. Jacobi H, Bauer P, Giunti P, Labrum R, Sweeney MG, Charles P, Durr A, Marelli C, Globas C, Linnemann C, Schols L, Rakowicz M, Rola R, Zdzienicka E, Schmitz-Hubsch T, Fancellu R, Mariotti C, Tomasello C, Baliko L, Melagh B, Filla A, Rinaldi C, van de Warrenburg BP, Verstappen CCP, Szymanski S, Berciano J, Infante J, Timmann D, Boesch S, Hering S, Depondt C, Pandolfo M, Kang J-S, Ratzka S, Schulz J, Tezenas du Montcel S, Klockgether T. The natural history of spinocerebellar ataxia type 1, 2, 3 and 6. Neurology. 2011;77:1035–41.
2. Ashizawa T, Figueroa KP, Periman SL, Gomez CM, Wilmot GR, Schmahmann JD, Ying SH, Zesiewicz TA, Paulson HL, Shakkottai VG, Bushara KO, Kuo S-H, Geschwind MD, Xia G, Mazzoni P, Krischer JP, Cuthbertson D, Holbert AR, Ferguson JH, Pulst SM, Subramony SH. Clinical characteristics of patients with spinocerebellar ataxias 1, 2, 3 and 6 in the US; a prospective observational study. Orphanet J Rare Dis. 2013;8:177: 1172-8.
3. Tezenas du Montcel S, Durr A, Rakowicz M, Nanetti L, Charles P, Sulek A, Mariotti C, Rola R, Schols L, Bauer P, Dufaure-Garé I, Jacobi H, Forlani S, Schmitz-Hübsch T, Filla A, Timmann D, van de Warrenburg BP, Marelli C, Kang JS, Giunti P, Cook A, Baliko L, Melegh B, Boesch S, Szymanski S, Berciano J, Infante J, Buerk K, Masciullo M, Di Fabio R, Depondt C, Ratka S, Stevanin G, Klockgether T, Brice A, Golmard JL. Prediction of the age at onset in spinocerebellar ataxia type 1, 2, 3 and 6. J Med Genet. 2014;51:479–86.
4. Jacobi H, Hauser TK, Giunti P, Globas C, Bauer P, Schmitz-Hübsch T, Baliko L, Filla A, Mariotti C, Rakowicz M, Charles P, Ribai P, Szymanski S, Infante J, van de Warrenburg BP, Dürr A, Timmann D, Boesch S, Fancellu R, Rola R, Depondt C, Schöls L, Zdzienicka E, Kang JS, Ratzka S, Kremer B, Stephenson DA, Melegh B, Pandolfo M, Tezenas du Montcel S, Borkert J, Schulz JB, Klockgether T. Spinocerebellar ataxia types 1, 2, 3 and 6: the clinical spectrum of ataxia and morphometric brainstem and cerebellar findings. Cerebellum. 2012;11:155–66.
5. Moscovich M, Okun MS, Favilla C, Figueroa KP, Pulst SM, Perlman S, Wilmot G, Gomez C, Schmahmann J, Paulson H, Shakkottai V, Ying S, Zesiewicz T, Kuo SH, Mazzoni P, Bushara K, Xia G, Ashizawa T, Subramony SH. Clinical evaluation of eye movements in spinocerebellar ataxias: a prospective multicentre study. J Neuroophthalmol. 2014;35:16–21.
6. Schulz JB, Borkert J, Wolf S, Schmitz-Hübsch T, Rakowicz M, Mariotti C, Schöls L, Timmann D, van de Warrenburg B, Dürr A, Pandolfo M, Kang JS, Mandly AG, Nägele T, Grisoli M, Boguslawska R, Bauer P, Klockgether T, Hauser TK. Visualization, quantification and correlation of brain atrophy with clinical symptoms in spinocerebellar ataxia types 1, 3 and 6. Neuroimage. 2010;49:158–68.

Case 38

History

This 38 year old man was referred by his GP to the local ophthalmic service for evaluation of a 2 month history of blurring of vision on the left side and a feeling of oscillopsia in the primary position of gaze. He was found to have nystagmus and was referred to the Neuro-ophthalmology clinic of the Royal Free Hospital.

Previously well, he had not experienced any other neurological symptoms until that time. There was no family history of neurological disease and he took no treatment.

Examination

He saw 6/9 N6 on the right, 6/36 N18 on the left. Color vision was normal on the right and 3/17 on the left. There was a left sided relative afferent pupillary defect. Each disc showed a temporal pallor, more evident on the left. The ocular media were clear.

In the primary position of gaze both eyes vibrated with an upbeat nystagmus. This increased on upgaze and horizontal gaze to the left, and was present also on downgaze, and continued on horizontal movements. In addition the left eye rotated slowly at a frequency of around 3 Hz in a clockwise direction. The saccadic movements were hypometric and, on horizontal movement to the left, adduction on the left moved more slowly than abduction on the right.

The neurological examination revealed a moderate bilateral upper limb ataxia and brisk reflexes without weakness or spasticity.

D.P. Kidd, *Neuro-Ophthalmology*, DOI 10.1007/978-1-4471-2410-8_38

Clinical Evaluation

This man presents with oscillopsia and is found to have rather widespread neurological signs, involving the optic nerves, the brain stem and cerebellum, and the spinal cord. Clearly all the signs point to a single disorder, but not to a single location. A structural lesion caused by a tumor or a vascular disorder would be unlikely; a degenerative or inherited disorder would be uncommon at this age and the history is rather short; infective, inflammatory and metabolic disorders need to be considered first.

There are four neuro-ophthalmic syndromes in this case; first a slow downwards drift of the eyes in the primary position followed by a fast movement upwards. This is nystagmus, and because it is seen in primary position and in all directions of gaze it is a third degree nystagmus. The direction of the fast phase is up so it is an upbeat nystagmus. This is seen most often in lesions of the medulla in the paramedian position at the pontomedullary junction.

Secondly there is a left sided internuclear ophthalmoplegia; the horizontal saccadic movements are not conjugate and there is a delay in initiation, so-called adduction lag, and a partial failure of adduction on the left. This is seen in lesions involving the medial longitudinal fasciculus.

Thirdly there is evidence for bilateral, left greater than right, optic neuropathy. Each disc is pale, although there is a retention of color acuity on the right, and more clear signs of an optic neuropathy on the left. The distance and near acuity will be influenced by the optic neuropathies but also by the eye movement disorder.

Finally there is this curious rotatory movement of the left eye at 3 Hz in a circular and clockwise direction. This is a form of pendular nystagmus (discussed in Case 36), in which the vertical and horizontal phases of nystagmus equally counteract the other, leading to a circular motion. It is seen when the deep cerebellar nuclei and their connections are diseased, and is associated with poor vision. As seen in this case, the nystagmus is greater in the eye with the more poor vision, the Heimann-Bielschowsky phenomenon.

Investigation

His MRI (Fig. 38.1) showed numerous white matter lesions within the brain stem and elsewhere. The visual evoked potentials were delayed on both sides and examination of the CSF revealed the presence of oligoclonal bands. I diagnosed multiple sclerosis.

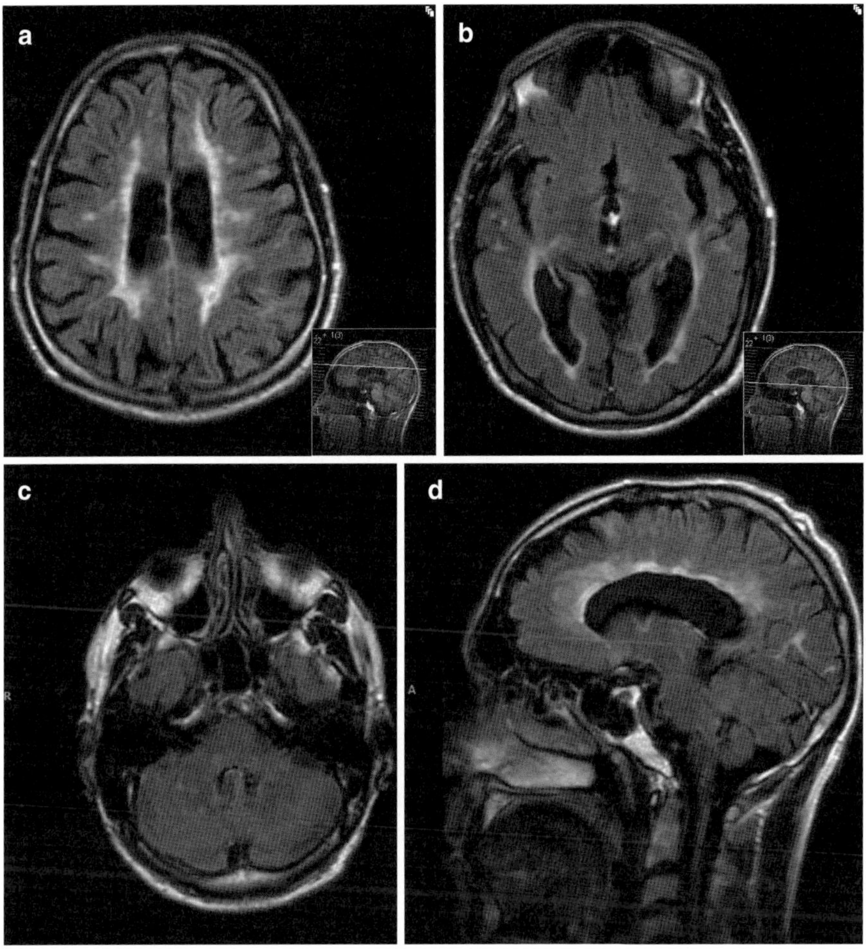

Fig. 38.1 FLAIR sequence (**a**–**c**) axial and (**d**) sagittal MRI showing numerous white matter lesions in a periventricular pattern within the brain and brain stem typical of that seen in multiple sclerosis. There are several lesions within the corpus callosum. Note the lesion seen medially at the pontomedullary junction (**d**)

Discussion

Upbeat Nystagmus

The slow phase is in a downwards direction and the direction of the fast phase determines the description. Unlike downbeating nystagmus the amplitude tends not to be increased in lateral gaze. Alexander's law states that the velocity of the slow phase is greater when the head is turned in the direction of the fast phase, and in upbeat nystagmus the velocity of the downwards movement therefore is quicker when the head moves up. In some cases convergence enhances the amplitude of the nystagmus (although in others it may do the opposite) [1]. It tends to be present in the primary position of gaze and varies with head position [2]. This and the obeying of Alexander's law makes it clear that the nystagmus is strongly influenced by otolith stimulation.

When single lesions are found they tend to be seen in the medial part of the medulla involving the perihypoglossal nuclei [2, 3]; it is supposed that the lesion interferes with connections between the vestibular nuclei and the interstitial nucleus of Cahal.

Table 38.1 Causes of upbeat nystagmus [1, 2]

Structural lesions at the medial pontomedullary and pontomesencephalic junction:
Inflammatory lesion: MS, sarcoidosis, Behçet's syndrome
Vascular lesions: infarction, hemorrhage, arteriovenous malformations
Tumors and infections
Cerebellar degenerations
Wernicke's encephalopathy (there are case reports of it being the only neurological sign)
Organophosphate poisoning
Anti-convulsant drug toxicity

Internuclear Ophthalmoplegia

Axons which form the medial longitudinal fasciculus (MLF) pass from the abducens nucleus to the oculomotor nucleus. This allows conjugate contraction of the ipsilateral lateral rectus and the contralateral medial rectus muscles on horizontal gaze. Lesions which affect the MLF therefore disrupt this pathway, leading to a failure of adduction or adduction lag on the side of the lesion, and nystagmus within the abducting eye (so-called ataxic or dissociated nystagmus) due to drift of the abducting eye with a corrective saccade.

Pathways between the vestibular nuclei in the pons and nuclei in the midbrain which control vertical gaze also pass within the MLF, and it is common to see skew deviation with INO. The hyperphoric eye is on the side of the lesion. Vertical and torsional nystagmus may also be seen [4].

The "one and a half syndrome" arises when the MLF and the adjacent parapontine reticular formation (PPRF) are both involved in a lesion of the pons on one side. This leads to a horizontal gaze palsy and an ipsilateral INO, with the result that the only remaining horizontal movement is the contralateral abducting eye. If the lesion is discrete vertical movements will not be affected.

The causes of these lesions are as noted before; vascular, inflammatory, infective and neoplastic lesions are the most common.

References

1. Leigh RJ, Zee DS. Diagnosis of central disorders of ocular motility. In: Leigh RJ, Zee DS, editors. The neurology of eye movements. 3rd ed. New York: Oxford University Press; 1999. p. 417–38.
2. Fisher A, Gresty M, Chambers B, Rudge P. Primary position upbeating nystagmus: a variety of central positional nystagmus. Brain. 1983;106:949–64.
3. Janssen JC, Larner AJ, Morris H, Bronstein AM, Farmer SF. Upbeat nystagmus: clinicoanatomical correlation. J Neurol Neurosurg Psychiatry. 1998;55:380–1.
4. Leigh RJ, Zee DS. Diagnosis of central disorders of ocular motility. In: Leigh RJ, Zee DS, editors. The neurology of eye movements. 3rd ed. New York: Oxford University Press; 1999. p. 502–10.

Case 39

History

This man presented at the age of 18 years with the abrupt onset of diplopia with pupillary dilatation on the right, which was painless. The diplopia was worse on looking down and there was a mild ptosis. This all improved quickly over the course of 10 days and when reviewed in the ophthalmic department all that remained was a slight pupillary inequality.

Nonetheless investigations were performed and the putative cause identified.

He presented again 2 years later with an identical clinical syndrome which too resolved over a few weeks. Over the following 6 years it recurred three times more, with an incomplete recovery, and a slight movement induced tremor of the left hand with loss of balance.

Examination

The anterior visual pathways and discs were normal. There was a partial right ptosis and slight pupillary mydriasis. There was a left over right hyperphoria in the primary position due to underaction of the elevators on the right, and medial rectus was also weak. The eye movements on the left were normal. There were no other abnormalities in the cranial nerves, nor in the limbs save for an intention tremor of the left upper limb with mild dysmetria and dysdiadochokinesis.

D.P. Kidd, *Neuro-Ophthalmology*, DOI 10.1007/978-1-4471-2410-8_39

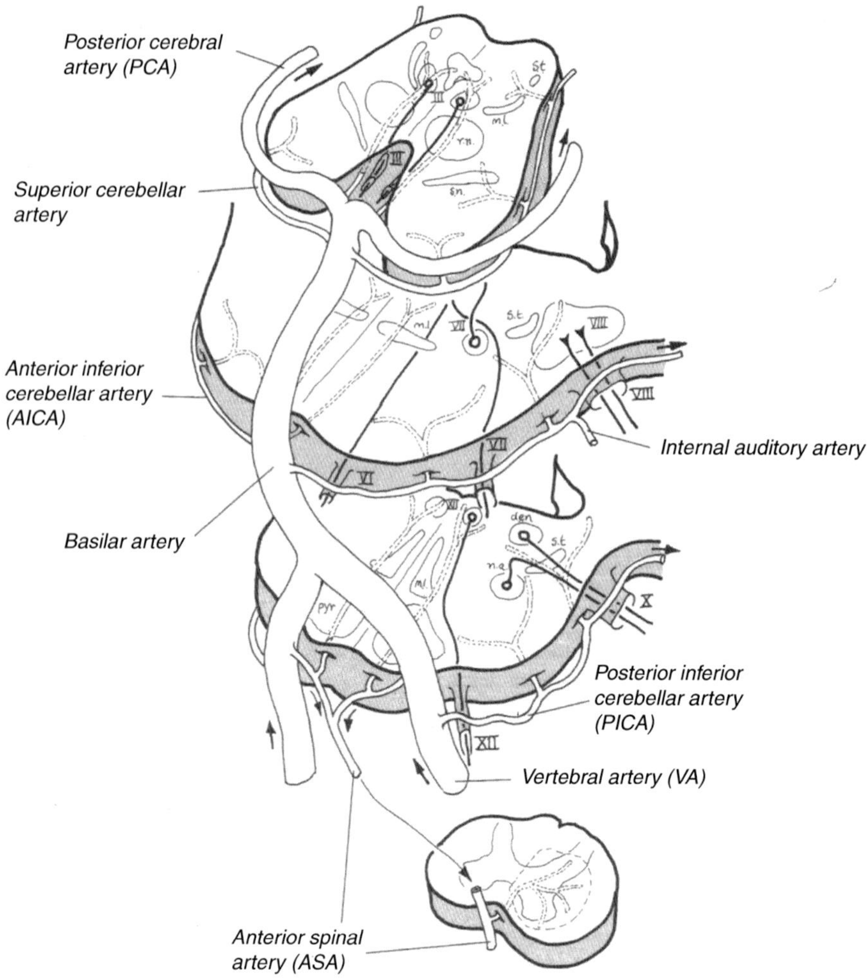

Fig. 39.1 The vascular supply of the brain stem (Reproduced with permission from Patten [6])

Evaluation

This young man has a relapsing remitting disorder which always affects the same area of the nervous system, which recovers but increasingly incompletely, leading to an accrual of impairments each time the event occurs. There is a right sided third nerve palsy which involves the pupil, and there is a contralateral ataxia. The lesion must be in the brain stem, therefore, and, because the ataxia is contralateral to the lesion (see Fig. 39.1) it must be in the midbrain, and on the right side.

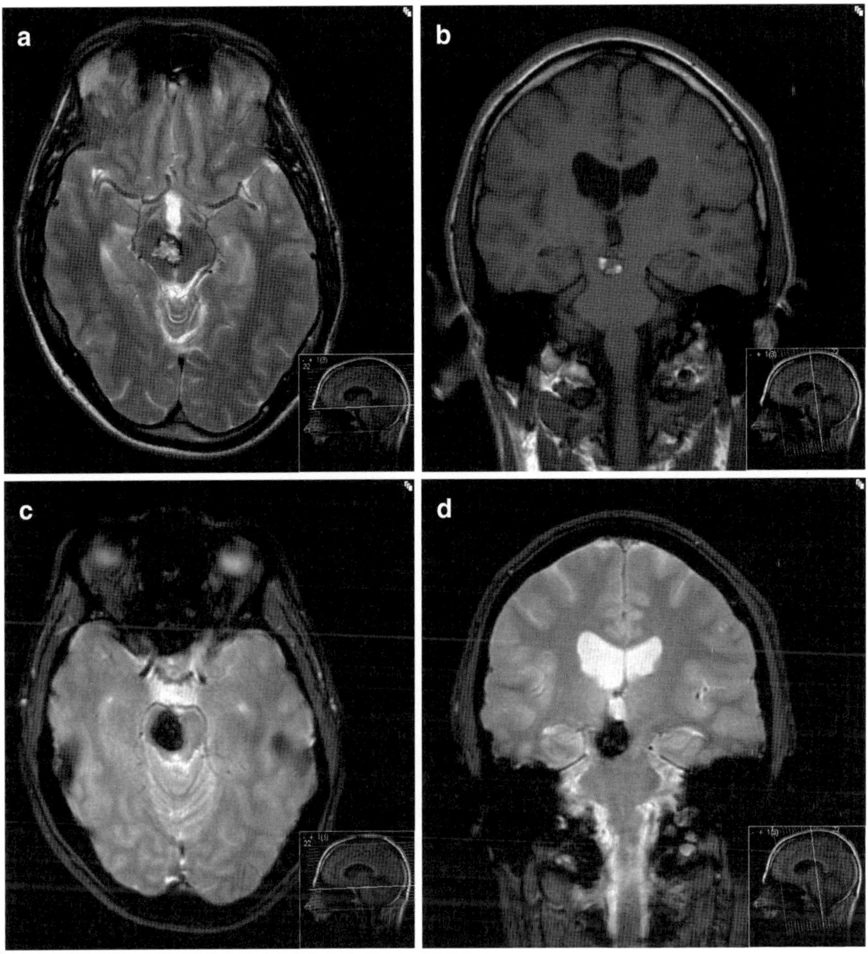

Fig. 39.2 (**a**, **b**) T2 weighted axial and T1 weighted coronal; (**c**, **d**) T2* weighted axial and coronal MRI showing the cavernous hemangioma with a mixture of signal characteristics and hemosiderin staining throughout

The MRI scan (Fig. 39.2) shows a lesion of the right side of the midbrain with prominent staining with hemosiderin. It is compatible with a cavernous hemangioma.

A vascular lesion of the midbrain situated thus produces an ipsilateral IIIrd and contralateral ataxia; when not associated with long tract signs it is known as Claude's syndrome (Table 39.1).

Table 39.1 Vascular syndromes involving the brain stem

Midbrain		
Dorsomedial	Ipsilateral IIIrd Contralateral ataxia	Claude syndrome
Paramedian	Ipsilateral IIIrd Contralateral hemiparesis	Weber syndrome
Paramedian	Ipsilateral IIIrd Contralateral ataxia and chorea Contralateral hemiparesis	Benedikt syndrome
Tectum	Ipsilateral IIIrd Contralateral ataxia Contralateral spinothalamic	Nothnagel syndrome
Pons		
Lateral	Contralateral hemiparesis Contralateral spinothalamic Ipsilateral ataxia Ipsilateral V Ipsilateral VII and VIII	Marie-Foix syndrome
Inferior medial	Contralateral hemiparesis (Including face) Contralateral proprioception Ipsilateral ataxia Ipsilateral gaze palsy	Foville syndrome
Inferior medial	Ipsilateral VI Contralateral hemiparesis	Raymond syndrome
Upper dorsal	Ipsilateral ataxia Contralateral hemisensory loss Contralateral hemiparesis Ipsilateral VI	Raymond – Céstan
Ventral	Ipsilateral V, VI and VII Contralateral hemiparesis (Spares face)	Millard – Gubler syndrome
Facial colliculus	Ipsilateral gaze palsy Ipsilateral VII	Facial colliculus syndrome
Medulla		
Lateral medulla	Ipsilateral V Ipsilateral Horner's syndrome Ipsilateral ataxia Contralateral spinothalamic Ipsilateral vestibular (with OTR and skew) Ipsilateral IX and X	Wallenberg
Medial medulla	Ipsilateral XII Contralateral hemiparesis Contralateral proprioceptive loss Upbeat nystagmus	Déjerine
Hemimedulla	Infarction of medial and lateral medulla	Babinski-Nageotte

Management

The cause was considered untreatable and careful monitoring undertaken. Over the next 5 years the condition recurred three times, resulting in a complete third neuropathy on the left side. The right side was normal. The tremor had not deteriorated. It was clear that repeated bleeding would endanger his life and inevitably be associated with the accrual of neurological impairments; the decision was made to proceed with surgery and the lesion removed successfully (Fig. 39.3), although the procedure was complicated by the development of a Parinaud's syndrome and a more prominent rubral type tremor with a severe left sided ataxia. This improved with rehabilitation over 5 years and he was able ultimately to return to work on a part time basis.

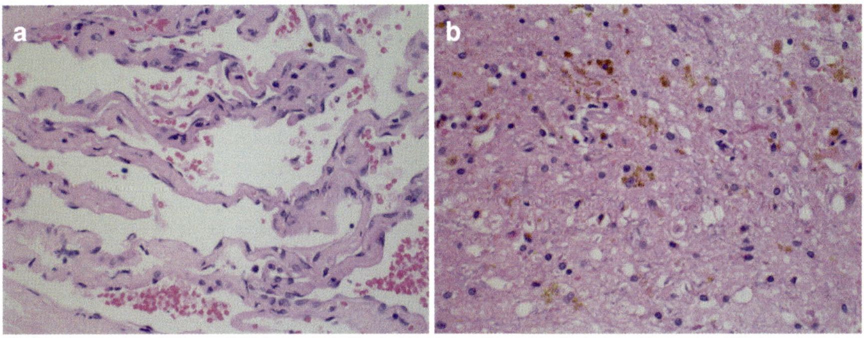

Fig. 39.3 Hematoxylin and eosin stained section showing a back-to-back arrangement of ectatic thin-walled vessels (**a**). This would favor a cavernous hemangioma. This section (**b**) shows gliotic brain tissue adjacent to the lesion. There is prominent brown hemosiderin pigment, as a consequence of previous hemorrhage (Curtesy of Dr Malcolm Galloway, Dept. Neuropathology, Institute of Neurology)

Discussion

Cavernous hemangiomas (cavernomas) of the brain are uncommon, accounting for less than 20 % of all neurological vascular malformations. They present with focal neurological deficits when they bleed, and when cortically situated often cause seizures.

Those which are found in the brainstem account for 25 % of all cavernomas. In one early series half were in the pons and the remainder equally divided between midbrain and medulla [1]. Bleeding is common and the risk of rebleeding after the first is increased, although different series have different results. Kupersmith et al. [2] found that bleeding was more common if it had occurred before, and if the lesion was large. However 67 % of his cohort did not exhibit an increase in lesion size over a 5 year follow up. A more recent series from China revealed an annual hemorrhage rate of 15 % [3] with substantial neurological recovery after the event, allowing 81 % to "live independently".

The literature is by far and away a neurosurgical one, and a recent meta-analysis of all the recent series published [4] concluded that with surgical treatment there is a 45 % change of substantial perioperative morbidity including a 12 % risk of requiring ventilatory support and/or gastrostomy but that long term results were that 84 % were the same or improved and the remainder of course worse. Importantly however one must note that 91 % of brainstem cavernomas are removed in entirety at surgery, with an attendant substantial reduction in the chance of further post-operative bleeding. It is obvious that lesions deep within the brainstem are more difficult to gain access to without causing neurosurgical morbidity; it is often recommended that surgeons wait until the lesion enlarges near to the ependymal surface of the brainstem before surgery is contemplated, and this is what we did in this case.

Non-surgical treatments such as radiosurgery appears also to reduce the risk of rebleeding; a recent series from Korea in patients considered to have unresectable lesions who were treated with gamma knife radiosurgery showed a significant reduction in rebleeding following treatment [5].

References

1. Fritschi JA, Reulen HJ, Spetzler RF, Zabramski JM. Cavernous malformations of the brain stem: a review of 139 cases. Acta Neurochir. 1994;130:35–46.
2. Kupersmith MJ, Kalish H, Epstein F, Yu G, Berenstein A, Woo H, Jafa J, Mandel G, De Lara F. Natural history of brain stem cavernous malformations. Neurosurgery. 2001;48:53–4.
3. Li D, Hao SY, Jia GJ, Wu Z, Zhang LW, Zhang JT. Hemorrhage risks and functional outcomes of untreated brainstem cavernous malformations. J Neurosurg. 2014;121:32–41.
4. Gross BA, Batjer HH, Awad IA, Bendok BR, Du R. Brainstem cavernous malformations: 1390 surgical cases from the literature. World Neurosurg. 2013;80:89–93.
5. Park SH, Hwang SK. Gamma knife radiosurgery for symptomatic brainstem intra-axial cavernous malformations. World Neurosurg. 2013;80:261–6.
6. Patten J. Neurological differential diagnosis. 2nd ed. London: Springer-Verlag Ltd; 1996.

Case 40

History

This 63 year old lady developed blurred vision with difficulty focusing for near, and her daughter spotted that her pupils had become larger on both sides. There were no headaches and no other neurological symptoms at the time, although there had been an upper respiratory tract infection 2 weeks previously, and she had been taking an over the counter cough remedy.

On the following day she awoke with double vision and an unsteadiness of gait. There was no vertigo, no numbness and no other neurological symptom. Over the following 2 days her pupils enlarged further and the double vision worsened. She became more unsteady. Her daughter brought her to the local hospital emergency department.

She had mild and treated hypertension, hypercholesterolemia and type II diabetes. Her past medical history was otherwise unremarkable.

Examination

The anterior visual pathways and discs were normal. Both pupils were fixed and dilated. There were no eye movements whatsoever. There was bilateral partial ptosis. Trigeminal and facial nerve function was normal. There was no dysarthria or dysphagia.

She walked with an unsteady gait but there was no limb ataxia. Power was unimpaired and reflexes were present. Plantar responses were flexor. Sensation was within normal limits.

The systemic examination was normal.

D.P. Kidd, *Neuro-Ophthalmology*, DOI 10.1007/978-1-4471-2410-8_40

Clinical Evaluation

This alarming set of symptoms when evaluated carefully can quickly be disentangled. The differential diagnosis involves the condition it turned out to be and a lesion of the brain stem. The absence of long tract or lateralising signs makes an extrinsic lesion of the cerebellopontine angle or the foramen magnum unlikely, so it would have to have intrinsic. The eye movements are absent, so both horizontal and vertical gaze systems are not working, and the pupillary responses are also affected. This a complete external and internal ophthalmoplegia.

In order for there to be a failure of horizontal gaze on both sides there would need to be a lesion (or two lesions) symmetrically disrupting the function of the abducens nucleus and the parapontine reticular formation (Fig. 40.1). This would cause a bilateral horizontal gaze palsy. Two lesions of the medial longitudinal fasciculus and the abducens nucleus would produce bilateral one and a half syndromes. In both cases it is possible that vergence would be preserved, since this relies on input from projections which pass directly to the medial rectus motor neurons [1].

Paralysis of upgaze comes about when the rostral interstitial nucleus of the medial longitudinal fasciculus is damaged. This also affects convergence; the association of an upgaze palsy, downgaze palsy and absence of convergence comprises Parinaud's syndrome. Some patients exhibit the phenomenon of convergence retraction nystagmus, in which a retraction of the eyes is seen on attempted upgaze or more often when stimulated by a downwards movement of the optokinetic drum. Parinaud's syndrome may be complete or partial, and cases of isolated upgaze paresis, down gaze paresis or asymmetry have been reported [2].

Patients with dorsal midbrain lesions also show pupillary abnormalities, in which there is light – near dissociation; the pupils fail to react to direct light but constrict on attempted convergence.

Such ocular motor disorders are most commonly caused by brain stem stroke or by brain stem glioma. Inflammatory lesions of the brain stem due for example to Behçet's syndrome, multiple sclerosis, lupus, neuromyelitis optica and a paraneoplastic encephalitis are also possible and imaging will help to identify them.

Whipple's disease is an important consideration, since when it affects the brain stem it may be associated with a variety of uncommon ocular motor and neurological abnormalities. These include the characteristic oculomasticatory myorhythmia, in which pendular vergence movements occur at a frequency of 1 Hz, accompanied by a concurrent contraction of the muscles of mastication. Such patients are usually systemically and neurologically unwell, with weight loss and confusion.

Other diseases should be considered, in particular Wernicke's encephalopathy, although it tends not to involve the pupils, and Botulism, in which pupillary disorders and ophthalmoparesis are common, although the disorder is almost always severe and life-threatening, involving swallowing and breathing muscles quickly, and of course a much greater weakness.

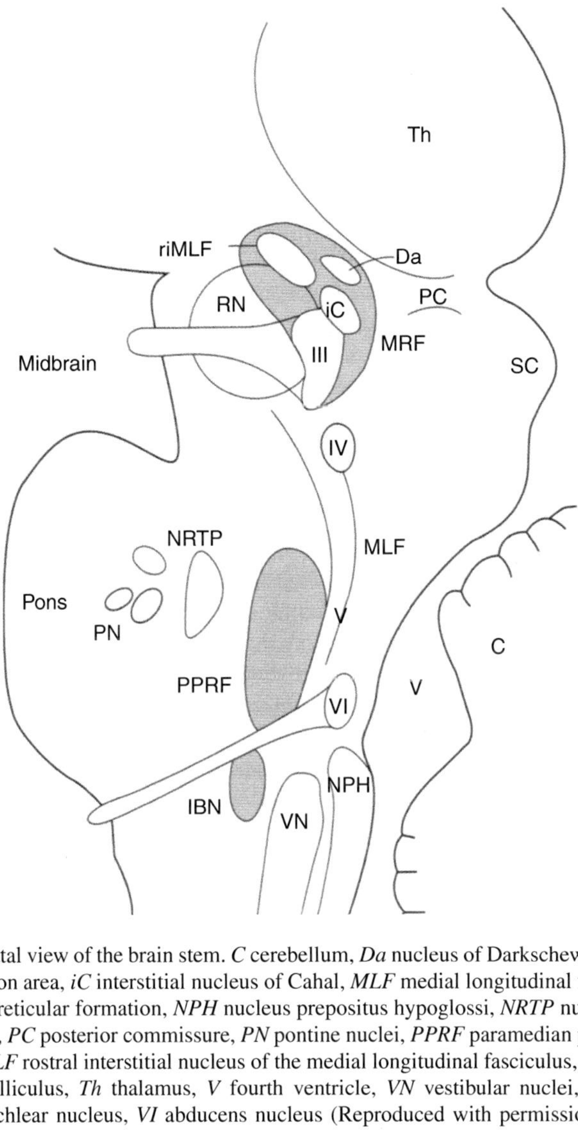

Fig. 40.1 Sagittal view of the brain stem. *C* cerebellum, *Da* nucleus of Darkschewitch, *IBN* inhibitory burst neuron area, *iC* interstitial nucleus of Cahal, *MLF* medial longitudinal fasciculus, *MRF* mesencephalic reticular formation, *NPH* nucleus prepositus hypoglossi, *NRTP* nucleus reticularis tegmenti pontis, *PC* posterior commissure, *PN* pontine nuclei, *PPRF* paramedian pontine reticular formation, *riMLF* rostral interstitial nucleus of the medial longitudinal fasciculus, *RN* red nucleus, *SC* superior colliculus, *Th* thalamus, *V* fourth ventricle, *VN* vestibular nuclei, *III* oculomotor nucleus, *IV* trochlear nucleus, *VI* abducens nucleus (Reproduced with permission from Peirrot-Deseilligny [6])

Finally degenerative disorders such a progressive supranuclear palsy would be considered, although the timing is out of keeping for this more slowly progressive disorder.

Urgent imaging, therefore, with screening blood investigations and a spinal fluid examination would be important and mandatory initial investigations.

Investigations

Blood count was normal, biochemical screening within normal limits, CRP raised at 31.

Chest X-Ray normal, blood cultures negative.

An MRI scan of the brain showed evidence for supratentorial small vessel disease but no brain stem lesion. A further MRI following gadolinium showed no evidence for meningeal enhancement around the brain stem.

A spinal fluid examination showed clear fluid under normal pressure (19 cm), protein was 0.53 g/dl and there were no cells.

A nerve conduction study was normal. EMG showed a few complex partial units in the right orbicularis oculi, and the blink reflex was delayed on the same side.

She was found to have anti-GQ1b antibodies, and a bioassay was negative for Botulinum toxin A.

She was treated with intravenous immunoglobulin and improved. Her eye movements and pupillary responses were normal when reviewed 3 months later.

Discussion

The disorder is compatible with a diagnosis of Miller Fisher syndrome. This is an uncommon condition, with a prevalence of around 5 % of all cases of Guillain-Barré syndrome, whose incidence is 2×10^5. It appears to be more common in Asian populations. The triad of ophthalmoplegia, ataxia and areflexia was first described by Collier in 1932, with a further three cases published by C Miller Fisher in 1956 [3].

The ophthalmoparesis may be mild and affect only single muscles or severe, as in this case. An internal ophthalmoplegia, in which the autonomic supply to the muscles of the iris is affected, as in this case, is uncommon but well recognized. Some patients only show an ophthalmoparesis. The ataxia is considered to be both cerebellar and proprioceptive. Areflexia is common but no longer a pre-requisite for the diagnosis. Many cases show an overlap with acute Guillain-Barré syndrome, and when drowsiness is present, an overlap exists with Bickerstaff's encephalitis.

In general imaging is normal, although there are reports of enhancement of the IVth and VIth nerves, and the brain stem and cerebellum.

Anti-ganglioside antibodies are common in Guillain-Barré syndrome, particularly GM-1, GD1a and GT1b. In Miller Fisher syndrome 90 % have anti-GQ1b antibodies. These antibodies have been shown to bind avidly to motor end plates of the muscles supplied by the IIIrd, IVth and VIth nerves [4] and presumably explains the clinical phenotype.

There is no evidence that treatment influences the outcome; it is most uncommon for patients to fail to recover well, with a return to independent living [5]. Nonetheless, as in this case, IVIg is often recommended, if only to speed up recovery.

References

1. Leigh RJ, Zee DS. Diagnosis of central disorders of ocular motility. In: Leigh RJ, Zee DS, editors. The neurology of eye movements. 2nd ed. Philadelphia: FA Davis; 1991.
2. Pierrot-Deseilligny C, Chain F, Gray F, Serdaru M, Escourolle R, Lhermitte F. Parinaud's syndrome: electro-oculographic and anatomical analyses of six vascular cases with deduction about vertical gaze organization in the premotor structures. Brain. 1982;105:667–96.
3. Teener JW. Miller Fisher's syndrome. Semin Neurol. 2012;32:512–6.
4. Liu JX, Willison HJ, Pedrosa-Domellof F. Immunolocalization of GQ1b and related gangliosides in human extraocular neuromuscular junctions and muscle spindles. Invest Ophthalmol Vis Sci. 2009;50:3226–32.
5. Overell JR, Hsieh ST, Odaka M, Yuki N, Willison HJ. Treatment for Fisher syndrome, Bickerstaff's encephalitis and related disorders. Cochrane Database Syst Rev 2007;(1):CD004761
6. Peirrot-Deseilligny C. Nuclear, internuclear and supranuclear ocular motor disorders. Handb Clin Neurol. 2011;102:321.

Case 41

History

This 40 year old man noticed increasing problems with visual blurring over the previous 5 years. There were no other or prior symptoms. The blurring was noticeable on looking down a flight of stairs or when reading, but not present when looking into the distance, or when looking upwards.

On further questioning he was able to recount that the blurring was not a defocusing but a shudder as he looked down, which resolved once his gaze was fixed in a downwards direction. There was no diplopia, no giddiness or vertigo and no unsteadiness of gait.

He was otherwise well and took no regular treatment. There was no family history of neurological disease.

Examination

The anterior visual pathways were normal. The fields were full and the discs and retinae showed normal appearances. The horizontal eye movements were normal. On upgaze the movements were also normal but as he scanned down in pursuit, the eyes shuddered with a downbeating nystagmus. It tended to be brought out by moving the eyes down and to either side. The saccadic velocities were normal and fast, and the saccades were not hypometric. Optokinetic nystagmus was the same in horizontal and vertical planes.

The neurological examination showed no evidence for ataxia, nor a vestibular asymmetry, nor other abnormal signs.

D.P. Kidd, *Neuro-Ophthalmology*, DOI 10.1007/978-1-4471-2410-8_41

Clinical Evaluation

The history provided is typical for a downbeating nystagmus. The absence of other features of brain stem or cerebellar dysfunction, and the otherwise normal examination, is reassuring. However investigations are nonetheless important, and he should undergo an MRI of the brain stem and foramen magnum.

Investigation

An MRI scan of the brain (Fig. 41.1) was normal.

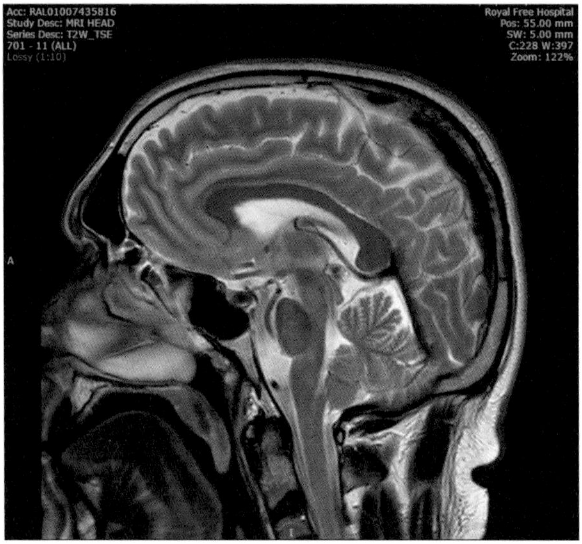

Fig. 41.1 T2 weighted sagittal MRI showing no evidence for cerebellar or brainstem atrophy, nor for a lesion at the foramen magnum

Table 41.1 Causes of downbeating nystagmus [1–3]

Congenital or inherited disorders	Acquired structural disorders	Metabolic disorders
Cerebellar degenerations	Cerebellar infarction	Anti-convulsant intoxication
Arnold-Chiari malformation	Multiple sclerosis	Lithium intoxication
Basilar invagination	Tumors of the cerebellum	Alcohol intoxication
Syringobulbia	Paraneoplasic cerebellar degeneration	Toluene intoxication
Congenital nystagmus	Alcohol-related cerebellar degeneration	Wernicke's encephalopathy
		B12 deficiency

Discussion

This is downbeating nystagmus; there is no nystagmus in the primary position and the nystagmus is in a downbeating direction on down gaze. Downbeat nystagmus is present in the primary position and indeed often also in all positions of gaze, even upwards. However the amplitude of the nystagmus tends to be greatest in downgaze (occasionally it may increase in upgaze, so it is important to identify accurately the direction of the fast phase of the movement).

The causes of downbeating nystagmus are noted in the Table 41.1. Lesions causing the disorder tend to involve the vestibulocerebellum and its connections, particularly within the medulla. Two reasonably large series have shown that around one third of patients have no identifiable cause and the remaining majority show cerebellar degenerations, Arnold-Chiari malformations or drug toxicity. Those without an identifiable cause were followed up and no change in the severity of the nystagmus was noted over a 5 year period [4].

The potassium channel blocker 4-aminopyridine has been shown to reduce the amplitude of downbeat nystagmus, allowing an improvement in near visual acuity [5].

References

1. Leigh RJ, Zee DS. Diagnosis of central disorders of ocular motility. In: Leigh RJ, Zee DS, editors. The neurology of eye movements. 2nd ed. Philadelphia: FA Davis and Co; 1991. p. 378–530.
2. Wagner JN, Glaser M, Brandt T, Strupp M. Downbeat nystagmus: aetiology and comorbidity in 117 patients. J Neurol Neurosurg Psychiatry. 2008;79:672–7.
3. Halmagyi GM, Rudge P, Gresty MA, Sanders MD. Downbeating nystagmus: a review of 62 cases. Arch Neurol. 1983;40:777–84.

4. Wagner J, Lehnen N, Glasauer S, Strupp M, Brandt T. Prognosis of idiopathic downbeat nystagmus. Ann N Y Acad Sci. 2009;1164:479–81.
5. Claassen J, Spiegel R, Kalla R, Faldon M, Kennard C, Danchivijiitr C, Bardins S, Reitlinger N, Schneider E, Brandt T, Jahn K, Tuefel J, Strupp M, Bronstein A. A randomised double-blind cross-over trial of 4-aminopyridine for downbeat nystagmus – effects on slow phase eye velocity, postural stability, locomotion and symptoms. J Neurol Neurosurg Psychiatry. 2013;84:1392–9.

Case 42

History

This 77 year old man developed pain within his right ear canal which he described as severe, burning and stinging. Three days later he developed hearing loss on the right side with high pitched tinnitus and a bubbling sound, with muffling leading over the course of hours to a total unilateral loss of hearing. On the following day he noted a facial weakness on the same side. He received treatment with oral antibiotics from his GP but failed to improve. When he noted double vision he referred himself to the emergency department of the Royal Free Hospital and was admitted.

The double vision initially was horizontal when looking only to the right. After a few hours he became nauseated and described episodes of visual disturbance and loss of balance in which he felt that suddenly the whole world had been tilted over to the left by 90°. At first this was momentary but by the following day he was experiencing this several times an hour and it was lasting about ten seconds at a time. There was nausea and during the tilt he felt particularly sick. He was unable to walk owing to imbalance.

His past medical history involved ischemic heart disease, hypertension and hypercholesterolemia. A pacemaker had been implanted following investigation of episodes of fainting. There had been no prior neurological symptoms.

D.P. Kidd, *Neuro-Ophthalmology*, DOI 10.1007/978-1-4471-2410-8_42

Examination

He was distressed and nauseated. The higher cortical functions were normal and he was not drowsy. The anterior visual pathways and discs were normal. Examination of the eye movements at an early stage revealed a right lateral rectus paresis but after the condition had worsened he was noted to have a right over left hyperphoria in all directions of gaze, an inability to move either eye to the right, but also a coarse horizontal beating nystagmus to the right in the right eye. There was diminishment of sensation in the ophthalmic division of the right trigeminal nerve and a right sided facial weakness which involved all muscles equally.

The lower cranial nerves were normal and there were no long tract signs in the limbs. His gait was exceedingly unsteady and he was unable to stand unsupported.

When he experienced the tilting motion, the junior staff noted that he tilted his head to the right and became distressed.

An ENT examination of the external auditory canal revealed encrusted vesicles in the skin.

Clinical Evaluation

This elderly man suffered pain in his ear then a rapidly evolving neurological syndrome involving hearing loss, vertigo and double vision. On admission to the emergency department there was evidence for a right sided lateral rectus weakness, deafness also on the right and a facial weakness which affected the upper half of the face as much as the lower; a lower motor neuron facial neuropathy. In summary he had a right VI, VII and VIII. There were other signs or symptoms at that time and so the syndrome is in keeping with Gradenigo's syndrome, in which suppurative middle ear disease extends out into the petrous bone, causing a petrous osteomyelitis. The original description refers to a sixth (since it passes through the petrous bone within Dorello's canal), but a seventh is often also seen, and of course the hearing loss would occur at an earlier point. The lesion cannot be situated within the cavernous sinus since the VIIth is also involved, so it must be either at the petrous apex or the cerebellopontine angle or within the brainstem, The subsequent evolution of the clinical features makes this more clear.

He describes clearly a paroxysmal vestibular symptom in which his world is tilted over by 90°; this is accompanied by nausea. This would be caused by torsion of the eyes conjugately, in this case to the left.

The examination findings on the second day of admission revealed an inability to look with either eye to the right, a right over left hypertropia (in which the right eye is seen to be higher than the left in the primary position of gaze) which remains the same in all directions of gaze, and a torsional nystagmus to the right. The first two disorders are a horizontal gaze palsy and a skew deviation.

Horizontal Gaze Palsy

A lesion of the parapontine reticular formation will lead to a horizontal gaze palsy. In the acute phase the eyes are held conjugately to the contralateral side. The important feature is that saccadic eye movements are lost on the ipsilateral side; pursuit and vestibular eye movements (such as the vestibulo-ocular reflex) may be lost too but may remain. When the lesion is on the right, movement of the eyes suddenly to the left will be normal, and movements from the left to the midline (*ie* in a rightward direction) will be slow, and the eyes will not cross the midline. Preservation of the function of the abducens nucleus can be tested using vestibular and pursuit eye movements.

Skew Deviation

This is a prenuclear disorder which results from a disturbance of otolithic input to the ocular motor system, that is, there is a disturbance of the control of balance of the eyes which is brought about from information supplied to the brain stem by the vestibular system, the semicircular canals, the utricle and saccule. It may be seen, therefore, in acute vestibulopathies arising within the vestibular organ or the vestibular nerve, and when the vestibular nuclei are damaged, for example in the lateral medullary syndrome of Wallenberg, in which infarction of the lateral medulla occurs through thrombosis of the posterior inferior cerebellar artery.

Lesions higher up within the brainstem, involving the medial longitudinal fasciculus, which carries axons from the vestibular nuclei to the ocular motor nucleus, may cause both internuclear ophthalmoplegia and skew deviation, in which the hypertropia is ipsilateral to the lesion. Lesions of the interstitial nucleus of Cahal may also be associated with skew deviation as well as vertical gaze palsies and nystagmus, including seesaw nystagmus. Lesions here are commonly associated with an ocular tilt reaction; when tonic the hypertropia is ipsilateral to the lesion and the head tilt contralateral.

The right PPRF is involved in this case and the right over left skew would if on the right also be located low; that is, before the tracts decussate …….. What about the tilting disorder which affects him? This is a paroxysmal ocular tilt reaction.

Ocular Tilt Reaction

This disorder is usually tonic, *ie* sustained, but may rarely, as in this case, be paroxysmal. What happens is the opposite of what happens with an intact vestibular system when the head is voluntarily tilted over (Fig. 42.1). When the head tilts towards the right shoulder the eyes turn (cyclodeviate) towards the left, so allowing the world to remain upright. In an ocular tilt reaction the opposite occurs; the cyclodeviation continues to the right [1].

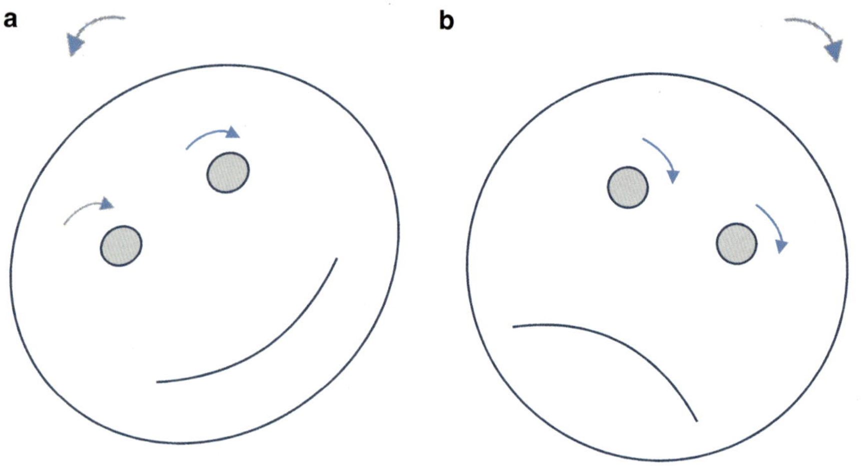

Fig. 42.1 Cartoon showing (**a**) normal eye movement when the head is tilted to the right and (**b**) cyclodeviation to the left in an ocular tilt reaction to the left

The pathway involved rises from the vestibular organ to the vestibular nuclei and up to the interstitial nucleus of Cahal in the midbrain. It decussates in the pons, and so tonic tilt reactions due to lesions in the lower pons are ipsiversive (the lower eye is on the same side as the lesion) whereas higher up the tilt is contraversive [2]. This implies a deficit of function (Fig. 42.2).

Paroxysmal disorders imply an irritation of retained or partially retained function and are in the opposite direction [3]. In this case, and in the interesting case reported in [3] in which there is a tonic tilt reaction alongside a superimposed paroxysmal tilt reaction, the lesion on the right causes a contraversive tilt reaction leading to the leftward head tilt lasting for 10 Seconds at a time.

Investigations

An MRI would have been very helpful in this case but was contraindicated by his pacemaker; a CT scan revealed periventricular small vessel disease and no clear abnormality within the brain stem, such as infarction, hemorrhage, abscess or tumor. The presence of vesicles within the ear canal strongly suggested Herpes Zoster, and we assumed that he had suffered an inflammatory lesion within the pons associated with zoster. Ramsay Hunt syndrome is the association between Herpes Zoster oticus, deafness and an ipsilateral facial neuropathy, but this is clearly a more central disorder. There are case reports which show this, including one from the author in his training days [4, 5].

He was treated with intravenous acyclovir, and improved.

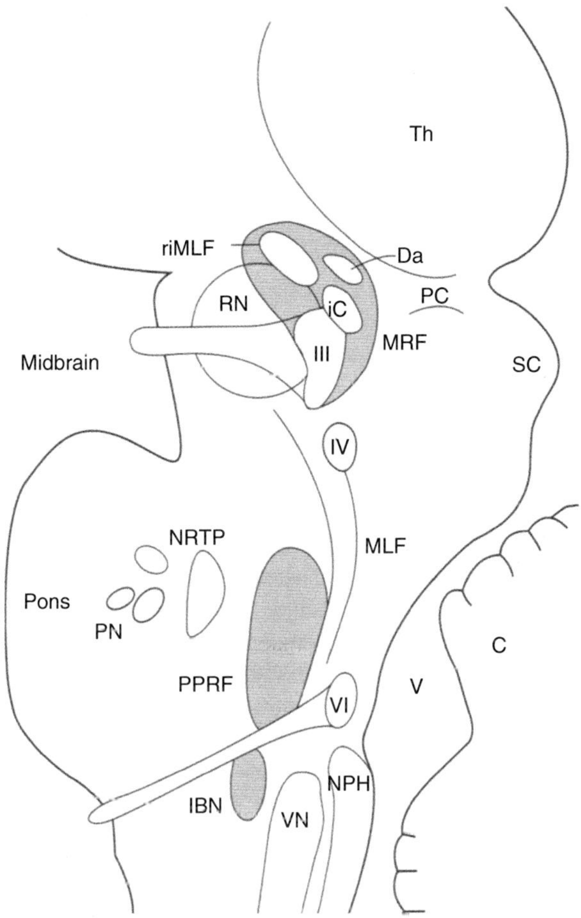

Fig. 42.2 Sagittal view of the brain stem. *C* cerebellum, *Da* nucleus of Darkschewitch, *IBN* inhibitory burst neuron area, *iC* interstitial nucleus of Cahal, *MLF* medial longitudinal fasciculus, *MRF* mesencephalic reticular formation, *NPH* nucleus prepositus hypoglossi, *NRTP* nucleus reticularis tegmenti pontis, *PC* posterior commissure, *PN* pontine nuclei, *PPRF* paramedian pontine reticular formation, *riMLF* rostral interstitial nucleus of the medial longitudinal fasciculus, *RN* red nucleus, *SC* superior colliculus, *Th* thalamus, *V* fourth ventricle, *VN* vestibular nuclei, *III* oculomotor nucleus, *IV* trochlear nucleus, *VI* abducens nucleus (Reproduced with permission from Peirrot-Deseilligny [7])

Discussion

This is a complicated case and most unusual, but the clinical signs are interesting and understandable. The diagnosis made was a brain stem lesion in the right pons related (either by inflammation or by arteritis) to Varicalla-Zoster oticus.

The neurological complications of Varicella-Zoster reactivation are more common in immunosuppressed patients, with HIV infection, lymphoreticular disorders and following bone marrow transplantation but also occur in otherwise healthy people [6]. Optic neuritis, myelitis, orbital apex syndrome and isolated cranial neuropathies have all been described, as well as brain stem lesions as noted above. Isolated meningitis, meningoencephalitis and encephalitis (including the cerebellitis seen with primary infection in children) are less common.

VZV vasculopathy causes cerebral infarction and hemorrhage; arteriograms show focal arterial stenosis with occlusion, and there is pathological evidence for an arteritis.

References

1. Leigh RJ, Zee DS. Diagnosis of central disorders of ocular motility. In: Leigh RJ, Zee DS, editors. The neurology of eye movements. 3rd ed. New York: Oxford University Press; 1999. p. 463–5.
2. Halmagyi GM, Brandt T, Dieterich M, Cuthoys IS, Stark RJ, Hoyt WF. Tonic contraversive ocular tilt reaction due to unilateral meso-diencephalic lesion. Neurology. 1990;40:1503–9.
3. Rodriguez AR, Egan RA, Barton JJS. Pearls & Oy-sters: paroxysmal ocular tilt reaction. Neurology. 2009;72:e67–8.
4. Kidd D, Duncan JS, Thompson EJ. Pontine inflammatory disorder due to shingles. J Neurol Neurosurg Psychiatry. 1998;65:208.
5. Mizock BA, Barn R, Aghemazdo B. Herpes zoster oticus with pontine lesion: segmental brainstem encephalitis. Clin Infect Dis. 2000;30:229–30.
6. Gilden D, Nagel MA, Cohrs RJ. Varicella-zoster. Handb Clin Neurol. 2014;123:265–83.
7. Peirrot-Deseilligny C. Nuclear, internuclear and supranuclear ocular motor disorders. Handb Clin Neurol. 2011;102:321.

Part V
The Cortex

Case 43

History

This 27 year old lady was admitted through the emergency department very unwell with high fever and drowsiness. She was found to have a pneumonia and her renal function declined rapidly.

She complained of a sudden onset headache on the second day of admission, then progressively became disorientated, anxious and rather paranoid. She reported visual hallucinations. She became more drowsy and complained that she could no longer see clearly. She then had a series of generalized tonic clonic seizures.

Examination

She was drowsy, disorientated, suspicious and frightened. There was poor vision on both sides, appreciating hand movements only, but with normal pupillary responses. Neither disc was swollen. The ocular media were clear and the retinae normal. The BP was 200/115.

D.P. Kidd, *Neuro-Ophthalmology*, DOI 10.1007/978-1-4471-2410-8_43

Evaluation

This medical emergency was characterized neurologically by drowsiness with encephalopathy, visual problems and a seizure. It is clear that the disorder is one which has affected the brain widely, including the cortices. Worsening uremia, drug intoxication and metabolic acidosis should all be considered first.

The visual disorder, difficult to characterize when she was unable to perform a visual field examination, was in keeping with a cortical visual loss when the pupillary responses were observed to be unimpaired. Imaging is warranted.

The differential diagnosis would include infective disorders, most particularly bacterial (including tuberculous) meningitis and viral encephalitis. Fungal and parasitic disorders including Cryptococcus are important in this unwell, generally immunosuppressed lady. Inflammatory disorders such as lupus, NMDAR-associated and paraneoplastic encephalitis would also be considered. Neoplastic causes would include carcinomatous meningitis, pituitary apoplexy and glioma of the corpus callosum. Vascular causes would involve consideration of a venous sinus thrombosis with bilateral lobar hemorrhage, ischemic infarction and arterial hemorrhage related to hypertension.

The differential diagnosis is exceedingly wide.

Investigations

ESR, CRP and blood counts were all raised. She had a metabolic acidosis. The CSF was clear, with a normal sugar differential and no white cells. An echocardiogram showed no evidence for endocarditis. A renal biopsy revealed evidence for acute tubular necrosis. A CT scan of brain revealed bilateral low density in the occipital regions. MRI (Fig. 43.1) showed bilateral regions of high signal in the occipital and frontal white matter and cortex. Diffusion weighted imaging showed restriction in some but not in other lesions (Fig. 43.2). MRA of the neck arteries was normal; that of the circle of Willis showed a beading appearance (Fig. 43.3); this was considered to be in keeping with the uncommon condition reversible cerebral vasoconstriction syndrome (RCVS).

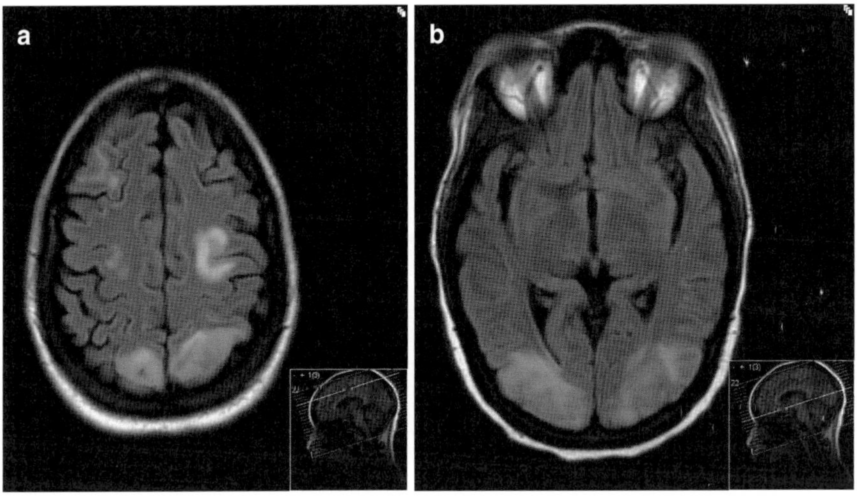

Fig. 43.1 FLAIR sequence MRI showing high signal within the occipital lobes, the precentral gyri and the left frontal white matter. The cortex is swollen. Note that the occipital high signal does not obey the boundary of the territory of the posterior cerebral artery

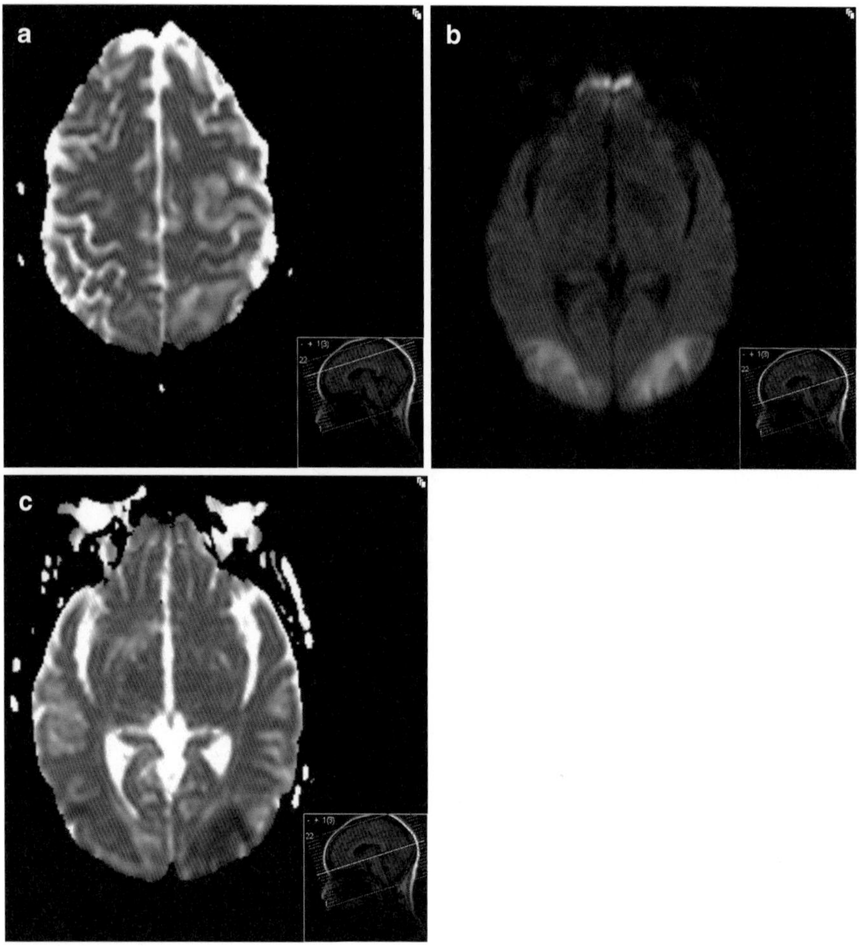

Fig. 43.2 ADC map and DWI showing restricted diffusion and a low apparent diffusion coefficient (ADC) in the occipital regions, but not in the frontal ones

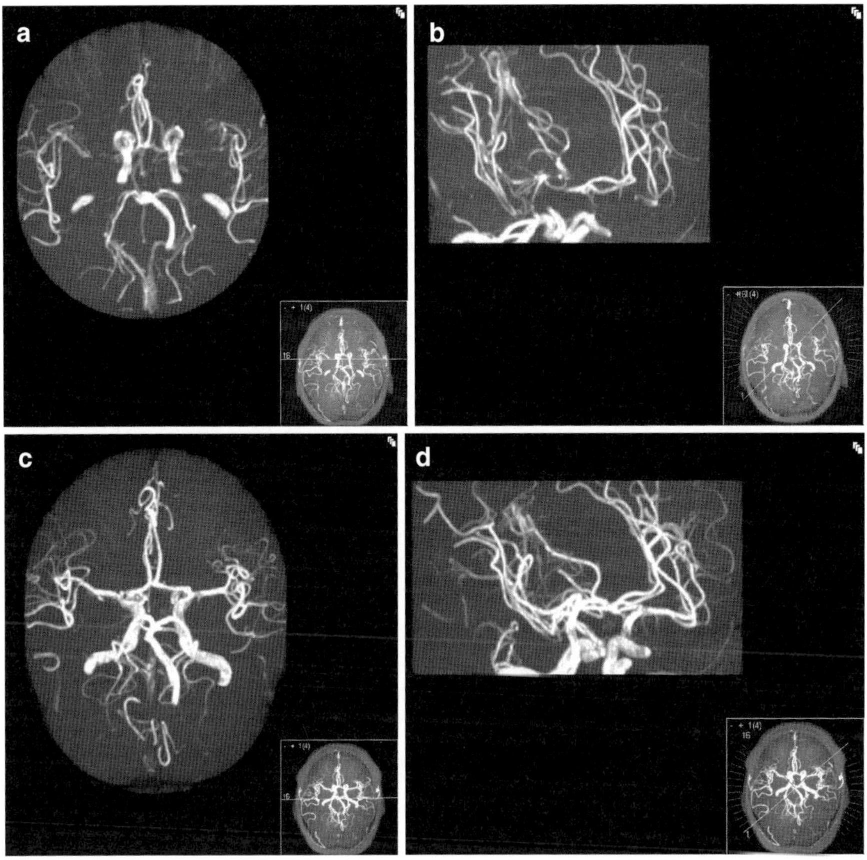

Fig. 43.3 MR angiogram: (**a**, **b**) there is abnormal focal narrowing of both A1 segments of the anterior cerebral arteries, and both P1 segments of the posterior cerebral artery are diminutive and thread-like; focal narrowing is also seen within the distal (P3 and P4) segments of the left posterior cerebral artery; (**c**, **d**) resolution of the abnormalities after 4 months

Management

She was treated in the renal department for fluid overload and with anti-hypertensive medication. She underwent renal dialysis. Her cardiovascular state improved. She became less drowsy and her vision improved. Her right hemifield enlarged but the left was slow to improve and she has a small residual left inferior quadrantic scotoma (Fig. 43.4).

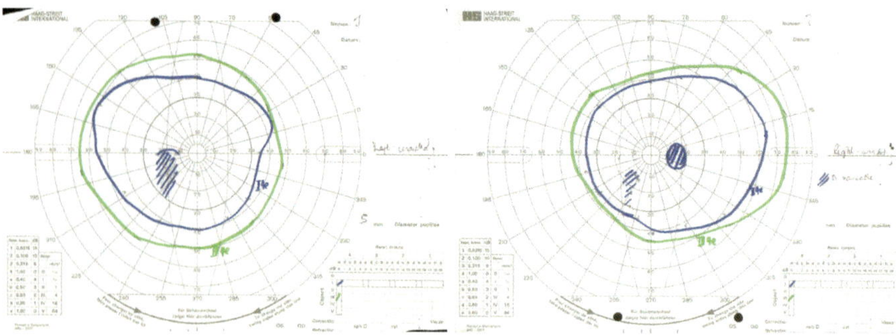

Fig. 43.4 Goldman visual fields after recovery showing a left sided inferior quadrantic scotoma

Discussion

Posterior reversible encephalopathy syndrome (PRES) is an uncommon condition associated with reversible cerebral vasoconstriction (RCVS), itself exceedingly rare [1–3]. Patients present acutely with a severe sudden onset "thunderclap" headache with vomiting which simulates subarachnoid hemorrhage. The encephalopathy may be severe causing coma, but can also be mild leading only to drowsiness. Seizures arise in 70% and visual symptoms in 40%. These include blurring due to field defects, visuospatial disorders and visual hallucinations. Some develop cortical blindness.

The imaging abnormalities are characteristic: high signal on FLAIR and T2 weighted MRI is seen in the parieto-occipital regions usually symmetrically. Sparing of the calcarine cortices helps to distinguish this from bilateral posterior cerebral artery occlusion. There are important differences in diffusion weighted imaging in addition; an increased apparent diffusion coefficient (ADC) does not occur in cerebral infarction, and implies the presence of vasogenic edema. The ADC map can be quantified; those with very high coefficients are more likely to recover than those with lower values [3]. Most show beading of the large vessels and the circle of Willis, which resolves as the condition disappears. Convexity subarachnoid hemorrhage is seen in around 30% (Table 43.1).

It is common after bone marrow transplantation and in renal disease complicating connective tissues diseases and vasculitis. It is also a feature of cerebral hyperperfusion syndrome, following carotid dissection and treatment of carotid stenosis, and during arterial catheterization. It has also complicated the autonomic dysregulation in Guillain Barré syndrome. It has been seen to occur in pheochromocytoma and carcinoid syndrome, and following head injury.

In one series of 67 [1] most were related to use of vasoactive drugs, including cocaine, ephedrine and SSRIs. All presented with thunderclap headache and hemorrhagic complications such as cortical subarachnoid hemorrhage occurred within the first week, whereas ischemic complications arose in the second. PRES arose in 9% of that series.

Table 43.1 Causes of RCVS

Hypertension
Postpartum and eclampsia/pre-eclampsia
Exposure to drugs: Cannabis, cocaine, LSD, Ecstasy, methamphetamine, alcohol
Prescribed drugs: SSRI, nasal decongestants, ephedrine, ergotamine, bromocriptine, triptan, calcineurin inhibitors, cyclophosphamide, vincristine, cisplatin, cytarabine, IVIg, blood products, interferon alpha

The cardinal feature is the development of a reversible multifocal segmental narrowing of the cerebral arteries (Fig. 43.3), often misinterpreted as vasculitis.

RCVS is a self-limiting condition, resolving over 1–3 months after onset; treatment with calcium channel blockers has been shown to help in some cases [1] although no evidence for this was found in another series [2]. The cause when identified should be treated or withdrawn quickly.

The pathogenesis has not yet been proven, but is considered to be a disorder of cerebral arterial blood flow autoregulation, in which the vessels constrict then dilate, and T cell activation leads to endothelial cell dysfunction, both of which lead to extravasation of fluid leading to vasogenic edema [3].

The neurological outcome is thought to be related to the duration of the abnormal vascular changes, although there appears not to be a formal study in the literature. One study found a "good" outcome in 90 % [2].

References

1. Ducros A, Boukobza M, Porcher R, Sarov M, Valade D, Bousser MG. The clinical and radiological spectrum of reversible cerebral vasoconstriction syndrome. A prospective series of 67 patients. Brain. 2007;130;3091–101.
2. Singhal AB, Hajj-Ali RA, Topcuoglu MA, Fok J, Bena J, Yang D, Calabrese LH. Reversible cerebral vasoconstriction syndromes: analysis of 139 cases. Arch Neurol. 2011;68:1005–12.
3. Lamy C, Oppenheim C, Mas JL. Posterior reversible encephalopathy syndrome. Handb Clin Neurol. 2014;121:1687–701.

Case 44

History

This 63 year old lady presented with a 6 month history of a gradually worsening problem with visual recognition. Initially there was insomnia and intermittent agitation, then over the following months there were increasing problems with topographical disorientation. She noticed no problem with her memory but problems recognizing people's faces and then also recognizing objects, for example in kitchen cupboards.

She had to give up her job, running her catering company, and became no longer able to drive or to shop.

A few months prior, she had developed an abrupt onset of numbness on one side of the face and she went to the stroke clinic of her local hospital. They performed a Doppler of the carotid arteries and a CT scan of brain which were normal. Later, she developed a urinary disturbance and a feeling of tingling and numbness up her legs, to the abdomen, which had persisted. There were no other or prior neurological symptoms.

Examination

She was seen first in outpatients; the neuro-ophthalmic examination showed normal central acuities, but she was unable to process color vision. There was a left-sided hemianopia and there was a visuospatial disorder, ignoring lines presented to her left visual field whilst recognizing them within the right. She had problems recognizing objects and her geographical orientation was impaired but not very poor. She was able to dress skillfully. Mental arithmetic was normal and memory tests were satisfactory.

It was recommended that she be admitted for further urgent investigations. Over the course of the ensuing 2 weeks she continued to deteriorate, and was found by then to have developed complete cortical blindness. There were signs of spasticity in the limbs, and there were occasional myoclonic jerks.

D.P. Kidd, *Neuro-Ophthalmology*, DOI 10.1007/978-1-4471-2410-8_44

Evaluation

This lady presents with an alarming clinical syndrome which is rapidly progressive. Her first symptoms were non-specific in isolation, with difficulty sleeping and anxiety, and were followed by a deteriorating cognitive disorder which undoubtedly was not recognized by her or her family initially, then when a focal neurological symptom was identified a TIA investigation pathway was followed which did not allow for an understanding of the deteriorating problem, with the added distraction of the false reassurance that a brain scan was seen to be normal.

She then develops problems with geographical orientation, both within the home and outside, and in particular with very familiar tasks such as working in her kitchen, topographagnosia. She and the family realized the seriousness of the problem when it became clear that she had difficulties recognizing familiar objects, visual object agnosia, and faces, prosopagnosia.

The examination in my clinic room revealed a left hemianopia, acquired achromatopsia, and visuospatial disorganization, with visual neglect. This constellation of features points to dysfunction of the right side, in particular the striate cortex (for the field defect), the ventral occipital lobe anteriorly (for the prosopagnosia), the lingual and fusiform gyri (for the achromatopsia and the visual agnosia), but because the deficits, in particular the disorders of recognition, were so pronounced I assumed that the lesion was bilateral. A normal CT does not rule out a degenerative process nor indeed a neoplastic one; infiltrative gliomas may have the same density as normal brain and not therefore show up as an abnormality.

Differential Diagnosis

Clearly the differential is vast, ranging from structural lesions occupying space to degenerations leading to loss of volume. Inflammation, including multiple sclerosis, sarcoidosis and cerebral vasculitis is possible; perhaps more likely would be a progressive immune based encephalitis for example due to a paraneoplastic disorder with anti-neuronal or NMDAR antibodies. Infection, due to HIV or to tuberculosis or a parasitic infection for example cysticercosis should be considered, heavy metal poisoning and poisoning with carbon monoxide could cause these symptoms as well. Neoplastic disorders such as glioma particularly that which infiltrates the corpus callosum, lymphoma and metastatic tumors should also be on the list. Finally degenerative disorders such as posterior cortical atrophy, Alzheimer's disease and of course Creutzfeldt-Jakob disease would in many ways, in view of the normalcy of the previous imaging and the time course of the clinical syndrome, be the most likely cause.

Imaging first, then other investigation proportionate to its result.

Investigations

An MRI scan of brain was reported to be within normal limits (Fig. 44.1).

Screening blood investigations including heavy metals, thyroid function and antibodies, anti-NMDAR antibodies, anti-neuronal antibodies and voltage gated potassium channel antibodies were all normal.

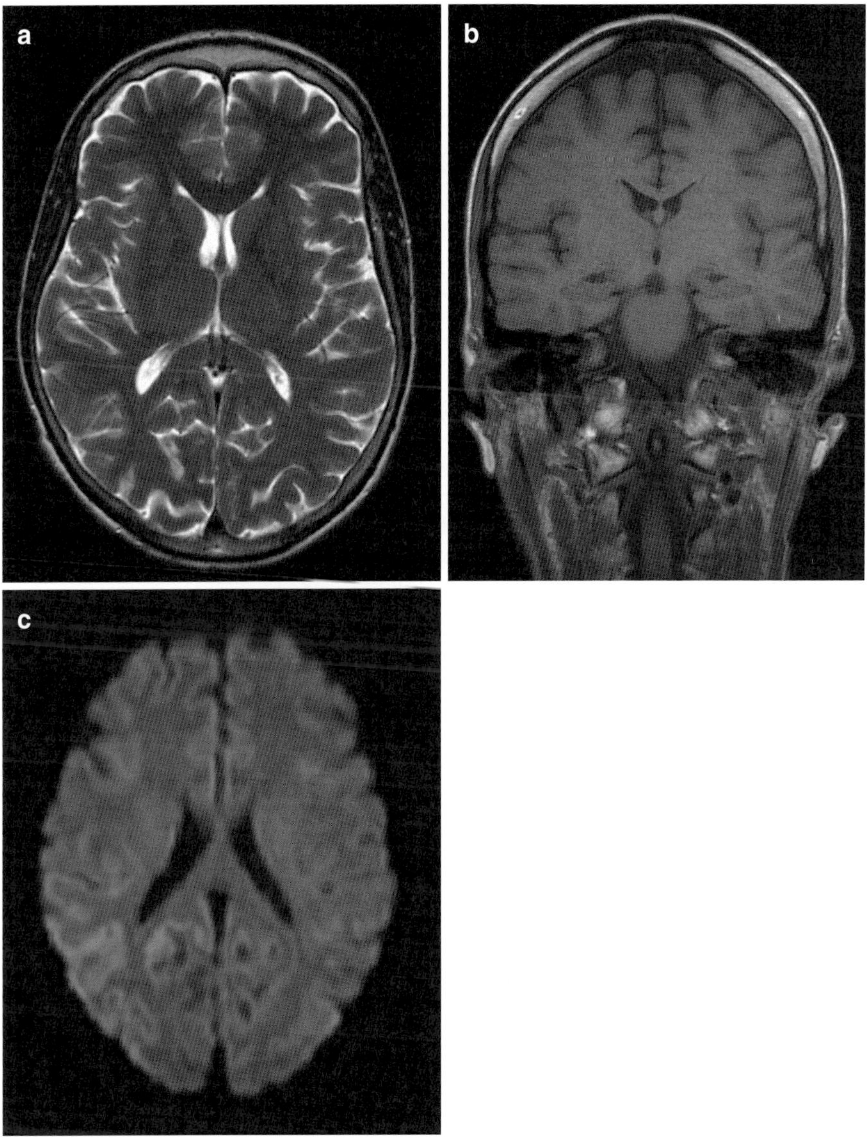

Fig. 44.1 (**a**, **b**) T2 weighted axial and T1 weighted coronal MRI which are within normal limits; (**c**) notice a subtle restriction in diffusion in the right hemisphere cortex posteriorly on diffusion weighted imaging

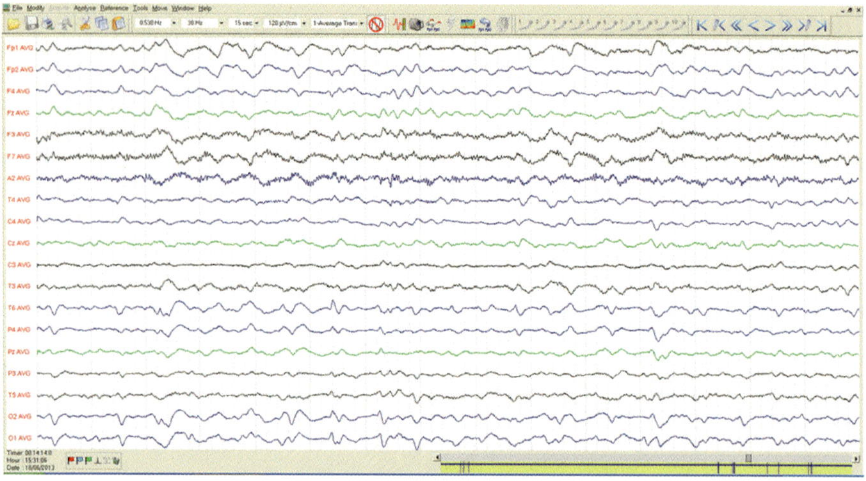

Fig. 44.2 EEG showing slow background rhythm with semi-periodic sharp waves over the right hemisphere (courtesy of Dr Tom Tidswell, Consultant Neurophysiologist, Royal Free Hospital)

An EEG showed a marked slowing of the EEG background, compatible with a severe encephalopathy. Runs of sharp waves were seen over the right temporal and occipital regions, with variable, semi-periodic frequency (Fig. 44.2). The Neurophysiologists felt this to be in keeping with a profound encephalopathy with a reduced seizure threshold.

A spinal fluid examination was not performed.

Clinical Course

The clinical features, disease course and imaging and neurophysiological findings were considered typical of a rapidly evolving degenerative process. We considered it unnecessary to proceed to other investigations, including a spinal fluid examination and brain biopsy, and merely consulted with the MRC prion unit and the UK Creutzfeldt-Jakob disease surveillance unit, who agreed with the diagnosis of the Heidenhain variant of Creutzfeldt-Jakob disease. She continued quickly to deteriorate; she was transferred to a hospice nearer home and died there within a month of diagnosis.

Discussion

The Heidenhain variant of CJD shows characteristic neuro-ophthalmic clinical features and a more rapid disease course. Common visual symptoms include visual blurring with rapidly progressive visual field defects, metamorphopsia, visuospatial deficits and hallucinations [1, 2]. It is uncommon, affecting only 4 % of those reported to the UK CJD register between 1990 and 2005 [1] although accounted for 20 % of a smaller cohort in Germany [3].

It is common for the MRI to be normal in the early stages of the disease, but diffusion weighted imaging may reveal hyperintensity in the occipital and parietal regions (Fig. 44.1c), and 99 m Tc-SPECT shows often profound hypometabolism in the same regions [4]. The CSF contains the 14-3-3 marker of neuronal loss, and the EEG shows focal then generalized slowing then later on the characteristic triphasic slow wave complexes at 1 Hz.

All are homozygous for the Methionine polymorphism at codon 129 of the PrP gene.

Prion diseases are caused by a conformational change of the prion protein PrP^{C} into an abnormal variant termed PrP^{SC}, which is partially protease-resistant, which leads to increased production of the variant protein which accumulates within the brain [5]. Eighty-five percentage of prion diseases are sporadic, as in this case, 15 % are genetic through inheritance of mutations of the prion protein gene PRNP (genetic CJD (gCJD), Gerstmann Straussler Scheinker disease (GSS) and familial fatal insomnia (FFI)), and less than 1 % are acquired (variant CJD (vCJD), iatrogenic and kuru).

The neuropathology of sporadic CJD varies with the clinical features; macroscopic signs of atrophy (except in the cerebellum) are uncommon, and the microscopic abnormalities are often patchy. Most show the characteristic (although not specific) spongiform changes within the cortex, with neuronal loss, astrocyte activation and microglia. Amyloid plaques are seen in only 10 % (but greatly more prevalent in kuru and in variant CJD). Immunohistochemical staining for PRP^{SC} is specific; there is dense deposition around the spongiform change (Fig. 44.3) [6].

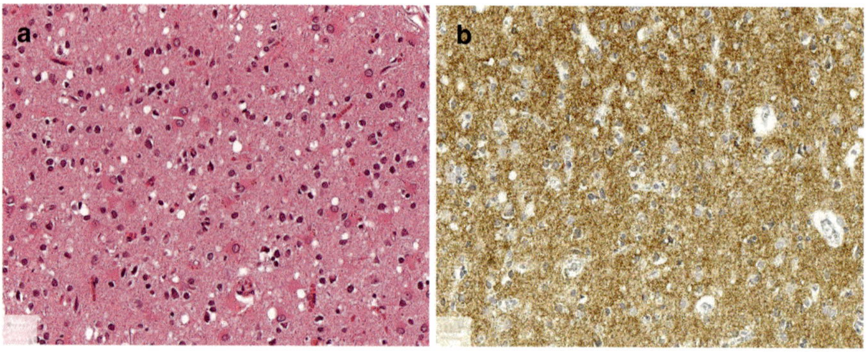

Fig. 44.3 Morphological appearances of Heidenhain variant of sporadic Creutzfeldt-Jakob disease in occipital lobe (with grateful thanks to Prof Tamas Revesz); haematoxylin and eosin stained section reveals pan-cortical microvacuolar degeneration in the neuropil accompanied by prominent reactive astrogliosis and neuronal loss (**a**). Immunostaining for abnormal prion protein with ICSM35 antibody shows characteristic diffuse synaptic labeling in the neuropil (**b**) (courtesy of Prof Sebastian Brandner and Dr Zane Jaunmuktane, Department of Neuropathology, Institute of Neurology)

References

1. Cooper SA, Murray KL, Heath CA, Will RG, Knight RSG. Isolated visual symptoms at onset in sporadic Creutzfeld-Jakob disease: the clinical phenotype of the "Heidenhain variant". Br J Ophthalmol. 2005;89:1341–2.
2. Parker S, Gujrati M, Pula J, Zallek SN, Kattah JC. The Heidenhain variant of Creutzfeld-Jakob disease – a case series. J Neuroophthalmol. 2014;34:4–9.
3. Kropp S, Schulz-Schaeffer WJ, Finkenstaedt M, Riedemann C, Windl O, Steinhoff BJ, Zerr I, Kretzschmar HA, Poser S. The Heidenhain variant of Creutzfeld-Jakob disease. Arch Neurol. 1999;56:55–61.
4. Prasad S, Lee EB, Woo JH, Alavi A, Galetta SL. Photo essay: MRI and positron emission tomography findings in Heidenhain variant Creutzfeld-Jakob disease. J Neuroophthalmol. 2010;30:260–2.
5. Kim MO, Geschwind MD. Clinical update of Jakob-Creutzfeldt disease. Curr Opin Neurol. 2015;28:302–10.
6. Ironside JW, Head MW. Biology and neuropathology of prion diseases. Handb Clin Neurol. 2008;89:779–97.

Case 45

History

This 33 year old lady was sitting at home at around five in the evening when she became aware of an abrupt onset of right-sided visual loss affecting both eyes as well as right arm and leg weakness. The right arm and leg weakness resolved after 20 min, but the visual loss persisted and she attended the hospital's Accident & Emergency Department at around eight that evening. There were no other or prior neurological symptoms and she was otherwise well. She smoked cigarettes.

Examination

The central acuities and color vision were normal. The discs showed normal appearances. She was seen to have a right sided visual field defect (Fig. 45.1).

It was recommended that she be admitted for investigations in the hyperacute stroke assessment unit, but she was unable to do this because of her young child at home and she discharged herself against medical advice. She agreed to be referred to the Neuro-ophthalmology unit.

D.P. Kidd, *Neuro-Ophthalmology*, DOI 10.1007/978-1-4471-2410-8_45

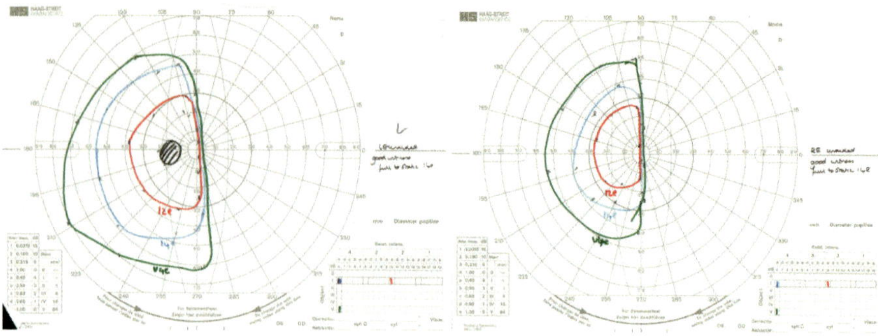

Fig. 45.1 Goldman visual field showing a complete congruous righted sided hemianopia

Clinical Evaluation

Were the cause of the disorder to be a cerebral infarction she had presented within the time window which would have allowed us to give her thrombolytic agents and to determine the risk of stroke recurrence quickly, but she returned instead two days later and the investigations were carried out then.

The cause in such a young person would be considered to be vascular first, then neoplastic, then infective or inflammatory. As noted below inherited disorders would also be considered.

Investigations

Screening blood investigations were normal; specifically FBC, clotting screen, glucose, lipids. ANA, ENA, ANCA and anti-cardiolipin and beta-2 glycoprotein antibodies were negative. JAC-2 and α-galactosidase assays were normal.

An MRI of the brain revealed high signal and restricted diffusion within the left occipital lobe corresponding precisely to the vascular territory of the posterior cerebral artery (Fig. 45.2).

A CT angiogram of the aortic arch, vertebral arteries and circle of Willis revealed no evidence for large vessel vasculitis, atheromatous disease or dissection of the main arteries.

A transoesophageal echocardiogram showed normal chambers and valves, no patent foramen ovale or atrial septal defect. A 24 hours cardiac monitor revealed sinus rhythm throughout.

A spinal fluid examination was normal.

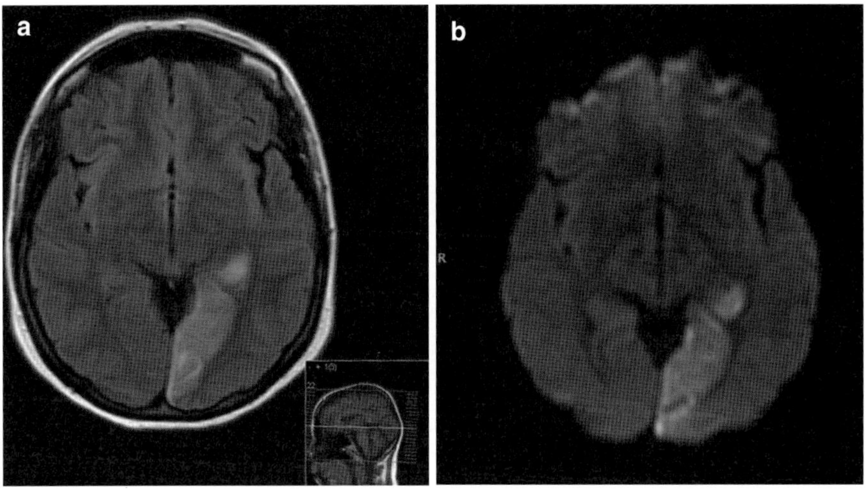

Fig. 45.2 (**a**) T2 weighted axial MRI showing high signal within the left occipital lobe, and (**b**) diffusion weighted MRI showing restricted diffusion within the same area, in keeping with a recent onset infarction

Discussion

Cerebral infarction in a young person

In a recent series of 3331 patients aged 18–49 with first stroke, the etiology was undetermined in 40 % of cases [1]. Embolism from a cardiac source was found in 17 % and from carotid dissection in 13 %. Large and small vessel disease accounted for 21 %.

The cardiac disorders included valvular and muscle disease and patent foramen ovale. Of the 720 with "other" causes, carotid dissection arose in 426 cases, and other causes always considered in young people, such as cerebral vasculitis (42 cases), Moyamoya disease (which is more common in Asian populations) and fibromuscular dysplasia (which is more common in young Caucasian women) (20 cases) were uncommon. Inherited thrombophilia accounted for 59 cases and antiphospholipid antibody syndrome for 39.

The incidence of stroke increases from 4.5 per 10^5 for people aged 30–34 to 32.9 per 10^5 for people age 45–49; this is related to an increase in the incidence of stroke related to atherosclerosis. Smoking is related, and increases with duration and exposure to cigarettes [2]. The incidence of stroke in women who take the contraceptive pill is 4 per 10^5 [2].

The risk of stroke with a patent foramen ovale is 5.1 in young people, although closing these shunts is not associated with a reduction in second stroke compared with those who have medical therapy (aspirin, clopidogrel or warfarin) alone [3].

Causes of posterior circulation stroke

In one large series of 117 patients, embolism from the heart or from a large vessel was responsible in 54 % of cases. 67 % had hemianopia, 22 % quadrantic field defects and 7 % bilateral field defects. 25 % were associated with addition motor or sensory signs, 10 % had visuospatial neglect, and dyslexia and/or dysgraphia in a further 13 % [4].

A recent MRI study of 205 patients with posterior cerebral artery territory infarction revealed embolic infarction accounted for 49 % of strokes and 43 % had large vessel atheromatous disease. A cardiac source of embolism was seen in 20 %, and 79 patients had evidence for more widespread cerebrovascular disease [5].

Eighty-seven had large vessel atheromatous disease of whom 38 had PCA disease without distal atheroma and 49 had vertebrobasilar and/or aortic arch disease without PCA disease. In the latter group embolic stroke was more common and in the former in situ thrombosis and embolization to branch arteries was more common. In these patients the ventrolateral thalamus was more often affected than the occipital cortex. Hence large vessel atheromatous disease is uncommon in the PCA, and around 40 % with PCA territory infarction have widespread cerebrovascular disease.

Cerebral infarction associated with migraine

Several studies have proven the association of cerebrovascular disease and migraine in young women [6–8]. In a French study of 72 women under the age of 45 the odds ratio for stroke was 3.0 for migraine without aura and 6.2 for migraine with aura. The risk increased to 10.2 in migrainous women who smoked more than 20 cigarettes per day and to 13.9 in those who took the contraceptive pill.

Another multicentre study of 291 women aged 20–44 with stroke revealed a similar association between migraine and stroke, which increased with hypertension, cigarette smoking and use of the contraceptive pill. The odds ratio of stroke in women with a history of migraine who took the contraceptive pill and who smoked was 34.4 compared with those who did not have migraine and did not take the contraceptive pill and who didn't smoke. The odds ratio of stroke in women who took the contraceptive ill and who did not have migraine was 1.19 [7]. The risk appeared further to be increased if the women had suffered more than 12 attacks of migraine in the previous year [8].

A meta-analysis of all papers published to 2005 revealed a risk of 2.16 (2.27 with aura, 1.83 without) and 8.72 for migraine and use of the oral contraceptive pill [9].

A clinical and MRI study of 17 patients out of 8137 seen in a stroke unit in Germany revealed that 70 % had lesions within the territory of the posterior circulation, and only 35 % had large infarctions; the remainder had small lesions seen on DWI, of whom 41 % had small multiple lesions. MRA studies were mostly normal; a minority showed flow abnormalities in the artery concerned. Patent foramina ovale were seen in 65 %. All but one patient had risk factors for stroke; 47 % had hypertension and 41 % had taken the oral contraceptive pill. At a telephone review 6 patients reported residual symptoms [10].

Other cases have shown cortical MRI abnormalities with the characteristic of oedema or cortical laminar necrosis which may be reversible [11] or permanent [12]. MRA studies in each case were normal.

Cortical disorders associated with posterior circulation infarction

These are noted in Appendix 4.

References

1. Yesilot Barlas N, Putaala J, Waje-Andreassen U, Vassilopoulou S, Nardi K, Odier C, Hofgart G, Engelter S, Burow A, Mihalka L, Kloss M, Ferrari J, Lemmens R, Coban O, Haapaniemi E, Maaijwee N, Rutten-Jacobs L, Bersano A, Cereda C, Baron P, Borellini L, Valcarenghi C, Thomassen L, Grau AJ, Palm F, Urbanek C, Tuncay R, Durukan Tolvanen A, van Dijk EJ, de Leeuw FE, Thijs V, Greisenegger S, Vemmos K, Lichy C, Bereczki D, Csiba L, Michel P, Leys D, Spengos K, Naess H, Tatlisumak T, Bahar SZ. Aetiology of first-ever ischaemic stroke in European young adults: the 15 cities young stroke study. Eur J Neurol. 2013;20:1431–9.
2. Ferro JM, Massaro AR, Mas J-L. Aetiological diagnosis of ischaemic stroke in young adults. Lancet Neurol. 2010;9:1085–96.
3. Furlan AJ, Reisman M, Massaro J, Mauri L, Adams H, Albers GW, Felberg R, Herrmann H, Kar S, Landzberg M, Raizner A, Wechsler L. Closure or medical therapy for cryptogenic stroke with patent foramen ovale. N Engl J Med. 2012;366:991–9.
4. Cals N, Devuyst G, Afsar N, Karapanayiotides T, Bogousslavsky J. Pure superficial posterior cerebral artery territory infarction in The Lausanne Stroke Registry. J Neurol. 2002;249:855–61.
5. Lee E, Kang DW, Kwon SU, Kim JS. Posterior cerebral artery infarction: diffusion-weighted MRI analysis of 205 patients. Cerebrovasc Dis. 2009;28:298–305.
6. Tzourio C, Tehindrazanarivelo A, Iglésias S, Alpérovitch A, Chedru F, d'Anglejan-Chatillon J, Bousser MG. Case-control study of migraine and risk of ischaemic stroke in young women. BMJ. 1995;310:830–3.
7. Chang CL, Donaghy M, Poulter N. Migraine and stroke in young women: case–control study. The World Health Organisation Collaborative Study of Cardiovascular Disease and Steroid Hormone Contraception. BMJ. 1999;318:13–8.
8. Donaghy M, Chang CL, Poulter N. Duration, frequency, recency and type of migraine and the risk of ischaemic stroke in women of childbearing age. J Neurol Neurosurg Psychiatry. 2002;73:747–50.
9. Etminan M, Takkouche B, Isorna FC, Samii A. Risk of ischaemic stroke in people with migraine: systematic review and meta-analysis of observational studies. BMJ. 2005;330(7482):63.
10. Wolf ME, Szabo K, Griebe M, Förster A, Gass A, Hennerici MG, Kern R. Clinical and MRI characteristics of acute migrainous infarction. Neurology. 2011;76:1911–7.
11. Resnick S, Reyes-Iglesias Y, Carreras R, Villalobos E. Migraine with aura associated with reversible MRI abnormalities. Neurology. 2006;66:946–7.
12. Liang Y, Scott TF. Migrainous infarction with appearance of laminar necrosis on MRI. Clin Neurol Neurosurg. 2007;109:592–6.

Case 46

History

This 46 year old lady developed episodes of visual disturbance lasting seconds. These were odd shaped flashes of light; sometimes like sheet lightening, and sometimes a less bright but white circular blob in one side of her vision. These would be momentary, and she would be well afterwards. There was no color, no scintillation or silver lining, no zig-zags or kaleidoscopic disturbance of the visual field. She would feel fine in between. There were no headaches.

She had mild and treated hypertension. Her past medical history was otherwise unremarkable.

Examination

The anterior visual pathways and discs were normal. The visual fields were full to confrontation.

D.P. Kidd, *Neuro-Ophthalmology*, DOI 10.1007/978-1-4471-2410-8_46

Clinical Evaluation

Is this just migraine? Should we reassure this lady and tell her that no investigation is required? No; the history is reminiscent of but not at all typical of a visual aura seen in migraine. It has a recent onset, is frequently recurrent, and there are no headaches. There is no prior history of migraine or headache for example in adolescence. Imaging most certainly is warranted.

Investigations

The MRI (Fig. 46.1) showed a lesion within the left occipital cortex which occupied space and compressed the underlying occipital lobe. There was a strong pattern of enhancement following injection of Gadolinium. The appearances were considered typical of a meningioma.

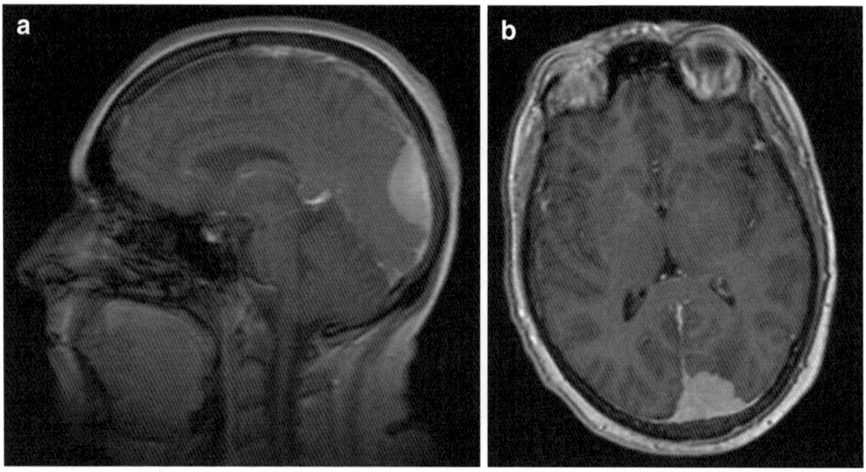

Fig. 46.1 T1 weighted axial MRI showing an enhancing mass lesion indenting the occipital pole on the left side

Management

The mass was removed through an occipital craniotomy (Fig. 46.2). A visual field defect arose (Fig. 46.3), which improved incompletely over the following 12 months, sufficient to allow her to drive legally. On treatment with Lamotrigine there were no further seizures. The mass has not recurred.

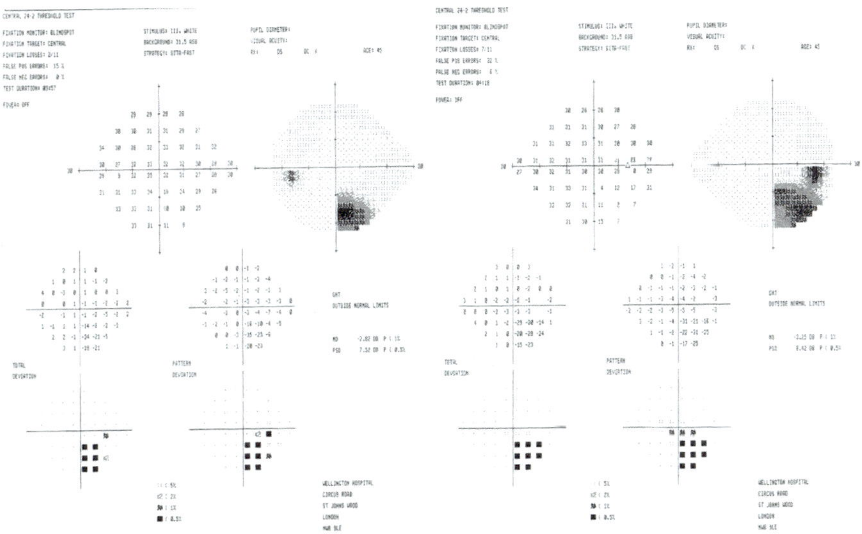

Fig. 46.2 Humphrey visual fields after surgery

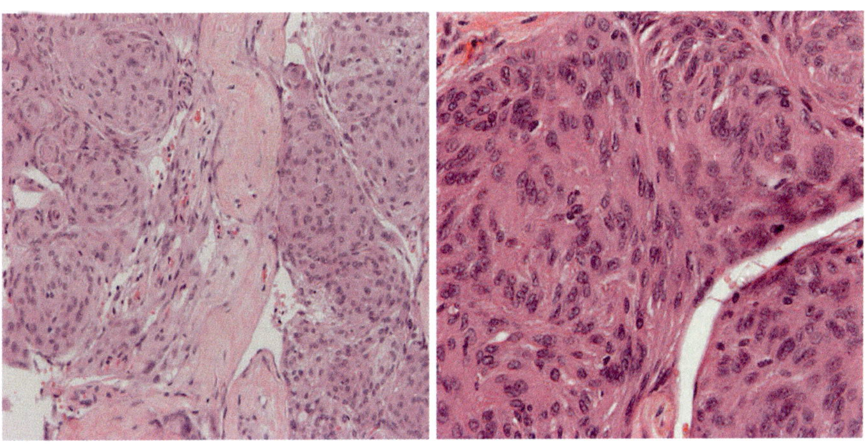

Fig. 46.3 Histological examination of the mass removed. This shows a tumor whose cells are arranged in sheets and lobules with whorl formation separated by collagenous tissue and hyalinized thickened blood vessels. The cells have elongated, slightly pleomorphic nuclei. There are only occasional mitotic figures. The appearances are of a grade 1 meningioma (Curtesy of Dr Nick Francis, Consultant Pathologist, HCA laboratories)

Discussion

Occipital Simple Partial Seizures

Simple partial seizures arising from occipital cortex are colored (usually multi-colored) and circular; other shapes, such as squares and stars are most uncommon. They arise in the temporal hemifield on one side, and can appear in a seeing or an unseeing or disorganized hemifield. Flashing or flickering is common, and the hallucination may enlarge but tends not to move.

They tend to develop rapidly, within seconds, and are brief, lasting seconds and rarely longer than 2 or 3 min. If interictal vision is normal it may take some time for normal vision to return. Headache is said to arise in 50 % of cases. The eyes may move, but not in a clonic way, more like a pursuit movement, and eyelid flickering may occur.

Occipital seizures may arise due to any disease process affecting the cortex, for example primary or secondary tumor, abscess or parasitic cyst, infarction, hemorrhage or arteriovenous malformation, and inflammatory lesion. It may be associated with disorders of neuronal migration, and in childhood with epilepsy syndromes such as idiopathic childhood occipital epilepsy of Gastaut, idiopathic photosensitive occipital lobe epilepsy and with Panayiotopoulos syndrome [1].

During a seizure paroxysmal fast activity with spiking is seen on surface electrode EEG [1]. Spread to the other side and the temporal regions is common.

The Visual Aura of Migraine

The so-called classic visual aura of migraine begins with the development of an enlarging shimmering central scotoma which arises at or near to the point of fixation. As it increases in size it changes into an arc, with scintillating or zig-zag lines at its leading edge. The arc gradually moves peripherally to the edge of the hemifield and as it does so the size of the zig-zags increase (in line with cortical magnification). Over the course of several minutes this scintillation is replaced by an absence of vision; either a blank scotoma or hemianopia.

This cortical event is considered to be cortical spreading depression, a slowly propagating wave of neuronal depolarization leading to suppression of cortical activity, which spreads across the cortex at a rate of 3 mm per minute (and which corresponds to the rate at which the scintillating scotoma passes across the visual field [2, 3].

It is untrue that lesions in the occipital cortex cause seizures and patients with migrainous visual auras will inevitably show normal imaging; Shams and Plant in a helpful paper discuss the relationship between a secondary form of migrainous aura and various lesions (predominately arteriovenous malformations of the cortex, although benign tumors also presented thus) may lead to a state of neuronal hyper-excitabilty which in turn may induce the same pattern of spreading cortical depression which occurs in migraine [3].

References

1. Adcock JE, Panayiotopoulos CP. Occipital lobe seizures and epilepsies. J Clin Neurophysiol. 2012;29:397–407.
2. Schott GD. Exploring the visual hallucinations of migraine aura: the tacit contribution of illustration. Brain. 2007;130:1690–703.
3. Shams PN, Plant GT. Migraine-like aura due to focal cerebral lesions: case series and review. Surv Ophthalmol. 2011;56:135–61.

Case 47

History

This 65 year old man became unwell 2 weeks prior to an emergency admission to the referring hospital. There were flu-like symptoms and headache, which increased in severity. A week later he had noticed blurring of his vision, then some numbness, and when he began vomiting his daughter brought him to the emergency department of their local hospital.

Previously well, he took no regular medication. He was an ex-smoker. There were no other symptoms on systematic enquiry.

Examination

On admission he looked unwell but was afebrile. The general examination was normal. The neurological examination was also considered to be normal; the central acuities within normal limits and the discs not swollen. There was a left sided upper quadrantinopia (Fig. 47.1).

He was admitted for further investigations, including a CT scan of his head. This showed a large mass within the occipital lobe on the right (Fig. 47.2). He was referred to the Royal Free Hospital.

D.P. Kidd, *Neuro-Ophthalmology*, DOI 10.1007/978-1-4471-2410-8_47

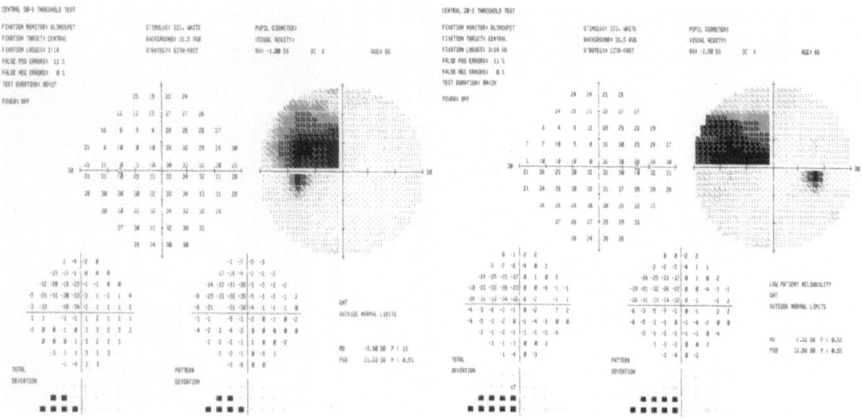

Fig. 47.1 Humphrey visual fields showing an upper quadrantinopia on the left side

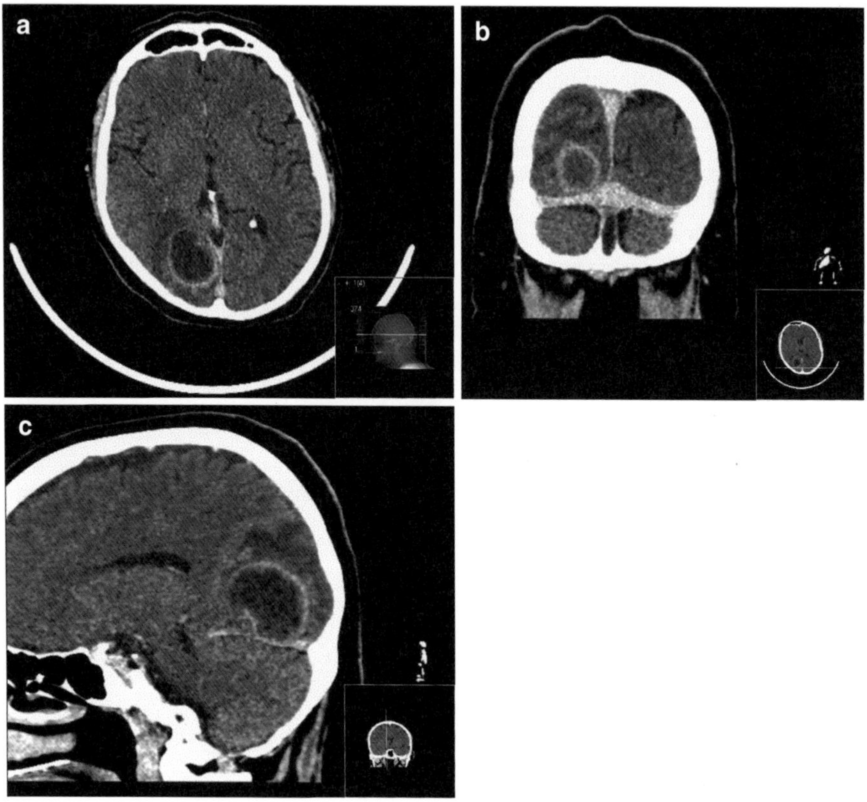

Fig. 47.2 CT scan of brain showing a spherical lesion with ring enhancement in the right occipital lobe

Evaluation

A 65 year old man previously well develops a flulike illness then increasing headache, then visual blurring and numbness and finally vomiting. This constellation of symptoms which have evolved quickly over a 2 week period strongly imply a disorder associated with increasing intracranial pressure and it was right to order the CT scan straightaway. This showed a mass lesion within the right occipital lobe surrounded by edema. The neurological signs were of a left sided homonymous hemianopia with a mild ipsilateral sensory loss but no pyramidal signs (because the lesion involved the ascending sensory white matter but not the descending motor tracts). The radiological differential diagnosis would be infection including abscess and protozoal disease, neoplasia which would be more likely secondary than primary in view of the ring enhancement and the surrounding mass effect, and would include primary and secondary lymphoma, and tumefactive inflammatory lesions for example sarcoidosis, vasculitis and Behçet's syndrome. If a primary cause for the disorder cannot be found then a biopsy should be undertaken.

Investigations

Screening blood tests were undertaken which were unremarkable save for a neutrophil leucocytosis of 11.5. The ESR was normal but the CRP was 16. The sodium was low at 127 mmol/l. The CT scan was reviewed and an MRI recommended (Fig. 47.3). The features were considered to be either that of an abscess or a metastasis. A CT scan of the chest abdomen and pelvis revealed no primary source for either possibility, and blood cultures were negative. An echocardiogram showed no evidence for infective vegetations on the valves.

The Neurosurgeons performed a biopsy and decompression with a stealth guided aspiration through a burr hole. Turbid green/yellow "smelly" fluid was aspirated and sent for analysis.

The cytological analysis revealed necrotic debris and numerous polymorphs. Microbiological analysis revealed gram positive cocci and they grew Streptococcus anginosis-constellatus, sensitive to Ceftriaxone.

He received treatment with 6 weeks of intravenous Ceftriaxone and recovered well. The infectious diseases physicians recommended a further 4 week course of oral Amoxicillin after. His visual field defect improved (Fig. 47.4) but did not resolve. The CT showed residual cavitation and surrounding gliosis.

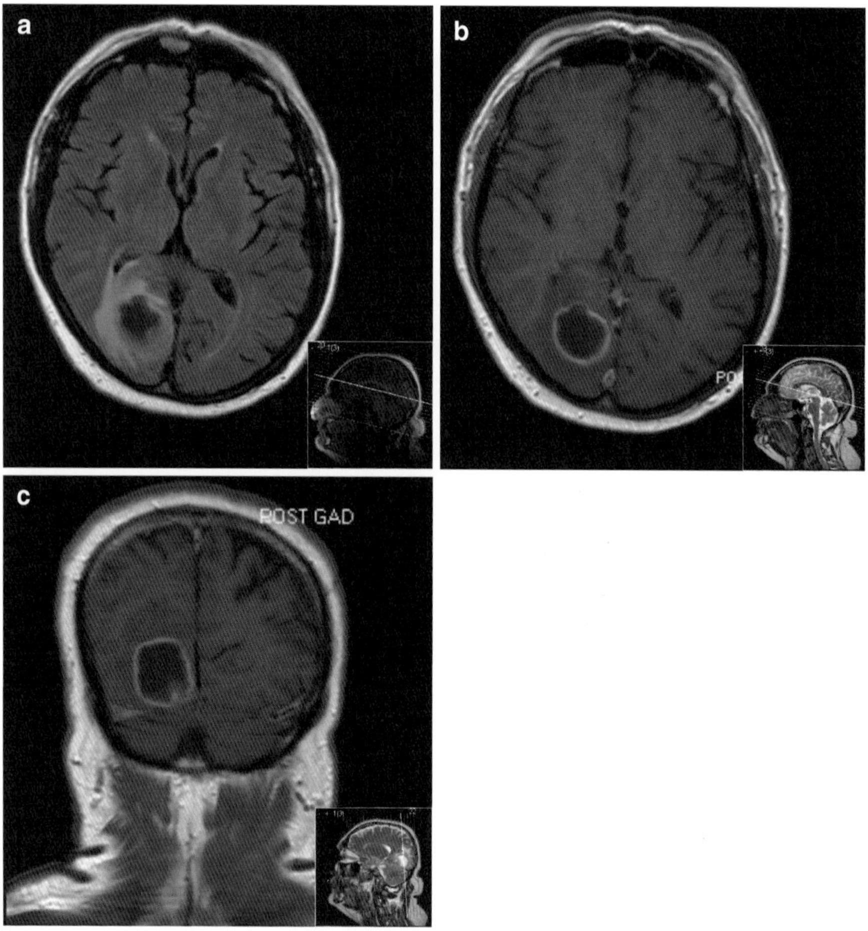

Fig. 47.3 MRI scan of brain showing the lesion with central necrosis and ring enhancement. There is surrounding vasogenic edema

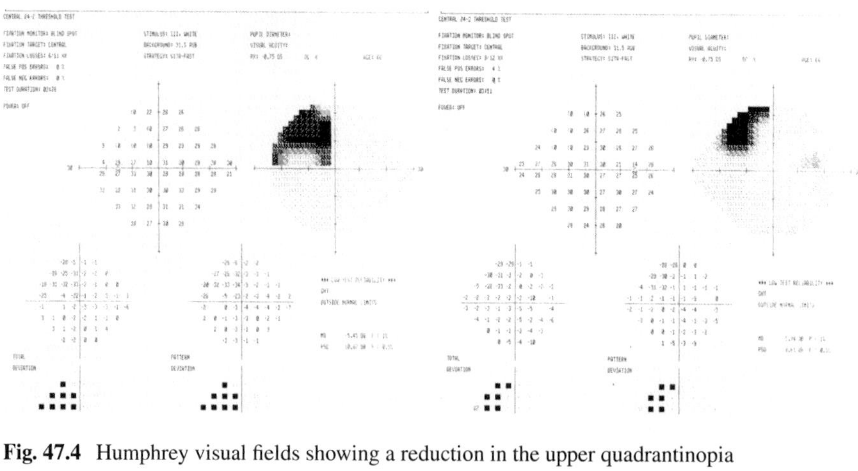

Fig. 47.4 Humphrey visual fields showing a reduction in the upper quadrantinopia

Discussion

Cerebral Abscess

Brain abscess due to bacterial infection is now rare, with an estimated annual incidence of 1×10^5. The majority is caused by gram positive aerobic bacteria such as streptococcus and staphylococcus. Gram negative species such as E Coli, Haemophilus, Pseudomonas and Acinetobacter are less common, and anaerobic species rare. The mortality rate remains high at around 10 %.

The infection arises from adjacent structures such as the paranasal air sinuses or middle ear, or though veins from the oral cavity and pharynx, or through arteries from elsewhere including the heart valves. Obviously an infection may also arise locally following trauma or neurosurgery. In children, congenital heart disease, especially those in which shunting occurs, is a recognized risk factor.

A focal cerebritis develops, leading to influx of inflammatory cells including neutrophils and macrophages. Edema develops and an enlarging capsule with a necrotic core develops quickly. Gliosis develops as the inflammatory response subsides.

Patients present with headache and drowsiness; focal neurological signs and signs of raised intracranial pressure develop later. Fever may only be present in around half the cases, and the patients may appear at the onset not to be systemically unwell.

Most are managed with a stereotactic aspiration as in this case, followed by prolonged antibiotic therapy empirically then specifically once organisms and sensitivities are learned.

Seizures arise in 50 % of patients at onset and in 90 % after treatment; most therefore need to continue anticonvulsant treatment after recovery. The prevalence of residual neurological impairments is around 50 %.

Reference

1. King N. Cerebral abscess. Handb Clin Neurol. 2010;96:65–74.

Case 48

History

This 42 year old lady was admitted through the emergency department following a generalized seizure. Perfectly well until the day before, she had noticed episodes of visual blurring in which she felt her vision darkening through both fields for a few seconds before returning to normal. This increased in frequency throughout the day, accompanied by headache and then drowsiness. Her condition worsened overnight and she had three tonic clonic seizures in succession in the early morning.

She had been treated for tuberculosis in 1992 for a year. Her past medical history was otherwise unremarkable.

Examination

She was drowsy, but afebrile. Her central acuities were 6/12, 6/9 with normal color vision and symmetrical pupillary responses. There was a right paracentral defect within the visual fields (Fig. 48.1). The ocular media were clear and the discs were normal. The remainder of the neurological examination was normal.

The systemic examination was normal, in particular the chest was clear.

D.P. Kidd, *Neuro-Ophthalmology*, DOI 10.1007/978-1-4471-2410-8_48

a

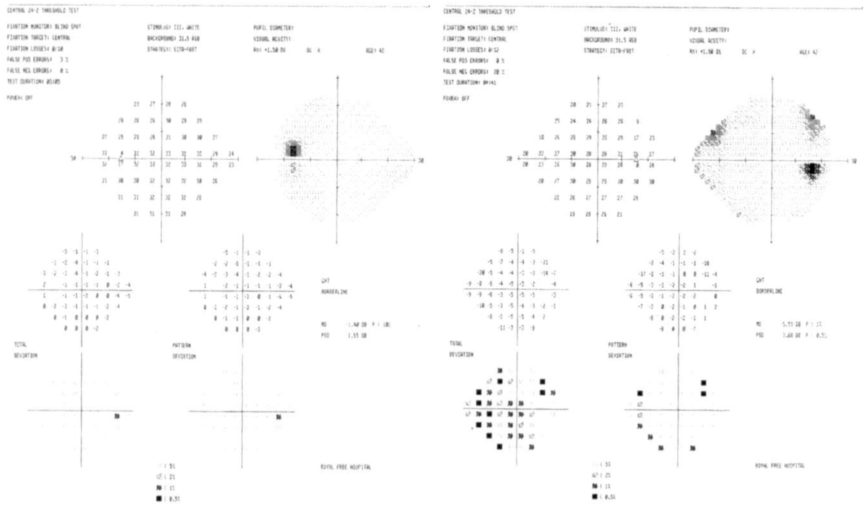

b

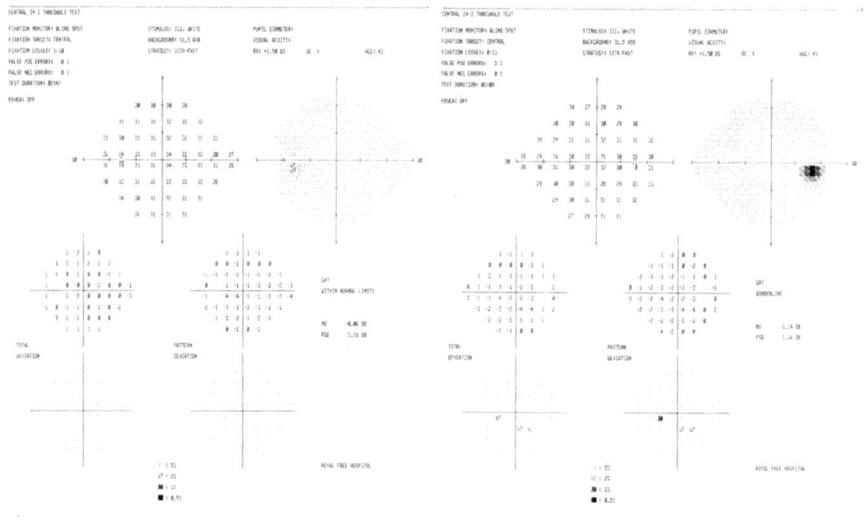

Fig. 48.1 Humphrey visual fields showing (**a**) right sided field defect which (**b**) resolved following treatment

Investigations

The CRP was <1, FBC showed a neutrophil leucocytosis of 13.3, biochemical screening was normal and blood gases within the normal range.

A chest X-ray was normal.

A CT of the lungs revealed lymphadenopathy and a patchy consolidation in the right upper lobe (Fig. 48.2).

A CT of the head showed an area of edema within the left occipital lobe, closely associated with a small area of calcification within the adjacent cortex (Fig. 48.3).

An MRI of the brain showed a single left occipital lesion with ring enhancement and surrounding vasogenic edema (Fig. 48.4a, b).

Induced sputum samples were negative for AAFB.

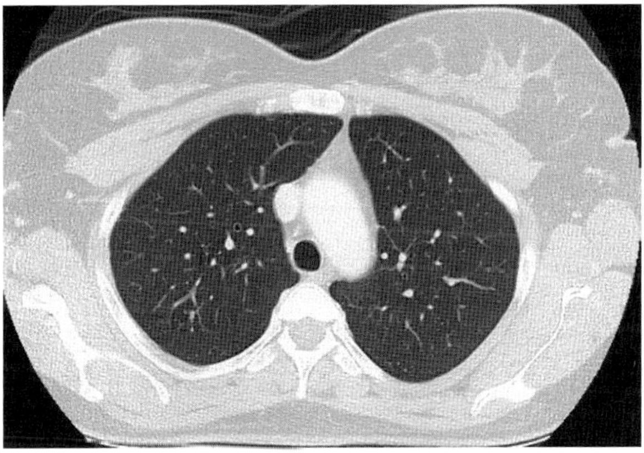

Fig. 48.2 CT thorax: there are multiple calcified hilar and mediastinal lymph nodes, and inflammatory nodules with an adjacent ground glass appearance in the right upper lobe

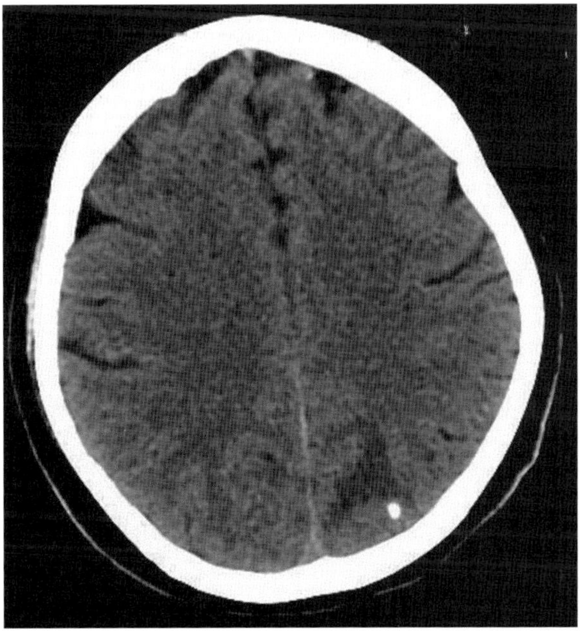

Fig. 48.3 CT head showing an area of vasogenic edema within the left occipital lobe, with a calcified spot within the cortex adjacent to it. The differential diagnosis of this appearance is infection such as TB, cysticercosis, toxoplasma; cavernous hemangioma, and metastasis

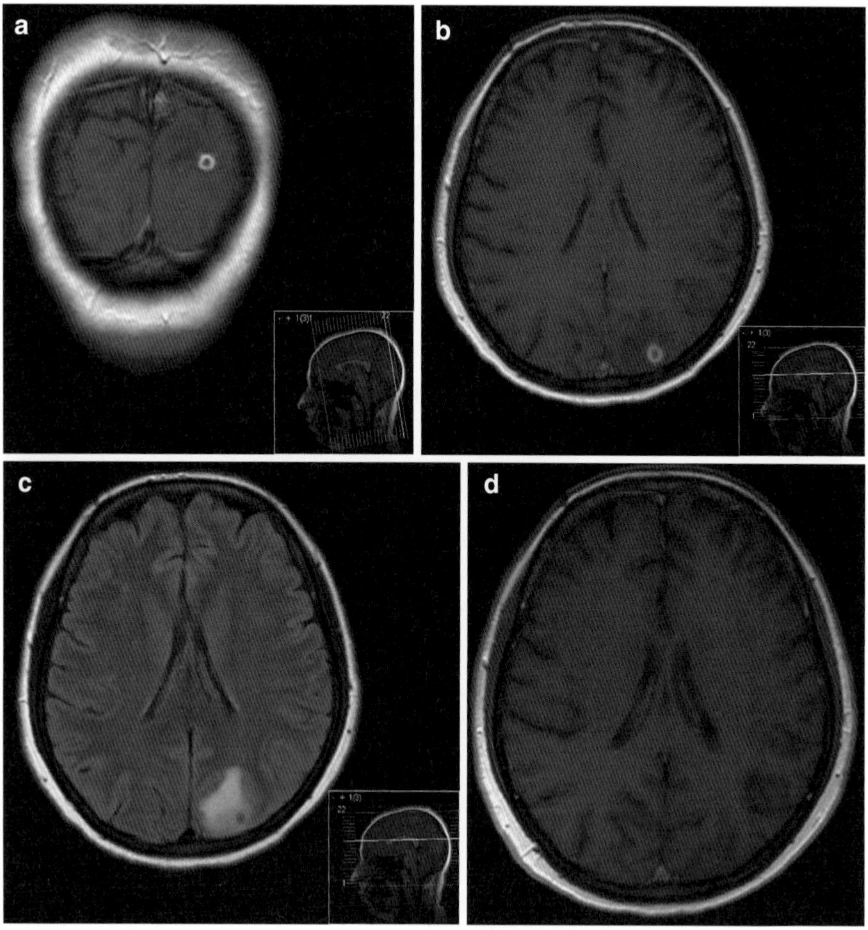

Fig. 48.4 (**a**, **b**) T1 weighted MRI showing left sided ring enhancing lesion within the occipital cortex, (**c**) axial T2 weighted MRI showing edema around the lesion, and (**d**) T1 weighted MRI showing reduction in the lesion following treatment

Clinical Evaluation

This lady with a history of TB presents with a series of generalized seizures and a visual field defect due to a solitary ring enhancing lesion in the occipital lobe. There is calcification on a CT, implying that the lesion is not new, but a reactivation of a previous disorder. Constitutionally she is well, and her screening blood tests confirm this. The differential diagnosis is as the radiologists have given, an infection, including TB and pyogenic abscess, cysticercosis, a neoplastic lesion, either primary or secondary and including lymphoma, inflammatory lesion such as seen in sarcoidosis, Behçet's syndrome, cerebral vasculitis and rarely in MS. The presence of calcification would make an infective disorder or tumor much more likely.

Management

She was treated with anticonvulsants and underwent the investigations noted above. There were no further seizures. Review of the previous investigations in 1992 revealed an abnormal chest X-ray with diffuse shadowing, evidence for TB meningitis with a raised CSF protein at 0.76 g/dl, CSF white cell count 25, and reduced CSF glucose at 1.9 mmol/l. She developed a VIth neuropathy which resolved. She was treated with Streptomycin for 2 months and Rifinah, Pyrazinamide and pyridoxine for a year. Her chest X-ray was reported to have returned to normal.

A brain biopsy was requested by the ID team but correctly the Neurosurgeons felt that this would pose a risk to vision, and she was treated for TB again, for a year. The MRI improved (Fig. 48.4c) and she has remained well, with normal visual fields and no seizures, since then.

Discussion

Tuberculosis affected 8.7 million people in 2011, of whom 1.4 million died (1). The incidence is highest in sub-Saharan Africa, then in Asia. It is the leading cause of death in people infected with HIV.

Neurological involvement occurs with tuberculous meningitis, tuberculous abscess and tuberculoma. Tuberculous meningitis (TBM) is a subacute illness with depression of consciousness, hydrocephalus and cranial nerve palsies. Seizures and hemiparesis may occur. The MRI shows meningeal enhancement and the CSF is active with a low CSF/blood sugar ratio.

A tuberculoma is a focus of infection which arises in the brain and grows in size but does not rupture into the subarachnoid space. They are composed of lymphocytes, giant cells and macrophages with central caseation; the caseous granuloma They may be single or multiple and present as space occupying lesions. They may be so large as to appear on CT or MRI to be tumors. Tuberculomas do not contain pus whereas tuberculous abscesses do. Mycobacteria can persist for years, and can reactivate if the host immune system becomes compromised (2). They occur anywhere but are more common in the infratentorial region in children. Imaging shows spherical lesions of 1–8 cm in size, which are hypodense in the center with ring enhancement on CT, and on MRI there is ring enhancement and hypointensity within. Spectroscopy and MTR techniques have failed to allow specific differentiation from other infections and from tumors, leading to a need for biopsy in most cases.

In a recent series from France, India and Mexico (3) 24 cases of solitary tuberculoma were reviewed and 92 previously reported cases discussed. Evidence for systemic infection was common (in 54 %) but not invariable, with abnormal thoracic radiological infections or lymphadenopathy. The CSF was active in the majority of patients, and clinical outcome was "good" in 83 % following treatment.

Treatment is with full anti-tuberculous chemotherapy; the response rate is cited as 87 % (1, 2). Rifampicin (10–20 mg/kg) and Isoniazid (10–15 mg/kg) for 9–12 months and Pyrazinamide (25–30 mg/kg) and Ethambutol (15–20 mg/kg) for 2 months, or Streptomycin 20–30 mg/kg also for 2 months. Drug resistance is becoming an increasing problem. Concomitant use of steroids in TBM is associated with a reduction in inflammation (and vasculitis) which improves outcome.

References

1. Chin JH, Mateen FJ. Central nervous system tuberculosis: challenges and advances in diagnosis and treatment. Curr Infect Dis Rep. 2013;15:631–35.
2. DeLance AR, Safaee M, Oh MC, Clark AJ, Kaur G, Sun MZ, Bollen AW, Phillips JJ, Parsa AT. Tuberculoma of the central nervous system. J Clin Neurosci. 2013;20:1333–41.
3. Psimaras D, Bonnet C, Heinzmann A, Cardenas G, Hernandez JLS, Tungaria A, Behari S, Lacrois D, Mokhtari K, Karantoni E, Sokrab Taq E, Idris Mohammed N, Sonmez G, Caumes E, Roze E. Solitary tuberculous brain lesions: 24 new cases and a review of the literature. Rev Neurol. 2014;170:454–63.

Case 49

History

This 62 year old left handed man presented with an escalating headache disorder over 2 weeks then an abrupt onset left facial weakness, weakness and sensory loss in the left upper limb. He found that he had no control over his hand, although he was still able to move it. Within minutes he lost consciousness and was observed to have a generalized seizure preceded by focal clonic movements of the left upper limb.

He was admitted to hospital and a peripherally placed right parietal hemorrhage was identified (Figs. 49.1 and 49.2).

A catheter angiogram revealed extensive arteriovenous fistulae between both internal and external carotid arteries and the superior sagittal and right transverse and sigmoid sinuses and the torcula (Fig. 49.3). That communicating between the external carotid artery and the superior sagittal sinus was seen to be under high pressure and flow. There was evidence for widespread venous outflow obstruction.

He underwent embolization of the main fistulae in three separate procedures. Following the last he developed problems with vision and reading.

Examination

The central acuities were counting fingers on both sides. There was a left sided upper quadrantinopia (Fig. 49.4). There was no color vision but he could recognize faces. There was a prominent dyslexia in which he was unable to recognize words and to read out loud. He found reading single letters difficult; however, when prompted he was able quite easily to write a sentence. Calculation was normal. When a children's chart of figures was shown to him he was able to recognize and name them down to 6/9.

A psychometric assessment confirmed the dyslexic disorder, with a retained ability to write. He performed memory, visuospatial and orientation tests normally, and there was no prosopagnosia.

D.P. Kidd, *Neuro-Ophthalmology*, DOI 10.1007/978-1-4471-2410-8_49

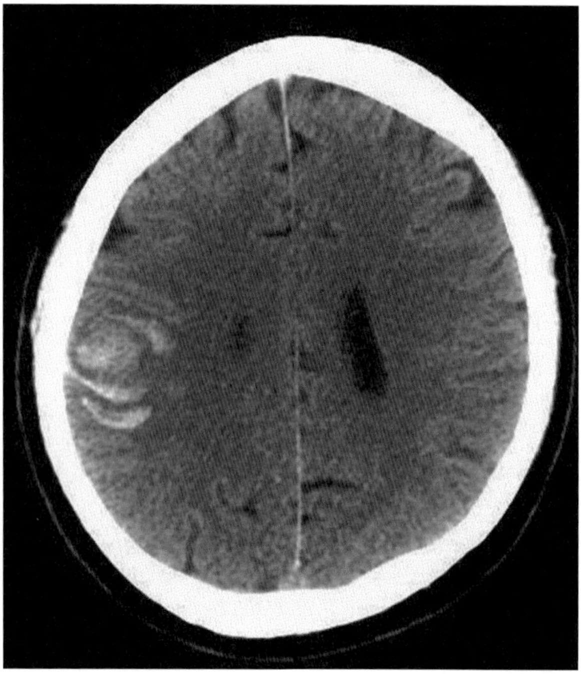

Fig. 49.1 CT scan of brain showing hemorrhage in the right parietal lobe including the cortex and adjacent white matter. The hemorrhage has the appearance of a series of layers, and is most unlike that seen in a lobar hemorrhage due to hypertension

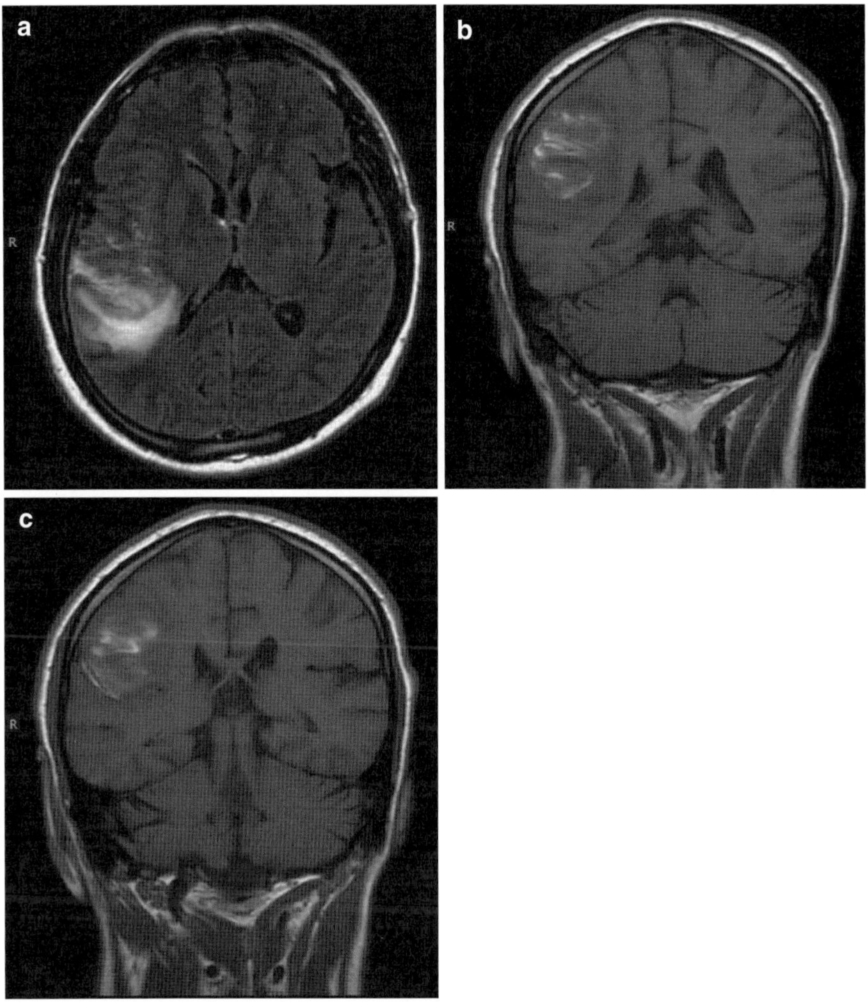

Fig. 49.2 (**a**) T2 weighted axial MRI scan at the same level showing heterogeneous T2 signal alteration edema of the parietal white matter, and some mass effect, and (**b**) coronal T1 weighted scan showing the same lesion, with T1 shortening inferiorly due to hemosiderin deposition (implying that the hemorrhage had occurred at various times in evolution)

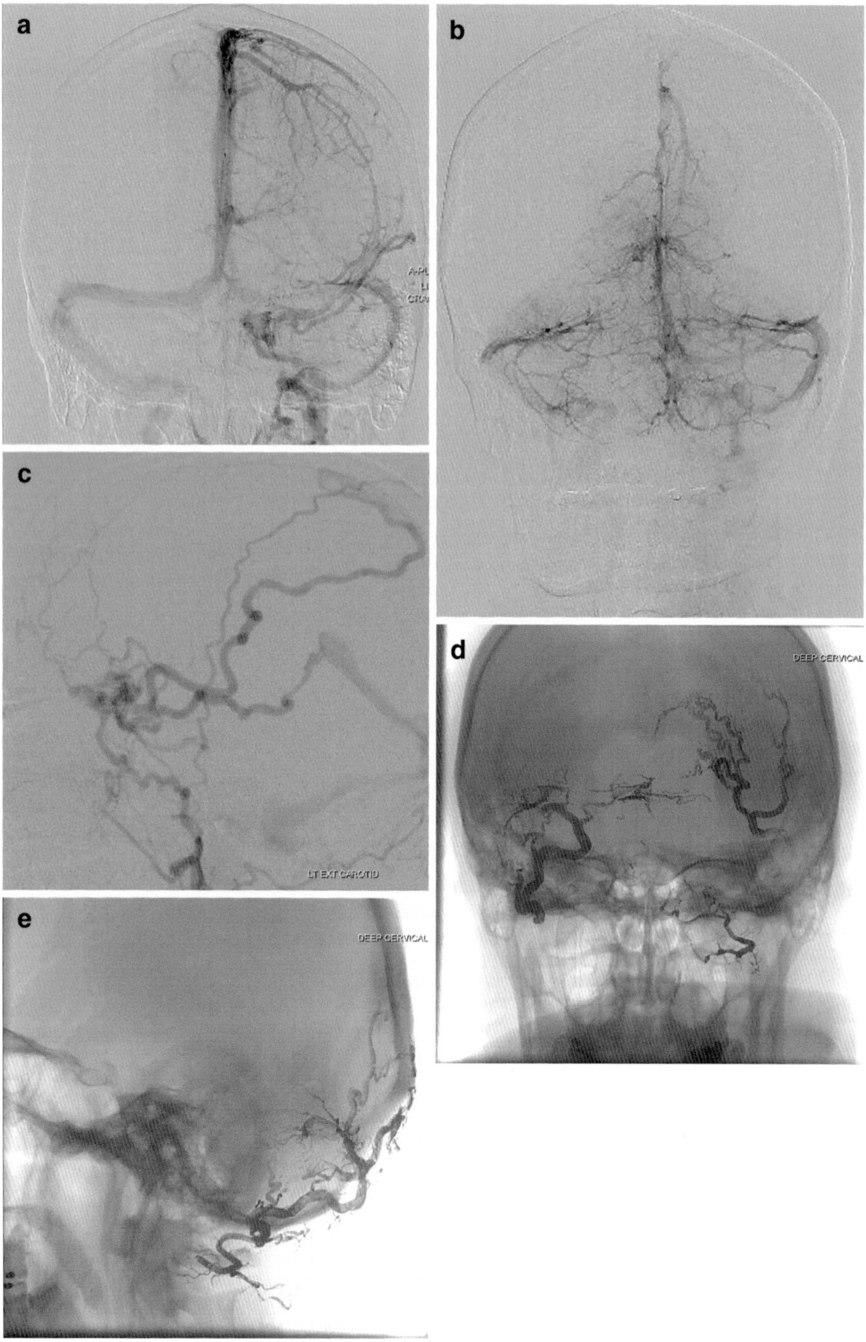

Fig. 49.3 Six vessel catheter angiogram showing occlusion of the middle third of the superior sagittal sinus with retrograde flow from the cortex into the anterior third (**a**, **b**). There are fistulae between the superior sagittal sinus and the external carotid artery on the left (**c**). High flow fistulae were seen at the torcula and transverse sinus on the right (**d**, **e**) (courtesy of Dr Peter Cowley Consultant Neuroradiologist, National Hospital)

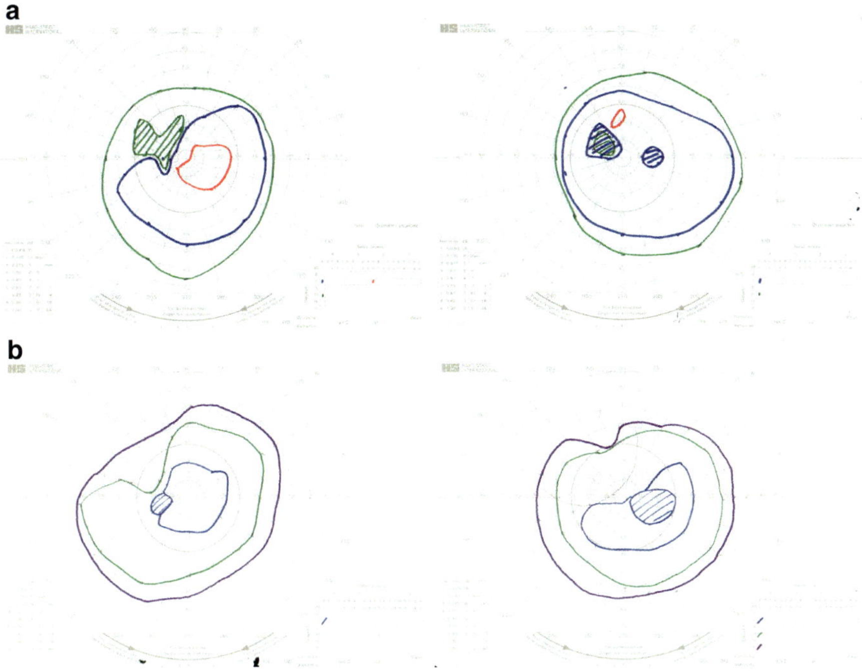

Fig. 49.4 Goldman visual field showing a left sided upper quadrantinopia

Evaluation

This left handed man presents with a left hemisensory loss and some weakness but a specific inability to control the movement of his left hand. This implies a proprioceptive disorder which would make the lesion placed within the cortex on the right side, and within the parietal lobe. This fits in well with the subsequent event; a focal motor seizure of the left side which generalized. It is of abrupt onset and associated with headache, and so it was not surprising that he was found to have had a hemorrhage in that region. It so happens that the hemorrhage shows features of a venous rather than an arterial origin, related to venous outflow obstruction as a result of the arteriovenous fistulae.

This, however, is not the reason for demonstrating the case; during treatment he developed a specific and uncommon problem with visual perception and reading.

He was found to have a profound acquired dyslexia with retained writing ability, achromatopsia and an upper quadrantinopia. This cannot be caused by a parietal lesion, which would in the first case be associated with a lower quadrantinopia. Secondly, a parietal lesion would be associated with so-called central alexia – an inability both to read and to write, alexia with agraphia. More anteriorly placed lesions would also be associated with dysphasia.

Alexia without agraphia is a peripheral alexia, the cause of which has to be situated more posteriorly and specifically within the occipital lobe. If the difficulty in

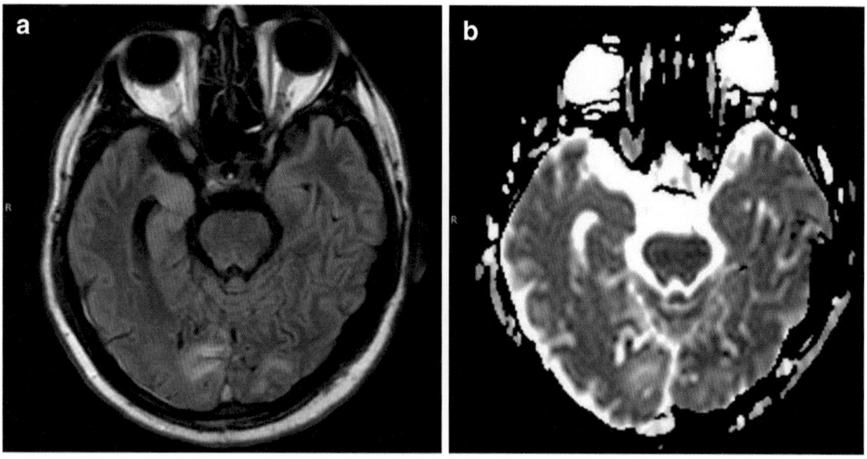

Fig. 49.5 T2 weighted (**a**) and diffusion weighted (**b**) axial MRI scan showing infarction of the right occipital lobe and posterior temporal (fusiform) gyrus

reading color plates is related to achromatopsia (it may not be, being related more to a difficulty in reading single numbers and therefore part of the dyslexia) then this to would put the lesion more posteriorly, and specifically at the occipito-temporal junction (see appendix 4). Finally the field defect is an upper quadrantinopia, placing the lesion either in the temporal or the ventral occipital pole.

A further MRI scan was undertaken which showed an infarction of the right medial occipital lobe, extending anteriorly into the posterior temporal region (Fig. 49.5).

Discussion

Alexia

Peripheral alexias are not associated with abnormal language function. Pure alexia refers to alexia without agraphia, and global alexia describes patients with this disorder who are also unable to recognize and name single letters. Recognition of words is unimpaired in patients with hemianopic dyslexia, but the hemianopia (particularly in left hemisphere dominant patients with right hemianopia) slows down left to right reading considerably. Its presence is related to the closeness of the field defect to the midline. A neglect alexia, related to non-dominant parietal lesions, occurs when the neglected half of the words are ignored and the word therefore makes little sense. In attentional alexia patients note that the letters overlap and therefore make no sense; this is associated with dominant parietal lesions.

This case describes a pure alexia with some global features. There was no evidence on the psychometric assessment for any neglect or attentional disorder as well. It has been reported before in left handed people [1].

fMRI and PET studies have shown that the lesions which cause pure and hemianopic alexias are found in the medial dominant occipital lobe. Those with a pure alexia usually also have involvement of the posterior fusiform gyrus in the temporal lobe [2, 3]. Patients with pure alexia may improve, and learn to read "LBL" (letter by letter), but tend to remain impaired and disabled, while those with hemianopic dyslexia may respond to treatment such as optokinetic reading training [4].

References

1. Pillon B, Bakchine S, Lhermitte F. Alexia without agraphia in a left-handed patient with a right occipital lesion. Arch Neurol. 1987;44:1257–62.
2. Leff AP, Crewes H, Plant GT, Scott SK, Kennard C, Wise RJ. The functional anatomy of single-word reading in patients with hemianopic and pure alexia. Brain. 2001;124:510–21.
3. Leff AP, Spitsyna G, Plant GT, Wise RJ. Structural anatomy of pure and hemianopic alexia. J Neurol Neurosurg Psychiatry. 2006;77:1004–7.
4. Schuett S. The rehabilitation of hemianopic dyslexia. Nat Rev Neurol. 2009;5:427–37.

Case 50

History

This 74 year old man was referred by the cataract clinic. He had been observed therein having been referred with a left sided visual field defect identified by his optometrist 2 years previously. His vision back then had been 6/9 and 6/6 and the cataracts had not been considered sufficiently severe to warrant surgery. The field defect evolved (Fig. 50.1) and he was referred to the Neuro-ophthalmology clinic for further investigation.

He did not volunteer any other or prior neurological symptoms, and his general health was good; he took medications for hypertension and tamsulosin for nocturia.

When interrogated specifically he admitted that he had noted some problems with getting around on his own; he was perfectly able to go out to the shops on his own, taking buses and the underground, but when on a holiday in Paris his wife had noticed that he was no longer able to work out where he was in the unfamiliar city, and how to manage a map to return to the hotel. Neither he nor his wife had noticed a change in his memory or behavior. Reading, writing and calculation were unaffected. There were no headaches.

Examination

The central acuities were 6/9 N8 with normal color vision and symmetrical pupillary responses. There was a non-congruous left sided hemianopia (Fig. 50.1). The discs were normal and there were no other abnormal neurological signs. His gait was normal.

D.P. Kidd, *Neuro-Ophthalmology*, DOI 10.1007/978-1-4471-2410-8_50

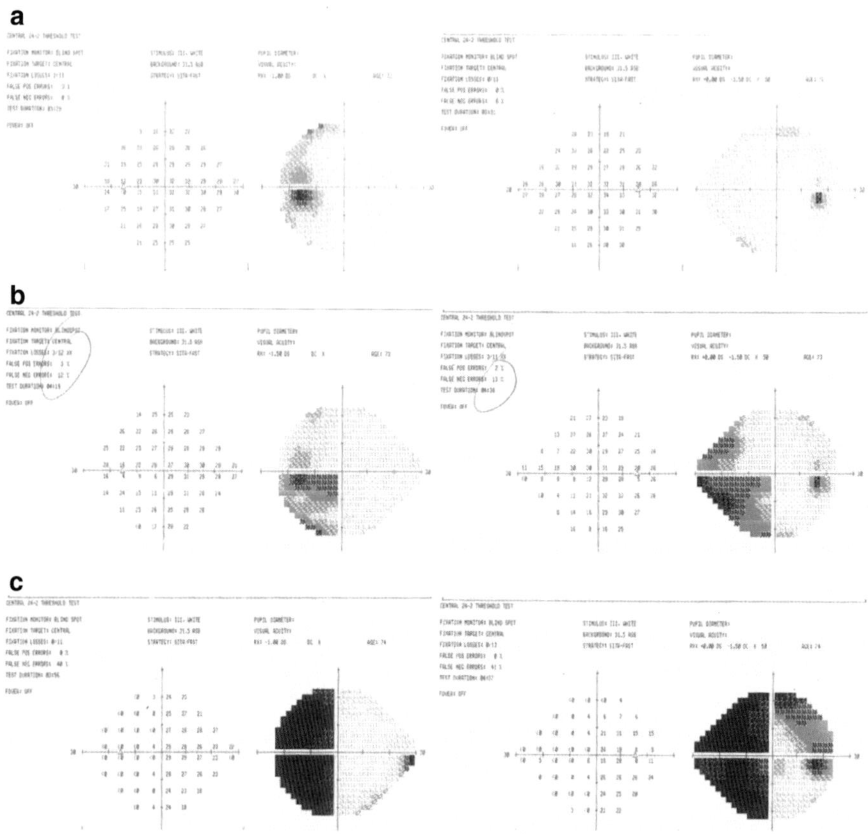

Fig. 50.1 Humphrey visual fields showing evolution of the visual field defect over a 2 year period. Notice that the field defect becomes complete then spreads to the other side

Clinical Evaluation

He presents with a documented slowly evolving left sided hemianopia seemingly without any other signs, aside from a new disorder of visuospatial perception. This implies a right hemisphere disorder, obviously involving the posterior visual pathway but the posterior parietal region too. Since it has evolved over a 2 year period it would not have a vascular basis, and, because it is seemingly unilateral, a metabolic or degenerative cause would be less likely. A neoplastic disorder, therefore, should be considered and obviously imaging would be the initial and urgent investigation of first choice.

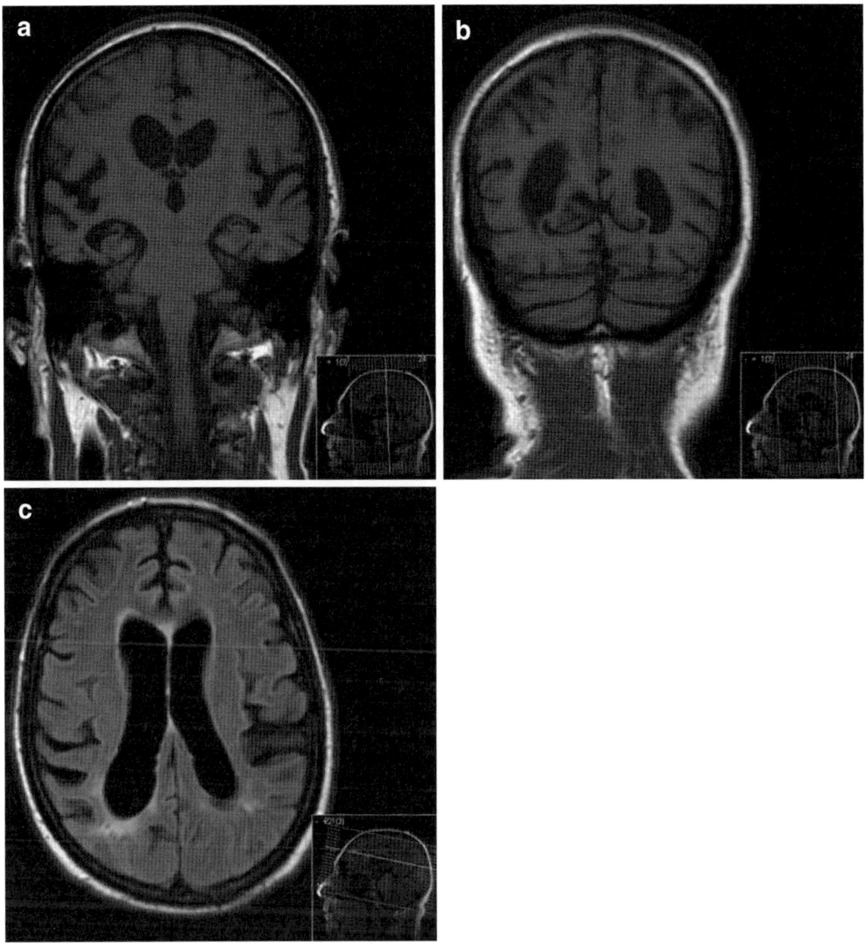

Fig. 50.2 (**a**, **b**) T1 weighted coronal and (**c**) axial FLAIR sequence MRI scans showing an asymmetric atrophy of the right temporal, parietal and occipital gray and white matter without any accompanying white matter disease

Imaging

An MRI scan of the brain showed a striking asymmetry of the occipital and parietal lobes, with atrophy on the right side. There was no evidence for a mass lesion, previous hemorrhage, infarction or abscess (Fig. 50.2).

A degenerative disorder would be the most likely cause, although asymmetric involvement by such a process is most uncommon. He was asked to undergo a formal neuropsychometric evaluation, which revealed a decline in intellectual abilities compared with his estimated pre-morbid optimal level of ability. There

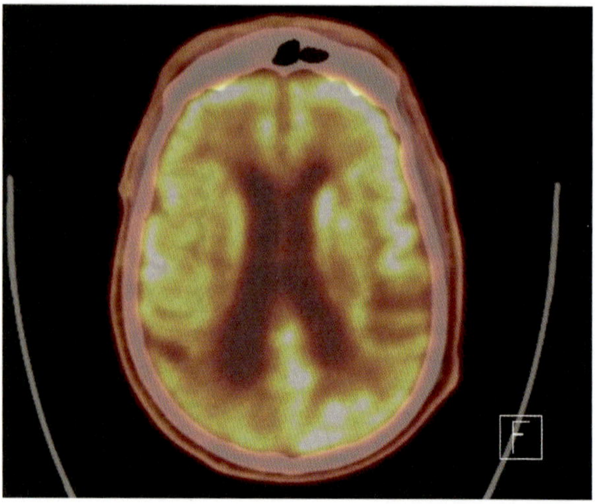

Fig. 50.3 SPECT scan showing marked hypometabolism in the right parietal cortex, right anterior, lateral and posterior temporal cortices and the right occipital cortex. Uptake within the frontal cortex, striati and cerebellum is within normal limits

were deficits on visuospatial tasks, visual perception and visual memory. He had anomia. Verbal memory was slightly impaired and working memory also affected.

An FDG SPECT scan of the brain revealed hypometabolism in the atrophic areas, in keeping with the diagnosis of posterior cortical atrophy (Fig. 50.3).

Posterior Cortical Atrophy

This is a clinical syndrome of different pathologies in which deficits in higher visual processing evolve with evidence on imaging for a degeneration in posterior cortical and subcortical structures within the brain [1, 2]. One study [3] found that 5 % of a series of 523 patients subsequently diagnosed with Alzheimer's disease presented with features of the disorder, so the prevalence appears to be rare (although highly likely to be underrecognized and therefore underreported). Patients with the typical syndrome tend to present in the sixth and seventh decades of life.

The cardinal features are the neuropsychometric impairments, most commonly visuospatial and visuoperceptual deficits such as Balint's syndrome and Gerstmann's syndrome (Table 50.1), but also with disorders of reading (alexia) [2].

These impairments increase and may become severe before evidence of a more widespread involvement of the brain develops. In the early stages memory, language function and executive skills may be surprisingly preserved, however with time these domains too begin to deteriorate and in some patients progression into a globally demented state develops.

Pathological studies have revealed that an Alzheimer pathology of neurofibrillary tangles and amyloid deposition is seen in 60 % of cases [4], with smaller proportions attributable to cortical Lewy body disease, corticobasal degeneration

Table 50.1

Balint's syndrome:	Simultanagnosia
	Oculomotor apraxia
	Optic ataxia
	Environmental agnosia
Gerstmann's syndrome:	Acalculia
	Agraphia
	Finger agnosia
	Left-right disorientation

and prion disease. In those with an Alzheimer pathology, there is a greater prevalence of plaques and tangles in the occipitoparietal regions than more anteriorly [4, 5]. In those with Lewy bodies the prevalence of visual hallucinations is said to be higher. In the two cases in which corticobasal degeneration was identified at autopsy, in which tau-positive astrocytes were seen, with no evidence for neurofibrillary tangles or Lewy bodies, case one went on to develop the usually asymmetric motor disorder seen in corticobasal ganglionic degeneration (CBGD) whereas case two had an asymmetric visuospatial disorder with frontal deficits later on [6]. A series of 6 patients who presented with homonymous hemianopia and visuospatial dysfunction [7] showed an asymmetric cortical atrophy as in this case, and SPECT scans in 4 revealed hypometabolism in the same areas. After follow up the disorder was attributed to Alzheimer's disease in 5 and CBGD in one.

No treatment exists, although some recommend the use of acetylcholinesterase inhibitors since the prevalence of Alzheimer and Lewy body pathologies is so high [2].

References

1. Benson F, Davis J, Snyder BD. Posterior cortical atrophy. Arch Neurol. 1988;45:789–93.
2. Crutch SJ, Lehmann M, Schott JM, Rabinovici GD, Rossor MN, Fox NC. Posterior cortical atrophy. Lancet Neurol. 2012;11:170–8.
3. Snowden JS, Stopford CL, Julien CL, Thompson JC, Davidson Y, Gibbons L, Pritchard A, Lendon CL, Richardson AM, Varma A, Neary D, Mann D. Cognitive phenotypes in Alzheimer's disease and genetic risk. Cortex. 2007;43:835–45.
4. Tang-Wai DF, Graff-Radford NR, Boeve BF, Dickson DW, Parisi JE, Crook R, Caselli RJ, Knopman DS, Petersen RC. Clinical, genetic and neuropathological characteristics of posterior cortical atrophy. Neurology. 2004;63:1168–74.
5. Levine DN, Lee JM, Fisher CM. The visual variant of Alzheimer's disease: a clinicopathological case study. Neurology. 1993;43:305–13.
6. Tang-Wai DF, Josephs KA, Boeve BF, Dickson DW, Parisi JE, Petersen RC. Pathologically confirmed corticobasal degeneration presenting with visuospatial dysfunction. Neurology. 2003;61:1134–5.
7. Formaglio M, Krolak-Salmon P, Tilekete C, Bernard M, Croisile B, Vighetto A. Homonymous hemianopia and posterior cortical atrophy. Rev Neurol. 2009;165:256–62.

Appendix 1

Visual Acuity[1]

The neurological examination of the visual system begins only after the ophthalmic examination has been completed. Corneal abnormalities, lens opacities and retinal problems can all cause blurring or distortion of vision which may be mistaken for a neurological disorder, and a sizeable minority of patients who are referred to a Neuro-ophthalmology clinic is found to have a refractive error as the only cause for the visual symptoms.

A Snellen 6 m distance chart is placed 6 m away from the patient in a brightly illuminated position; low luminance reduces visual acuity since foveal ganglion cells have high light thresholds. The patient is assessed with spectacles on and if the acuity is abnormal a pinhole is added to the lens and the assessment repeated. Near acuity can be assessed using Jaeger charts held by the patient at whatever distance is comfortable. Patients with refractive, corneal and lens problems may have better near than distance acuities, and patients with accommodative and convergence disorders may have better distance than near acuities. A more sensitive assessment of visual acuity involves the use of contrast sensitivity threshold measurements using wall charts or computer programs. These measure the sensitivity of minimum spatial resolution of gratings.

Patients with amblyopia will have normal ophthalmic examinations and no evidence for an optic neuropathy; a neutral density filter placed in front of the affected eye will cause a reduction in visual acuity (for example 6/9 to 6/60) when the visual loss is caused by an optic neuropathy; when it is due to amblyopia the reduction is much less.

Color vision is assessed using pseudoisochromatic plates such as Ishihara, Hardy-Rand-Ritter and Dvorine plates. These are all easy and quick to use although they are not quantitative, nor do they provide an adequate assessment of blue-yellow

[1] This has been adapted with permission from a previously published chapter in: *Neurology and Clinical Neuroscience*, Schapira AHV (editor). Philadelphia, Mosby Elsevier, 2007.

D.P. Kidd, *Neuro-Ophthalmology*, DOI 10.1007/978-1-4471-2410-8

Table 1 Signs of an optic neuropathy

Diminished central visual acuity
Proportionately reduced near acuity
Marked reduction in acuity when looking through a neutral density filter
Diminished color vision
Ipsilateral visual field defect
Afferent or relative afferent pupillary defect
The disc may not be abnormal

disorders. More complicated measurements such as the Farnsworth Munsell 100 hue test and others are better but greatly more time-consuming.

These tests are useful in the assessment of visual loss due to optic nerve and macular problems. Congenital color blindness occurs in 8 % of males and will be symmetrical; an asymmetric loss of color vision is always acquired.

Optic neuropathies which involve disruption of the papillomacular bundle (for example optic neuritis) will cause red-green color deficits whereas those which disrupt fibers arising from the perifoveal fields (for example glaucoma and papilloedema) will cause blue-yellow deficits (as well as a proportionately smaller reduction in visual acuity) (Table 1).

Visual Field Examination

Confrontation methods are adequate only if carried out very carefully indeed. Wiggling fingers will only detect field defects which are absolute *ie* there is no vision within that field, and some may have no vision within a hemianopic field but are nonetheless able to perceive movement. Finger counting is better, in which the patient must focus on the examiner's eye and say or copy the number of fingers presented to the four quadrants and the central field. Use of a small target such as a hat pin is more accurate; a white hat pin plots out the peripheral field and the red is used for central defects particularly optic nerve disorders in which, as noted above, red-green color deficits arise.

The principle behind dynamic perimetric methods of field analysis such as the Goldman (Fig. 1) is that the examiner is identifying successive boundaries of vision known as differential light sensitivities (DLS). These are the thresholds within which it is possible for that part of the retina to identify when a light projected is more bright than the background. The fovea is most sensitive and so a less contrasted ie less bright target will be seen, whereas away from the central field, at the periphery of vision, a much brighter target will be required. The temporal field changes slowly with distance from the fovea whereas the DLS on the nasal side reduces abruptly. The advantage of this method of field assessment is that the skilled

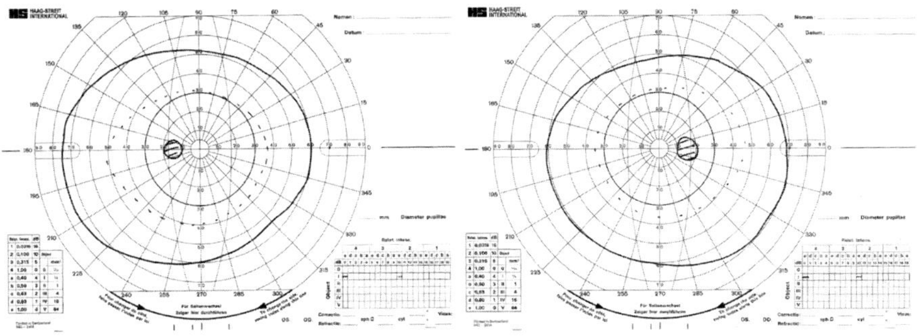

Fig. 1 Normal Goldman visual field

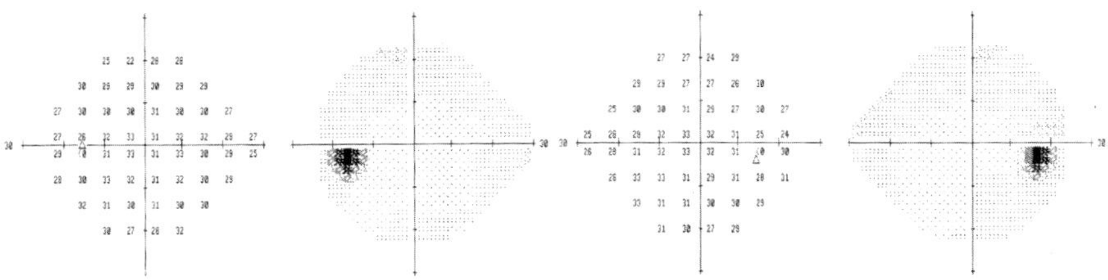

Fig. 2 Normal Humphrey automated visual field

examiner can plot very carefully visual field abnormalities and can return over and over again to check the boundaries of the field.

Automated static perimetry is available in all ophthalmic departments, can be carried out in around 10 min, is easy to administer and does not require so much skill to perform. It is however less sensitive a measure than the Goldman. Automated static field tests identify the threshold of accurate vision within the four visual quadrants within a 10, 24, 30 or 70° field (Fig. 2). Fields can be recorded for comparison with subsequent examinations; reliability can be assessed by noting fixation losses and false positive and negative errors. The gray scale indices note the mean or pattern deviation of the patient's responses to those of age-matched normal.

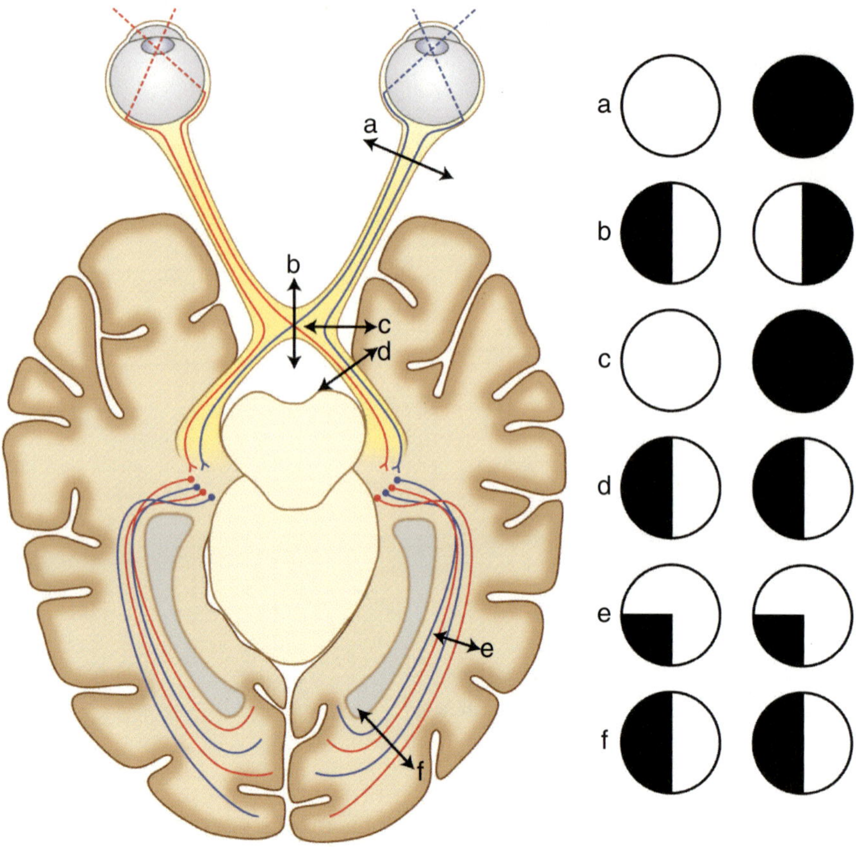

Common visual field defects and where they arise from

The Amsler grid is useful for plotting central field distortions, for example macular disorders, but also very small central field abnormalities due for example to optic neuropathy. The patient plots out the abnormality on the grid himself.

Tangent screen testing is also easy and rapid; a 1 m screen can be attached to the wall of a clinic room and a light source with different target sizes and luminances can be used very accurately to plot out a visual field. The contour of light sensitivity to the target of the same size and luminance is termed an isopter. Different target sizes and luminances give rise to different isopters and so the field is plotted.

Appendix 2

Examination of the Pupils[2]

Patients with recent onset pupillary mydriasis may complain of blurring of vision and photophobia but most patients have no symptoms.

The examination involves inspection of pupil size and shape at rest. Each should be round and the same size. Pupil size can be measured using a ruler or more easily using a pupil gauge such as that seen on a hand held pin hole – occluder. The pupils should then be inspected in light and dark. Physiological anisocoria is detectable in 20 % of young people and increases in prevalence with age to 33 % of people over the age of 60 years. The inequality increases in dark in the case of physiological anisocoria and to a greater degree in the case of Horner's syndrome. It may also be affected by anxiety which increases sympathetic drive, and by fatigue.

The Pupillary Reaction to Light

The pupil should be assessed by a bright light source such as a fully charged ophthalmoscope with low background illumination (just enough to see the pupil in darkness). The patient will be looking in to the distance in order to prevent meiosis in accommodation. The light source is applied to the pupil for two or three seconds and the response amplitude and reaction speed noted. This should be repeated several times. The latency of redilatation should also be observed; early pupillary

[2] The text and figures have been adapted with permission from a previously published chapter in: *Neurology and Clinical Neuroscience*, Schapira AHV (editor). Philadelphia, Mosby Elsevier, 2007.

escape, in which redilation occurs earlier on one side and sometimes even before the light source is removed, implies a mild afferent pupillary defect.

The Consensual Response

When light is applied to one eye the pupillary response in the other should be equal in amplitude and synchronous since the decussation of pupillary fibers in the midbrain is 50 %.

The Near Response

The patient is instructed to look into the distance then at a target held at the nearest point of distinct vision (25 cm in emmetropic people). A brisk and symmetrical meiosis should follow as convergence occurs. The speed and amplitude of the near response is noted and compared with the direct light response; light-near dissociation may arise in upper midbrain lesions due to compressive, infiltrative or inflammatory causes (including of course neurosyphilis), severe bilateral optic neuropathies and isolated parasympathetic nerve disorders.

Pupillary Dilatation

The pupil returns to its size appropriate for low levels of background illumination 12–15 s after a bright light source is removed from the eye. In patients with Horner's syndrome there will be dilatation lag, in which the affected side will dilate more slowly than the normal side, and an increase in anisocoria will be seen. This can be measured with infrared pupillography or by taking a photograph of the pupils after 15 seconds.

The Relative Afferent Pupillary Defect (RAPD)

A light source is applied in turn to each eye for 3–5 seconds repeatedly. The trick is to vary the time taken to move from one eye to the other; often the RAPD can be brought out thus. Great care should be taken not to apply the light source to one eye for longer than the other, that the light source is applied to the same amount of retina in each eye (this is particularly important if there is ocular misalignment) and that there is no accommodative meiosis. Provided the test is performed properly, the examiner will be able to see that there will be pupillary dilatation on the side of a unilateral optic neuropathy when the light source returns to that side.

Pharmacological Testing

Horner's syndrome: meiosis and ipsilateral partial ptosis, apparent enophthalmos and absence of sweating of the face ipsilaterally. The anisocoria is more evident in dark than light. The direct responses are normal. There is a failure of the affected pupil to dilate with 10 % cocaine solution. One percentage hydroxyamphetamine will dilate the affected pupil if the lesion is central or pre-ganglionic, and no response will occur if the lesion is post-ganglionic (Fig. 3). One percentage apraclonidine, which is more readily available in ophthalmic departments, will also cause the affected pupil to enlarge whilst the normal pupil is unaffected. The test cannot define the site of the causative lesion however.

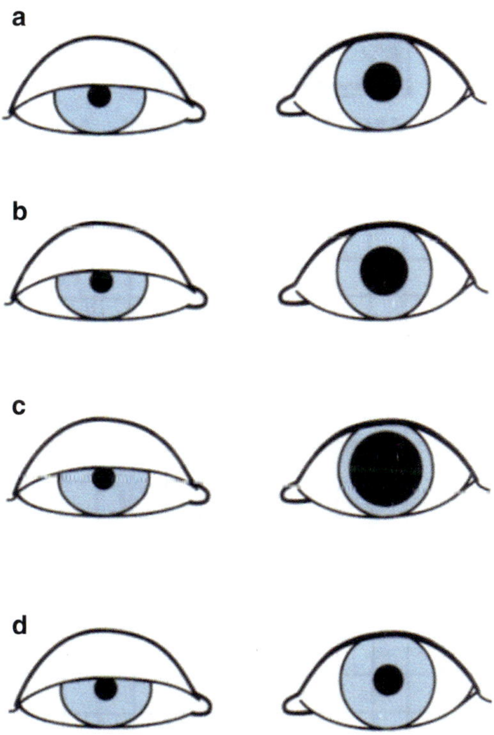

Fig. 3 Pupillary responses in Horner's syndrome (**a**) in light, (**b**) in dark, (**c**) following instillation of 10 % cocaine, (**d**) following instillation of 1 % hydroxamphetamine; the lesion is post-ganglionic

Holmes-Adie syndrome: subacute severe mydriasis which partially resolves over many months. It is associated with absent reflexes and rarely autonomic failure (Ross' syndrome). The anisocoria is more marked in light than dark. The pupils are tonic; denervation is rarely complete so vermiform movement (movements of the parts of the iris which have not been denervated) can be seen on slit lamp examination. 0.1 % pilocarpine will constrict the affected pupil more than the normal owing to denervation supersensitivity (Fig. 4). Tonic pupils may also be caused by trauma and more commonly to inflammation due to viral infections and uveitis.

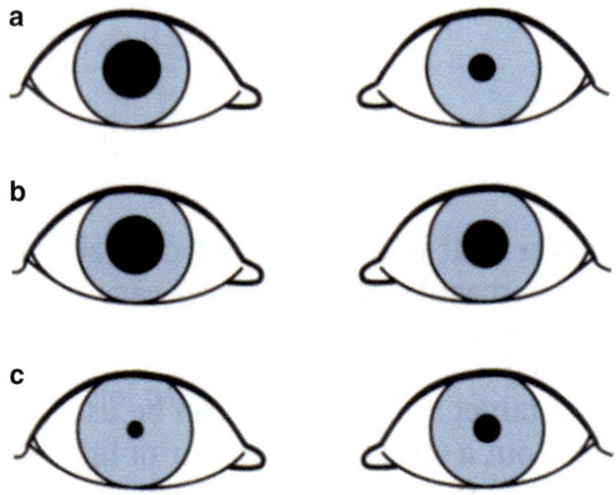

Fig. 4 Pupillary responses in Tonic pupil (**a**) in light, (**b**) in dark, (**c**) following instillation of 0.1 % pilocarpine solution

A partial IIIrd nerve palsy manifested only as mydriasis will not show denervation hypersensitivity and so will not constrict with 0.1 % pilocarpine but will do so with 1.0 %.

Finally a pharmacologically mediated mydriasis will fail to constrict with 1 % pilocarpine.

Essential anisocoria: The pupils are usually the same size in light and dark, although the disparity may be more apparent in dark (but not to the same degree as with Horner's syndrome). There are normal responses to cocaine (Fig. 5).

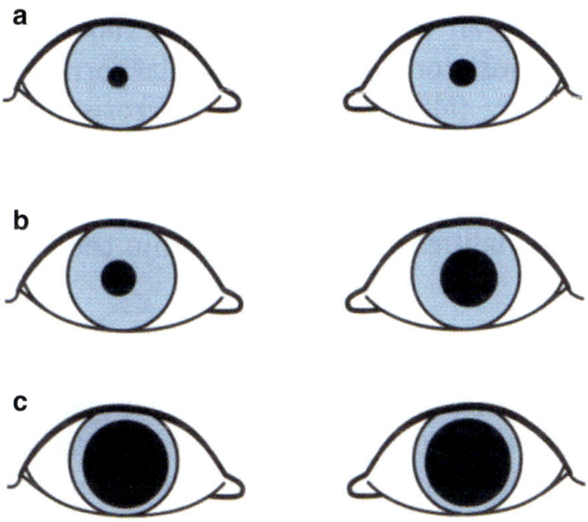

Fig. 5 Pupillary responses in essential anisocoria (**a**) in light, (**b**) in dark, (**c**) following instillation of 10 % cocaine

Appendix 3

The Ocular Motor Nerves

The Oculomotor Nerve

The oculomotor nuclei lie in the midbrain. Fibers from the Edinger-Westphal nuclei contain parasympathetic fibers, and from the caudal central nucleus fibers to the levator muscles on both sides. The fibers to each of the four muscles innervated by the nucleus arise separately; those to the superior rectus cross within the midbrain to the other side whilst those innervating the other three remain ipsilateral. The oculomotor nerve emerges on each side from the interpeduncular fossa of the midbrain anteriorly and passes between the superior cerebellar and posterior cerebral arteries to lie immediately below the posterior communicating artery before entering the cavernous sinus, where it lies in the lateral wall above the trochlear nerve. It passes through the superior orbital fissure and divides into superior and inferior divisions. The smaller superior division innervates the superior rectus and levator palpebrae superioris muscles. The inferior division divides into branches in the orbit then passes forward to innervate the remaining three muscles, and the parasympathetic supply to the ciliary ganglion.

The Trochlear Nerve

The trochlear nucleus lies adjacent to the oculomotor nucleus and the medial longitudinal fasciculus. The axons which arise from the nuclei pass caudally then converge and cross at the roof of the aqueduct. The trochlear nerve emerges from the dorsal surface of the midbrain just below the inferior colliculi then passes around the brain stem to enter the cavernous sinus where it lies in the lateral wall between the oculomotor nerve and the ophthalmic division of the trigeminal nerve. It crosses the oculomotor nerve and enters the superior orbital fissure outside the annulus of Zinn then passes in the supero-medial portion of the orbit to innervate the superior oblique muscle.

The Abducens Nerve

The abducens nucleus lies in the medial part of the pons, adjacent to the medial longitudinal fasciculus, and the genu of the facial nerve passes right over it. It passes laterally through the pons and emerges at the pontomedullary junction. It passes upwards within the subarachnoid space along the face of the clivus to the cavernous sinus where it lies medial to the other nerves, within the body of the sinus. The sympathetic nerves fuse briefly before joining the trigeminal nerve as the nasociliary nerve, and the abducens nerves enters the orbit through the annulus of Zinn to innervate the lateral rectus muscle.

Causes of Ocular Motor Paresis

IIIrd	
Nuclear	Infarction
	Infection/inflammation
	Tumor
Fascicular	Infarction/hemorrhage
	Inflammation
Subarachnoid	Aneurysm (PCA and basilar)
	Infarction (“microvascular”)
	Meningitis (infective, neoplastic and inflammatory)
	Tumor
Tentorial edge	Uncal hernaiation
	Hydrocephalus
	Cavernous sinus and orbital apex: see table 2
Orbit	Infection/inflammation
	Trauma

A nuclear IIIrd when unilateral will show a contralateral superior rectus underaction (because axons from each side innervate superior rectus bilaterally) and a bilateral partial ptosis (for the same reason to the levator muscles). When bilateral there will be an absence of ptosis and there may be an internal ophthalmoplegia.

IVth

Nuclear and fascicular	Infarction/hemorrhage
	Infection/inflammation
	Tumor
	Trauma
Subarachnoid	Trauma
	Infarction ("microvascular")
	Hydrocephalus
	Tumor
	Meningitis (infective and neoplastic)
	Mastoiditis
	Cavernous sinus and orbital apex
Orbit	Trauma
	Infection/inflammation
	Tumor
Congenital IVth	

VIth

Nuclear	Infarction
	Tumor
	Infection/inflammation
	Duane's syndrome
Fascicular	Infarction/inflammation
	Tumor
Subarachnoid	Aneurysm (AICA, PICA, basilar)
	Infarction ("microvascular")
	Trauma
	Meningitis (infective and neoplastic)
	CPA tumor
	Clivus tumor
Petrous	Infection of mastoid of petrous tip (Gradenigo)
	Thrombosis of inferior petrosal sinus
	Trauma
	Uncal herniation
	Cavernous sinus and orbital apex
Orbit	Trauma
	Infection/inflammation
	Tumor

Examination of Diplopia[3]

The patient is asked to follow a target through its range of movements in the nine directions of gaze. One eye is tested at a time (ductions) and then both are tested together (versions). The patient is asked to comment on the presence and severity of diplopia during version testing and the eyes examined for evidence for paresis. The patient will note that the diplopic image is displaced in the direction of the paresis when the direction of gaze is that of the paresis. Covering one eye with a red filter often helps to determine which image is which. Orthoptists use other tests such as the Maddox rod and the Lees screen chart.

The Alternate Cover Test

This is most helpful in subtle abnormalities of vergence since when one eye then the other eye is covered, the patient fixing on a target, the uncovered eye will be required to perform a corrective saccade in order to regain fixation, and so small movements in both horizontal and vertical directions may be seen. Esotropia and exotropia refer to outward and inward movement of the uncovered eye respectively when there is a horizontal deviation, and hypotropia and hypertropia when there is a vertical one. When the eyes appear not to be misaligned but nonetheless a refixation movement occurs at the alternate cover test the movement is termed a phoria.

The extent of the tropia can be measured in dioptres using a prism to correct the diplopia.

The Bielschowski Head-Tilt Test

This is undertaken in four stages:

1. identification of the site of the hyperphoria
2. Identification of the whether the deviation is greater in right or left gaze
3. Identification of whether the deviation is greater in up or down gaze
4. Measurement of the size of the deviation with the head tilted to the right or to the left.

Hence in Fig. 6, in the first stage the patient is examined with the alternate cover test in the primary position of gaze and this reveals a right over left hyperphoria, and so either the depressors of the right (superior oblique and inferior rectus) or the elevators of the left (inferior oblique and superior rectus) are weak

---

[3]This text has been adapted with permission from a previously published chapter in: *Neurology and Clinical Neuroscience*, Schapira AHV (editor). Philadelphia, Mosby Elsevier, 2007.

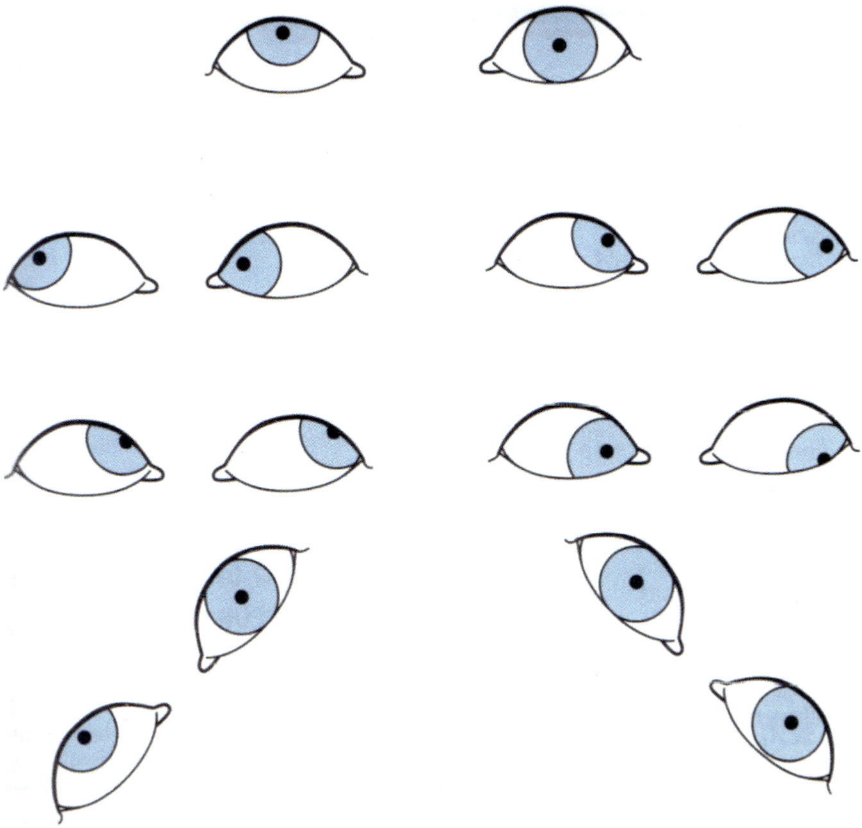

Fig. 6 Cartoon of the Bielschowski maneuver. This patient has a right IV neuropathy (This figure has been adapted with permission from a previously published chapter in: Schapira AHV, editor. Neurology and clinical neuroscience. Philadelphia: Mosby Elsevier; 2007)

(Fig. 6a). The second stage, in which the patient is examined again with the alternate cover test but in left and then right gaze, the right over left deviation increases on left gaze. Hence the oblique muscles, which exert a greater influence on vertical eye movements in adduction, and the recti, which exert a greater influence in abduction, can be differentiated. In this case the right hyperphoria increases in left gaze, so either the right superior oblique or the left superior rectus must be weak (Fig. 6b).

In the third stage the patient is asked to look up then down in left gaze; if the hyperphoria increases in downgaze then the oblique is weak, if in upgaze the rectus must be weak (Fig. 6c). Hence in this case the diagnosis is a right superior oblique palsy. The fourth stage measures its severity; the degree of head tilt to the left required to correct the vertical diplopia (Fig. 6d).

This works well for acute palsies, but in longstanding cases changes in the tone of the reciprocally innervated muscles may give differing abnormalities.

Superior Orbital Fissure, Orbital Apex and Cavernous Sinus Syndromes

Combinations of ocular motor and trigeminal dysfunction with optic neuropathy occur when a disease process involves the region of the skull base at the junction of anterior and middle cranial fossae. At the orbital apex cranial nerves III, IV, VI and the ophthalmic division of the trigeminal nerve lie so closely that a disease process may interrupt the function of some or all of these nerves (Fig. 7). If the optic nerve is not also involved the syndrome is called the superior orbital fissure syndrome (Rochon-Duvigneaud syndrome), when it is the lesion lies within the orbital apex itself. Because the maxillary division of the trigeminal nerve still lies within the middle cranial fossa it this point, in the inferior part of the lateral wall of the sinus (Fig. 8), a lesion of the cavernous sinus may involve that nerve as well (Table 2).

Published series and reviews reported that of 130 cases of superior orbital fissure syndrome, 71 % had an inflammatory cause whilst only 8 % were neoplastic [2]. In contrast in a series of 151 cavernous sinus disorders 35 % were caused by trauma or neurosurgery, 30 % were neoplastic, 23 % were inflammatory and 12 % had an infectious or vascular cause [3].

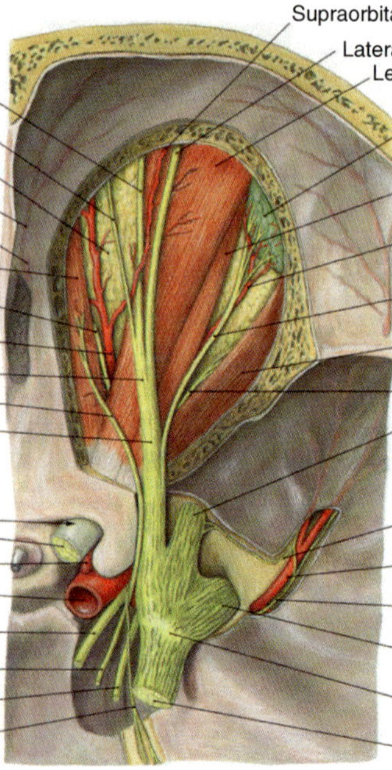

Fig. 7 The nerve and arteries of the orbit (From: Clemente CD. Reproduced with permissions from Paulsen, Waschke. Sobotta atlas of human anatomy. 15th ed. ©Elsevier GmbH, Munich: Urban & Fischer; 2011)

Table 2 Causes of disorders of the orbital apex and cavernous sinus

Inflammatory	Sarcoidosis	
	Idiopathic orbital inflammatory disease	
	IgG4 disease	
	Granulomatosis with polyangiitis	
	Churg-Strauss syndrome	
	SLE	
	Giant cell arteritis	
	Thyroid orbitopathy	
Infective	Bacterial:	tuberculosis, streptococcus, staphylococcus, actinomyces,
		Syphilis, pseudomonas, gram negative organisms
	Fungal:	aspergillus, mucormycosis
	Viral:	Varicella (through Herpes Zoster Ophthalmicus)
		Mucocoele of the sphenoid and ethmoid paranasal sinus
Neoplastic	Primary:	Meningioma
		Schwannoma
		Glioma
		Lymphoma
	Secondary:	Metastasis e.g., from lung, breast, skin
		Lymphoma, leukemia, nasopharyngeal carcinoma, squamous cell carcinoma
Vascular	Cavernous sinus thrombosis	
	Carotico-cavernous fistula	
	Intracavernous carotid aneurysm	
Trauma	Direct e.g., penetrating injury, surgery	
	Orbital fracture	

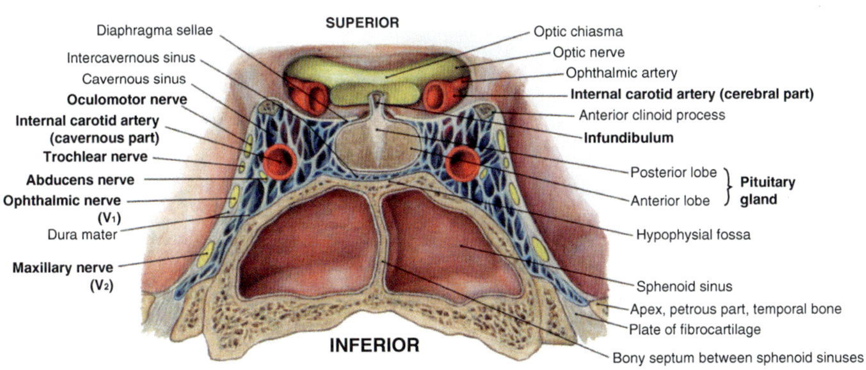

Fig. 8 The cavernous sinus (From: Clemente CD. Reproduced with permissions from Paulsen, Waschke, Sobotta atlas of human anatomy. 15th ed. ©Elsevier GmbH, Munich: Urban & Fischer; 2011)

References

1. Yeh S, Foroozan R. Orbital apex syndrome. Curr Opin Ophthalmol. 2004;15:490–8.
2. Lenzi GL, Fieschi C. Superior orbital fissure syndrome. Review of 130 cases. Eur Neurol. 1977;16:23–30.
3. Keane JR. Cavernous sinus syndrome; analysis of 151 cases. Arch Neurol. 1996;53:967–71.

Appendix 4

The Visual Pathway and Cortical Apperception of Vision

Figure 9 shows the same series of visual field defects seen in every ophthalmic and neurological text book. The anterior visual pathway extends from the retina to the lateral geniculate nucleus (LGN). The medial and lateral horns of the LGN serve superior and inferior visual fields on one side whereas the posterior horn serves macular vision. The medial and lateral horns are supplied by the anterior choroidal artery (supplied by the internal carotid artery) and the posterior horn by the lateral choroidal artery (supplied by the posterior cerebral artery). Non-vascular lesions of the LGN are associated with homonymous hemianopia but isolated vascular lesions may case homonymous sectoranopias; the horizontal sectoranopia when the lateral choroidal artery is involved, and a quadruple sectoranopia when the anterior choroidal artery is involved. The arteries supply adjacent structures so hemiparesis, hemisensory loss and visuospatial disorders are also seen; the "anterior and lateral choroidal artery syndromes".

The posterior visual pathway arises in post-synaptic fibers within the LGN and passes backwards as the temporal and parietal fascicles of the optic radiation to the striate cortex in the occipital lobe. Temporal lesions therefore cause superior quadrantinopias and parietal lesions inferior quadrantinopias [1]. They tend to be sloping and non-congruous, falling above or below the horizontal meridian [2].

The primary visual cortex forms the superior and inferior banks of the calcarine fissure and corresponds to Brodmann area 17. It is known as cortical area V1. A band of myelinated fibers (the stria of Gennari) crosses horizontally giving rise to the name striate cortex. It receives all of the afferent fibers from the lateral geniculate nucleus. The central 10° of the visual field is served by 60 % of the striate cortex, and the central 30° by 80 %, a feature known as cortical magnification, which clearly enhances the acuity and definition of central vision. There are luminance and orientation specific neurons, and some color and motion appreciation occurs. The

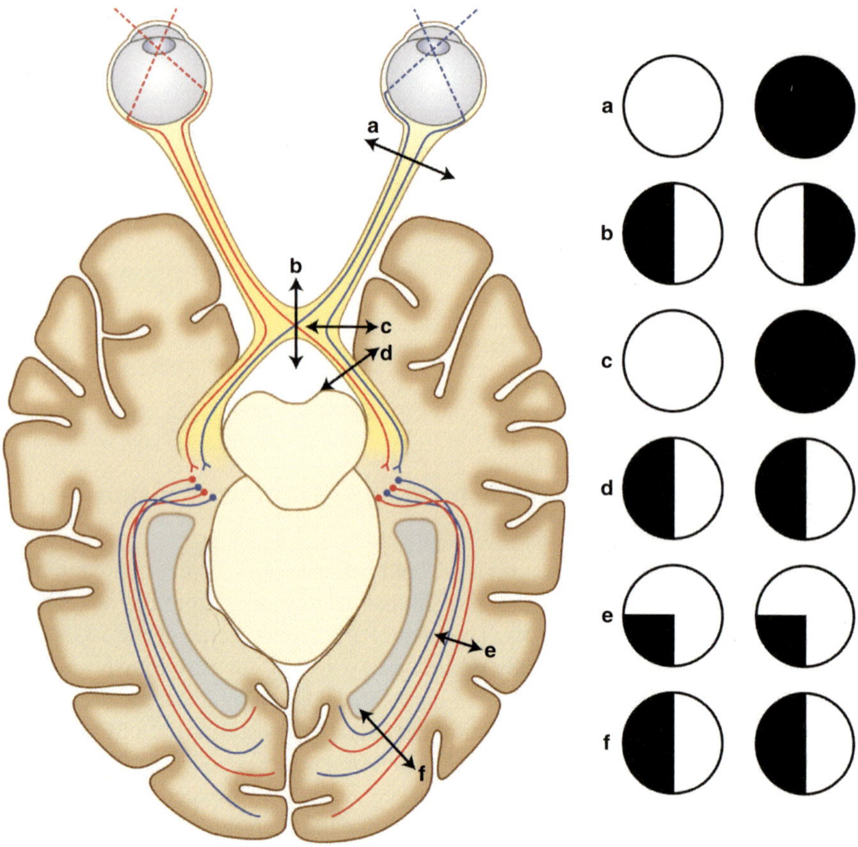

Fig. 9 Visual field defects and the site of their associated lesions

cells then project to cortical area V2, adjacent to V1 above and below the calcarine sulcus, corresponding to Brodmann area 18.

Cells in V2 project ipsilaterally to V4 and V5, contralaterally to V2 on the other side through the corpus callosum, and to and from pre-frontal motor and sensory areas, and to the superior colliculi where they aid in the regulation of eye movements.

Cortical area V3 lies above and below V2, and contains cells which serve motion direction, shape and color.

Visual "streams" are projecting pathways from V1 and V2 which send visual information to visual association areas. The ventral visual stream begins in V1 and passes through V2 to V4 thence to the inferior temporal cortex. It is associated with the understanding and recognition of shape, form and depth (the "what" pathways), whereas the dorsal visual stream passes through V5 and V6 to the posterior parietal cortex. This "where" pathway is associated with motion and spatial awareness (see Balint's syndrome below) [3].

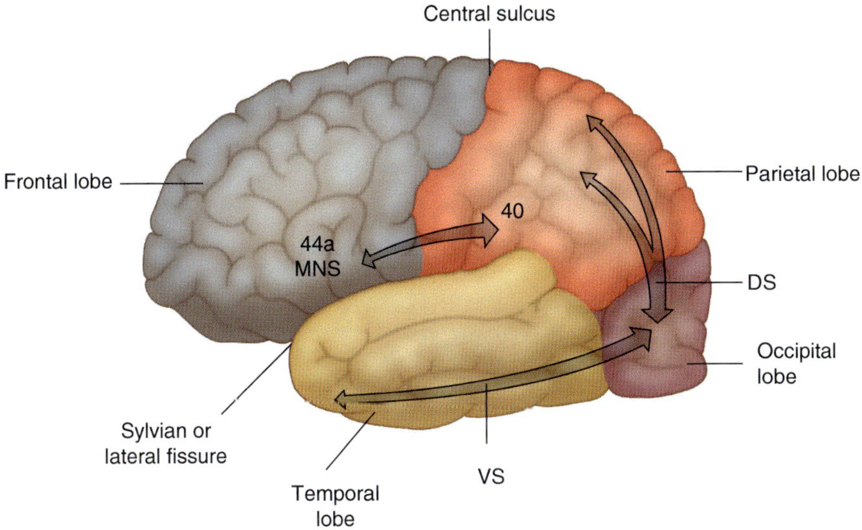

Fig. 10 Cartoon of the surface of the brain showing the Brodmann areas associated with vision, and the dorsal and ventral streams

Area V4 is located in the lingual and fusiform gyri of the anterior occipital and posterior temporal lobes and forms part of the ventral pathway. It contains a complete topographical representation of the contralateral visual field and serves visual recognition. Different parts serve object, face and place recognition and also color perception. The ventral stream pathways project to the inferior temporal cortex (visual area TE) and the posterior parietal cortex. Lesions in this area cause problems with face recognition, reading and color perception (see below).

The inferior temporal cortex is the end of the ventral pathway and allows an understanding of complex shapes and objects.

Visual area V5 lies at the junction of Brodmann areas 19 and 37 (Fig. 10); 90% of neurons are direction sensitive and so deal with the appreciation of movement. Lesions in this region cause problems with motion perception, and retention of function in lesions leading to cortical blindness allow an appreciation of movement known as blindsight (see below).

Other aspects of the appreciation of movement and recognition of visual stimuli rely on the function of deep nuclei such as the superior colliculus in the midbrain and the pulvinar nuclei of the thalamus. Neurons within the superior colliculus interact with the ventral and dorsal streams to activate eye movement in order to allow localization of objects in space, and may allow movement of the eyes into a blind hemifield.

Patients with hemianopia in whom a moving stimulus is applied within the blind hemifield show activation of the contralateral V5 area implying a recognition of movement therein, unless there is an ipsilateral lesion of the pulvinar, in which case no motion is perceived [4].

References

1. Kraft A, Grimsen C, Kehrer S, Bahnemann M, Spang K, Prass M, Irlbacher K, Kohnlein M, Lipfert A, Brunner F, Kastrup A, Fahle M, Brandt SA. Neurological and neuropsychological characteristics of occipital, occipito-temporal and occipito-parietal infarction. Cortex. 2014;56:38–50.
2. Horton JC, Hoyt WF. Quadrantic visual field defects; a hallmark of lesions in extrastriate (V2/V3) cortex. Brain. 1991;114:1703–18.
3. Goodale MA, Milner DA. Separate visual pathways for perception and action. Trends Neurosci. 1992;15:20–25.
4. Barleben M, Stoppel CM, Kaufmann J, Merkel C, Wecke T, Goertler M, Heinze HJ, Hopf JM, Schoenfeld MA. Neural correlates of visual motion processing without awareness in patients with striate cortex and pulvinar lesions. Hum Brain Mapp. 2015;36:1585–94.

Disorders of the Ventral Pathway

Color Recognition

Acquired achromatopsia describes the absence of color perception; patients find that everything appears gray.

Hemiachromatopsia affects only one hemifield and is not usually perceived until it is tested; it is not always picked up using isochromatic plates, but the patient will spot that the red hat pin becomes gray in the affected hemifield as it passes from one side to the other. Sometimes a patient with a superior quadrantinopia will have absent color vision in the seeing ipsilateral lower quadrant.

Achromatopsia is caused by bilateral lesions of the lingual and fusiform gyri and is often associated with adjacent perceptual deficits such as prosopagnosia and topographagnosia and, if the lesion is in the dominant hemisphere, alexia [1, 2].

Color agnosia is the inability to name colors when the patient is successfully able to discriminate between them. It occurs with left occipital lesions and is thought to be related to alexia.

In color agnosia patients are able to discriminate between colors but cannot color in a drawing or recognize whether or not it has been colored correctly. These lesions are also in the left occipito-temporal region, and may be associated with alexia.

Object Recognition

Visual agnosia is the inability to recognize previously recognized objects. Patients cannot relearn the knowledge. There are numerous subcategories, and patients tend to have widespread damage, so it seen in bilateral lesions and in degenerative disorders such as Alzheimer's disease and posterior cortical atrophy.

Prosopagnosia is the inability to recognize previously familiar faces. The lesion affects the fusiform gyrus and is either right sided or bilateral. As noted above it may be associated with achromatopsia and topographagnosia. The field defect is more often an upper quadrantinopia than a hemianopia. Patients may also have simultanagnosia, constructional dyspraxia, and visuospatial neglect [1].

Some patients can recognize faces familiar to them before the lesion arose but not when a person becomes familiar to them after; others can recognize if a context is provided, for example recognizing the Doctor in a hospital but not in the street outside. Patients learn to use other strategies to circumvent the problem, taking clues from characteristics of gait or hand gesturing, and of course the sound of the voice.

Reading

Literate people who lose the ability to read have an acquired alexia; "central" alexia refers to this inability in the absence of an impairment of visual acuity.

In pure alexia patients cannot read but do not lose the ability to write; severe forms include the inability to recognize symbols, road signs, numbers and single letters, whilst more mild forms show impairment in reading speed only for long or complicated words. It is associated with left sided lesions causing hemi- or upper quadrantinopia, and there may also be hemi-achromatopsia, and an anomia for colors and objects. Lesions involve the medial and inferior occipitotemporal region on the left side [2].

Alexia usually comes about as a result of disconnection of visual information from each hemifield with language areas in the left hemisphere, either with involvement of the left occipital cortex and the splenium of the corpus callosum or with bilateral occipital lesions. Less commonly a lesion of the white matter associated with the left angular gyrus may disconnect visual information from the language areas and in this circumstance there will not be a right sided hemianopia. In other cases the reading disorder is due to a visual agnosia for words with lesions of the left fusiform gyrus.

Hemialexia may arise with damage to the splenium of the corpus callosum; patients have difficulty reading in just the contralateral hemifield [1].

Alexia with Agraphia

Patients are unable to read and write but retain oral and auditory language. It is associated with lesions of the left angular gyrus.

Topographagnosia

An inability to recognize familiar places, patients get lost. It may arise as agnosia of landmarks, associated with prosopagnosia and achromatopsia caused by right ventral temporo-occipital lesions, as a failure to memorize routes with right parieto-temporal lesions, and as a "heading disorientation", a failure to understand direction using visual environmental clues, with lesions of the posterior cingulate gyrus.

Disorders of the Dorsal Pathway

Cerebral Akinetopsia

It is most uncommon to lose the appreciation of movement; most patients note a visual confusion when appreciating complicated and moving scenes, and in particular judging the speed of oncoming objects (such as cars on the street) or judging the direction of movement (and the relative speeds) in two or more objects traveling in different directions, but others can assess slow speeds, and determine the direction in which an object is traveling, until it speeds up. Bilateral lesions are seen in lateral occipito-temporal regions.

Unilateral lesions of the lateral temporal cortex may be associated with an impairment of motion understanding and processing within the contralateral hemifield. These disorders are seen in lesions on either side.

The Riddoch syndrome, or blindsight, in which cortically blind patients can nonetheless perceive moving objects within their visual field, occurs when the areas which motion perception remain unaffected by the lesion and receive stimulation from the lateral geniculate nuclei. This may also be seen in unilateral lesions, although the phenomenon is obviously more difficult to determine [3].

Balint's Syndrome

This is the visuospatial disorder of simultanagnosia, optic ataxia and ocular motor apraxia. It is caused by lesions on both sides involving the occipital and parietal cortices and white matter [1–3].

Simultanagnosia is the "inability to interpret the totality of a picture scene despite preservation of the ability to apprehend individual portions of the whole", and is seen in lesions of the dorsal occipital lobes. This also applies to words and letters in complex sentences, and to objects composed of many constituent parts. Patients are unable to describe a picture (such as the "cookie theft" picture) in entirety whilst being able to describe isolated parts of it.

Optic ataxia is a disorder of visually-guided movement in which patients are unable to grasp an object placed within the peripheral field, when there is no associated field defect or visuospatial or ocular motor disorder. Pure forms are associated with lesions of the superior parietal lobule and around the intraparietal sulcus which can be unilateral, in which case the disorder is worse on the contralateral side. Patients are asked to touch a finger held in a peripheral field without looking at it first, or touching coins or objects on a table again without looking at them.

Ocular motor apraxia (or "psychic paralysis of gaze") describes an inability to make voluntary saccades on command whilst retaining the ability to make them involuntarily, for example when looking to the source of an unexpected visual or auditory stimulation. So a patient will not look right or left on command but will do so if the examiner's hand is brought into the right or left hemifield suddenly.

Astereopsis

Bilateral or unilateral lesions of the occipito-parietal regions may impair the ability to discriminate depth (which object is below the other, or further away). Patients complain that their view is two dimensional. They often have other visuospatial deficits.

Visuospatial Neglect

This disorder is a common accompaniment of large right (non-dominant) hemisphere stroke. Patients fail to attend to stimuli presented to the contralateral side. It is associated with lesions throughout the parietal lobe on that side, most particularly the angular gyrus and parahippocampal region [4], but in others the superior temporal gyrus. It is always associated with a hemifield defect

Visual extinction refers to a neglect of one hemifield only when a simultaneous stimulus is presented to the ipsilateral side. A recent fMRI study has suggested that this is not a disorder of neglect but one of compensatory enhancement of the ipsilateral side [5]

Cortical Blindness

Patients with damage to both striate cortices will not be able to see. Some deny that this is the case; Anton's syndrome refers to denial of blindness. The etiology of this is unclear, and may be apperceptive in nature, or coincident with an amnesic disorder, or because of a residual appreciation of motion (as in the Riddoch phenomenon). Optokinetic nystagmus is absent, and is traditionally used to differentiate truly blind patients from those with a functional disorder. The pupillary responses are preserved.

Positive Visual Phenomena

Palinopsia refers to the abnormal persistence of an afterimage. It is may be transient or chronic. Often a single image is seen at the point of fixation but in other cases there may be replications of the image throughout the visual field. Others are contextually specific – for example a face seen is then replicated on all faces of the people around [2, 6].

It is common in metabolic disorders, for example illicit drug intoxication or with antipsychotics, and in psychotic illnesses as well. The localization of lesions is not clear since many case reports show lesions spread throughout the temporal, parietal and occipital lobes on either side. Visual field defects are common. It may be associated with other spatial illusions such as micropsia or metamorphopisia, and with prosopagnosia and achromatopsia. In other cases imaging is normal and an epileptic or migrainous etiology is hypothesized; indeed treatment with anticonvulsants has been seen to be helpful [6].

Polyopia may be related to palinopsia or may arise during recovery of vision from cortical blindness for example after encephalitis. It may also be associated with other visual sensory disorders.

Visual Hallucinations

Simple hallucinations are colors or flashes, simple shapes such as lines or patterns. Complex ones contains shapes, objects or animals, and even scenes. They are of course common in intoxicated states and in neurodegenerative diseases. Patients with cortical Lewy body disease, for example, will see people in the room, or sharing their bed, or children at the bottom of the garden.

Charles Bonnet syndrome occurs in elderly patients with poor vision from any source (even cataract). It is more common in patients socially isolated. The hallucinations are often of fine geometric shapes (like wall paper) or a branching pattern. Patients usually have insight that they are not real and are rarely disturbed emotionally by them. Oftentimes they can switch the hallucination off by closing then opening the eyes [7].

Peduncular hallucinations occur with rostal midbrain lesions and are dramatic and frightening. Patients suffer prolonged terrifying ordeals in which they feel themselves to be part of the hallucination, which may involve malevolent people, snakes and the like, or panoramic scenes with period costumes, or science fiction dramas. They tend to occur at night. When caused by brain stem infarction they tend to subside over a few weeks, having begun soon after the insult occurred, but they may be chronic [7].

The visual disorders of occipital epilepsy and migraine are discussed in case 46.

References

1. Barton JJS. Disorders of higher visual processing. In: Kennard C, Leigh RJ, editors. Handbook of clinical neurology, vol. 102; 2011. p. 223–61.
2. Rizzo M, Barton JJS. Central disorders of visual function. In: Miller NR, Newman NJ, editors. Walsh and Hoyt's clinical neuro-ophthalmology. 6th ed. Philadelphia: Lippincott, Williams & Watkins; 2005. p. 584–621.
3. Ffytche DH, Blom JD, Catani M. Disorders of visual perception. J Neurol Neurosurg Psychiatry. 2010;81:1280–7.
4. Mort DJ, Malhotra P, Mannan SK, Rorden C, Pambakian A, Kennard C, Husain M. The anatomy of visual neglect. Brain. 2003;126:1986–97.
5. Umarova RM, Saur D, Kaller CP, Vry MS, Glauche V, Mader I, Hennig J, Weiller C. Acute visual neglect and extinction: distinct functional state of the visuospatial attention system. Brain. 2011;134:3310–25.
6. Gersztenkorn D, Lee AG. Palinopsia revamped: a systematic review of the literature. Surv Ophthalmol. 2015;60:1–35.
7. Manford M, Andermann F. Complex visual hallucinations. Clinical and neurobiological insights. Brain. 1998;121:1819–40.

Printed by Printforce, the Netherlands